CASES IN INTERVENTIONAL CARDIOLOGY

CASES IN INTERVENTIONAL CARDIOLOGY

Michael Ragosta, MD, FACC, FSCAI

Professor of Medicine
Director, Cardiac Catheterization Laboratories
Cardiovascular Division
University of Virginia Health System
Charlottesville, Virginia

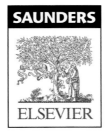

SAUNDERS

ELSEVIER

SAUNDERS
ELSEVIER

3251 Riverport Lane
St. Louis, Missouri 63043

CASES IN INTERVENTIONAL CARDIOLOGY   ISBN: 978-1-4377-0583-6

Notices

Knowledge and best practice in this field are constantly changing. As new research and experience broaden our understanding, changes in research methods, professional practices, or medical treatment may become necessary.

Practitioners and researchers must always rely on their own experience and knowledge in evaluating and using any information, methods, compounds, or experiments described herein. In using such information or methods they should be mindful of their own safety and the safety of others, including parties for whom they have a professional responsibility.

With respect to any drug or pharmaceutical products identified, readers are advised to check the most current information provided (i) on procedures featured or (ii) by the manufacturer of each product to be administered, to verify the recommended dose or formula, the method and duration of administration, and contraindications. It is the responsibility of practitioners, relying on their own experience and knowledge of their patients, to make diagnoses, to determine dosages and the best treatment for each individual patient, and to take all appropriate safety precautions.

To the fullest extent of the law, neither the Publisher nor the authors, contributors, or editors assume any liability for any injury and/or damage to persons or property as a matter of products liability, negligence or otherwise, or from any use or operation of any methods, products, instructions, or ideas contained in the material herein.

Library of Congress Cataloging-in-Publication Data

Cases in interventional cardiology/Michael Ragosta. – 1st ed.
      p. ; cm.
   Includes bibliographical references.
   ISBN 978-1-4377-0583-6 (hardback : alk. paper)   1. Heart–Surgery–Case studies. I. Title.
   [DNLM: 1. Cardiovascular Diseases–surgery–Case Reports. 2. Cardiovascular
   Diseases–diagnosis–Case Reports. 3. Cardiovascular Surgical Procedures–methods–Case Reports.
   4. Diagnostic Techniques, Cardiovascular–Case Reports. WG 168 R144c 2011]
   RD598.R343 2011
   617.4′12–dc22
                                                                            2010023240

Executive Publisher: Natasha Andjelkovic
Developmental Editor: Agnes Byrne
Publishing Services Manager: Anne Altepeter
Team Manager: Radhika Pallamparthy
Project Managers: Cindy Thoms/Antony Prince Dayalan
Text and Cover Designer: Steve Stave

To the memory of my father, Michele Ragosta, Jr. (July 20, 1928 – October 29, 2009), to whom I owe my deepest gratitude for the love and support he so freely gave and for the many lessons he taught me. He was the most generous, honest, and loyal man I know, and he will always be my hero.

Contributors

Loren Budge, MD
Cardiology Fellow
University of Virginia Health System
Charlottesville, Virginia

Jason T. Call, MD
Interventional Cardiologist
Winchester Cardiology and Vascular Medicine
Winchester Medical Center
Winchester, Virginia

Lawrence W. Gimple, MD, FACC, FSCAI
Donald C. Barnes Professor of Cardiology
Director of Clinical Cardiology
Cardiovascular Division
University of Virginia Health System
Charlottesville, Virginia

D. Scott Lim, MD, FACC, FSCAI
Associate Professor of Pediatrics and Medicine
University of Virginia Health System
Charlottesville, Virginia

M. Ayoub Mirza, MD
Cardiology Fellow
University of Virginia Health System
Charlottesville, Virginia

Michael Ragosta, MD, FACC, FSCAI
Professor of Medicine
Director, Cardiac Catheterization Laboratories
Cardiovascular Division
University of Virginia Health System
Charlottesville, Virginia

Angela M. Taylor, MD, MS
Assistant Professor of Medicine
Co-Director, Diabetes Cardiovascular Center
Cardiovascular Division
University of Virginia Health System
Charlottesville, Virginia

Preface

Interventional cardiology has transformed the practice of cardiovascular medicine. Since the first human balloon angioplasty by Dr. Andreas Gruentzig in 1977, cardiology has evolved from a purely diagnostic to a therapeutic specialty focused on cardiovascular procedures performed percutaneously. Armed with the knowledge acquired from more than three decades of research in vascular biology and from the results of large-scale clinical trials involving drugs, stents, and advanced techniques, today's interventional cardiologist confidently tackles complex coronary lesions considered untreatable just a short time ago. Initially confined to coronary artery disease, the field has expanded to include percutaneous treatment of vascular beds outside of the heart as well as nonatherosclerotic cardiovascular conditions such as valvular and congenital lesions, often described as "structural" heart disease.

Naturally, it is expected that interventional cardiology will continue to change rapidly. It is certainly challenging for the current practitioner to stay apace of these developments, and any publication attempting to teach interventional cardiology is at risk of becoming antiquated just as it is being published. Nevertheless, many underlying concepts and principles will endure through the years and require proficiency by the competent practitioner.

Currently, several outstanding interventional cardiology books provide comprehensive information in conventional textbook formats. *Cases in Interventional Cardiology* differs from these traditional books by focusing on a case-based approach to teach the core principles of interventional cardiology. Each case illustrates one or more important and enduring concepts that the competent interventional cardiologist is expected to master. This format was inspired by the Japanese woodblock artist Hiroshige, creator of "100 Views of Edo" (figure). Just as no single illustration can possibly capture all aspects of life in nineteenth-century Tokyo, careful study of numerous individual cases helps the practitioner appreciate the many nuances of interventional cardiology.

Each case presentation is formatted to include the relevant clinical background and representative images needed to understand the problem addressed. Still-frame images appear within the text, and when necessary, angiograms or ultrasound images are provided on the companion Expert Consult website. The outcomes of the case and management strategies are discussed, along with supportive didactic information and the most important and relevant literature. Key concepts are summarized at the end of the discussion.

Cases in Interventional Cardiology is designed principally for fellows enrolled in interventional cardiology training programs and for practicing interventional cardiologists preparing for board examination or recertification. In addition, general cardiology fellows, practicing cardiologists, cardiac catheterization laboratory nurses and technicians, cardiology nurse practitioners, physician assistants, and coronary care unit nurses will find this information highly relevant and of interest.

Michael Ragosta, MD, FACC, FSCAI

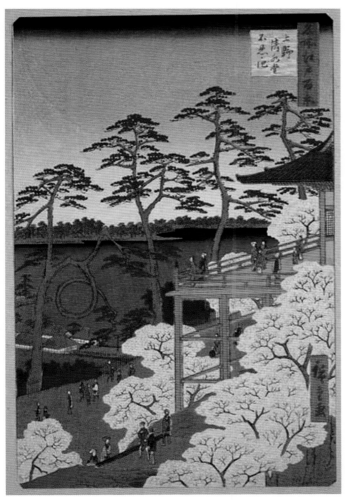

The Kiyomizu Temple and Shinobazu Pond at Ueno. From "100 Views of Edo" by Ando Hiroshige (1797–1858).

Contents

SECTION ONE

Complex Coronary Interventions

The pioneers of coronary intervention frequently faced devastating complications, great technical challenges, primitive equipment, and very high rates of restenosis. The performance of angioplasty without surgical back-up was unheard-of and nearly a criminal offense. The only devices were balloons, 10,000 units of heparin served as the universal "adjunctive pharmacology," and we understood very little of the pathobiology of the underlying disease. It is a wonder that the field of interventional cardiology was not banished, along with bloodletting and other barbaric practices, as a failed therapy. In fact, in 1987, when I was an internal medicine resident interested in the relatively new field of interventional cardiology, a prominent cardiologist advised me to reconsider my career choice, since he believed balloon angioplasty would likely be a passing fad, doomed to extinction because of the high complication rate and poor long-term success.

Thankfully, improvements in equipment, technique, and pharmacology, coupled with knowledge gained from the basic sciences and vascular biology, have established percutaneous coronary interventional procedures (PCI) as safe and effective methods of accomplishing coronary revascularization. The introduction of coronary stents and refinements in procedural anticoagulation are probably the two greatest triumphs that have allowed the field to advance and have made the outcomes of coronary interventional procedures highly predictable, thereby alleviating most of the operator's anxiety and uncertainty when facing a coronary lesion.

In the current era, a successful coronary intervention is defined in several ways. *Angiographic success* is often defined as achieving less than 30% stenosis following stenting and less than 50% stenosis after balloon angioplasty, with the attainment of TIMI-3 flow. *Clinical success* is defined as the presence of angiographic success along with the absence of major adverse events (death, myocardial infarction, or need for emergency bypass surgery). In the current era, the angiographic and clinical success rates are greater than 90%, with an in-hospital mortality of about 1.5% and a rate of emergency bypass surgery of less than 0.1% to 0.4%.

Revascularization decisions are often difficult. A physician faced with a choice between medical therapy, PCI, and coronary bypass surgery must take into consideration many important variables. Augmented by the lessons gleaned from randomized controlled trials, physicians often make a choice based on the therapeutic option they believe will result in the highest success at alleviating the patient's symptoms, with the lowest complication rate.

Several clinical variables (Table I-1) and numerous angiographic characteristics (Table I-2) are important predictors of an adverse outcome after PCI. Thus, there are both "high-risk" patients and "high-risk" lesions. Selection of patients for PCI should first focus on their clinical characteristics. Among the variables listed in Table I-1, the presence of cardiogenic shock is the most powerful predictor of an adverse event. Whenever possible, patient outcome is improved if these adverse variables can be modified or improved before undergoing PCI. Of course, it is understood that a PCI usually

TABLE I-1 Clinical Characteristics Associated with Increased Risk of PCI

Severe left ventricular dysfunction

Cardiogenic shock

Class IV congestive heart failure

Renal insufficiency

Evolving myocardial infarction

Female gender

Advanced age

Diabetes mellitus

Comorbid conditions

    Peripheral vascular disease

    Chronic obstructive pulmonary disease

    Bleeding disorder or coagulopathy

    Gastrointestinal bleeding

    Metabolic disarray

    Recent cerebrovascular accident

TABLE I-2 Angiographic and Lesion Characteristics Associated with Increased Risk of PCI

Multivessel coronary disease

Left mainstem disease

Large risk area subtended by treated artery

Eccentric lesion

Visible thrombus

Extensive coronary calcification

Ostial stenosis

Bifurcation stenosis

Degenerated saphenous vein graft

Chronic total occlusion

Excessive tortuosity

Excessive angulation of treated segment

Diffuse disease

Small caliber artery

cannot be postponed in the setting of an acute ST-segment–elevation myocardial infarction, cardiogenic shock, or recurrent ischemic pain; however, whenever possible, it is prudent to first treat heart failure, stabilize hemodynamics, improve renal function or metabolic derangement, and address active comorbid conditions before proceeding.

Several features identified on angiography are important predictors of an adverse event with PCI (see Table I-2). Particularly challenging lesion subsets include visible clot, bifurcation stenoses, degenerated vein graft lesions, and chronic total occlusions. In addition to these features, adverse outcomes are greater with certain devices such as rotational and directional atherectomy, as compared to balloons and stents.

Traditionally, coronary lesions were classified based on the ACC/AHA scheme as Type A, B, or C lesions.[1] This system was initially developed in the balloon era to assist operators select patients for PCI. Type A lesions were ideal for balloon angioplasty and were associated with the highest success rates and the lowest risk. Type A lesions involve native coronary arteries; are focal, concentric, and do not involve a bifurcation; and are without clot, angulation, or excessive tortuosity. Type B lesions have one (Type B1) or more (Type B2) unfavorable characteristics for PCI. Type B1 lesions also have a high success rate, but Type B2 lesions were traditionally associated with only modest acute success and moderate risk with balloon angioplasty. Type C lesions have the lowest success rates and the highest risk with balloon angioplasty. Type C lesions include degenerated saphenous vein grafts, lesions with excessive angulation and tortuosity, diffuse disease, prominent bifurcations, and chronic total occlusions.

With coronary stents, PCI of many "B" type lesions have a much more predictable outcome. Thus, the utility of the classic ACC/AHA classification system in the stent era has been called into question, and most operators now simply classify lesions as being either patent or occluded and either Type C or non-Type C.[2,3]

To assist the physician, practice guidelines describing the indications for percutaneous coronary intervention have been developed and are updated regularly.[4] These guidelines classify scenarios in which PCI is clearly indicated (Class I), probably indicated (Class IIa), probably not indicated (Class IIb), and generally not indicated or even contraindicated (Class III). In addition, professional societies have created "appropriateness" criteria for coronary revascularization procedures.[5] All practicing interventional cardiologists should be well-versed in their contents and remain current as they are modified and updated.

The cases chosen for this section include both high-risk patients and high-risk lesions, and all cases embody many of the features characteristic of the complex interventions regularly challenging the busy interventional cardiologist. The management of each case represents a single operator's opinion and is based on the best knowledge available when the case was performed. The author recognizes that alternative methods may have been as good or even superior to those chosen and, in addition, as new knowledge becomes available, the optimal strategies are subject to change.

Selected References

1. Ellis SG, Vandormael MG, Cowley MJ, DiSciasio G, Deligonul U, Topol EJ, Bulle TM: Coronary morphologic and clinical determinants of procedural outcome with angioplasty for multivessel coronary disease: Implications for patient selection. Multivessel Angioplasty Prognosis Study Group, *Circulation* 82:1193–1202, 1990.
2. Krone RJ, Laskey WK, Johnson C, Kimmel SE, Klein LW, Weiner BH, Cosentino JJA, Johnson SA, Babb JD: A simplified lesion classification for predicting success and complications of coronary angioplasty, *Am J Cardiol* 85:1179–1184, 2000.
3. Krone RJ, Shaw RE, Klein LW, Block PC, Anderson HV, Weintraub WS, Brindis RG, McKay CR: Evaluation of the American College of Cardiology/American Heart Association and the Society for Coronary Angiography and Interventions lesion classification system in the current "stent era" of coronary interventions (from the ACC-National Cardiovascular Data Registry), *Am J Cardiol* 92:389–394, 2003.
4. Kushner FG, Hand M, Smith SC Jr, King SB 3rd, Anderson JL, Antman EM, Bailey SR, Bates ER, Blankenship JC, Casey DJ Jr, Green LA, Hochman JS, Jacobs AK, Krumholz HM, Morrison DA, Ornato JP, Pearle DL, Peterson ED, Sloan MA, Whitlow PL, Williams DO: 2009 Focused updates: ACC/AHA guidelines for the management of patients with ST-elevation myocardial infarction (updating the 2004 guideline and 2007 focused update) and ACC/AHA/SCAI guidelines on percutaneous coronary intervention (updating the 2005 guideline and 2007 focused update): a report of the American College of Cardiology Foundation/American Heart Association Task Force on Practice Guidelines, *Circulation* 120:2271–2306, 2009.
5. Patel MR, Dehmer GJ, Hirshfeld JW, et al: ACCF/SCAI/STS/AATS/AHA/ASNC 2009 Appropriateness criteria for coronary revascularization, *J Am Coll Cardiol* 53:530–553, 2009.

Restenosis of a Drug-Eluting Stent

Loren Budge, MD, and Michael Ragosta, MD, FACC, FSCAI

CASE PRESENTATION

A 53-year-old man, with hypertension, dyslipidemia, and a history of multiple prior percutaneous coronary interventions involving the proximal left anterior descending artery, presented to his physician with a 3-month history of progressively worsening exertional chest pressure and left arm pain, similar to his previous episodes of angina.

Two years earlier, he first developed classic effort angina. An abnormal stress test led to a coronary angiogram, which revealed a severe stenosis in the proximal segment of the left anterior descending coronary artery (Figure 1-1 and Video 1-1). This was treated with a 3.0 mm diameter by 23 mm long sirolimus-eluting stent, with an excellent angiographic result (Figure 1-2 and Video 1-2). His angina completely resolved; however, 10 months after the procedure, he developed recurrent effort angina. Coronary angiography confirmed severe, focal, in-stent restenosis within the proximal edge of the drug-eluting stent (Figure 1-3). Balloon angioplasty using a 3.0 mm noncompliant balloon dilated to 16 atmospheres improved the angiographic appearance (Figure 1-4 and Video 1-3) and resolved the patient's symptoms. However, 6 months later (and 9 months before his current presentation) the development of recurrent angina prompted another angiogram. A second recurrence of in-stent restenosis within the proximal left anterior descending artery stent (Figure 1-5 and Video 1-4) was treated with a 3.0 mm diameter by 30 mm long zotarolimus-eluting stent, again with good angiographic result (Figure 1-6A). Intravascular ultrasound performed after this procedure demonstrated excellent stent apposition throughout the stented segment (Figure 1-6B). He remained symptom-free for 6 months until this presentation.

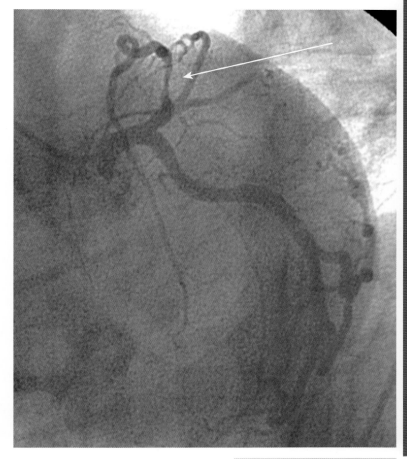

FIGURE 1-1. This is a representative left coronary angiogram in a left anterior oblique projection with caudal angulation, demonstrating the severely stenosed segment of the proximal left anterior descending artery prior to intervention (*arrow*).

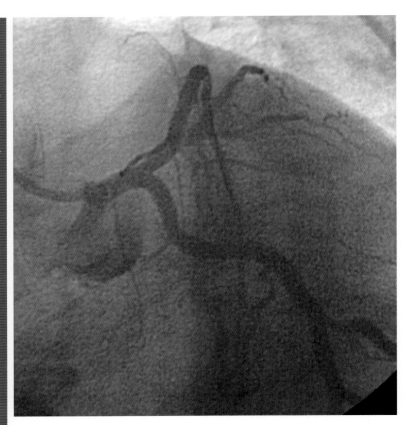

FIGURE 1-2. This angiogram shows the final angiographic result after insertion of a 3.0 mm diameter by 23 mm long sirolimus-eluting stent.

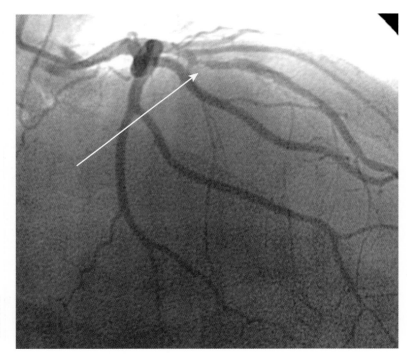

FIGURE 1-3. This angiogram was obtained after the patient developed recurrent angina, and reveals severe focal in-stent restenosis of the proximal edge of the sirolimus-eluting stent within the proximal left anterior descending artery (*arrow*) (right anterior oblique projection with cranial angulation).

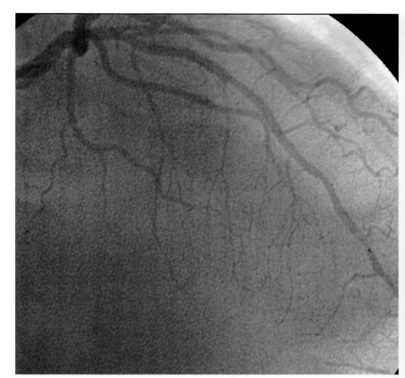

FIGURE 1-4. This is the result after balloon angioplasty of the restenotic lesion in the proximal left anterior descending artery shown in Figure 1-3.

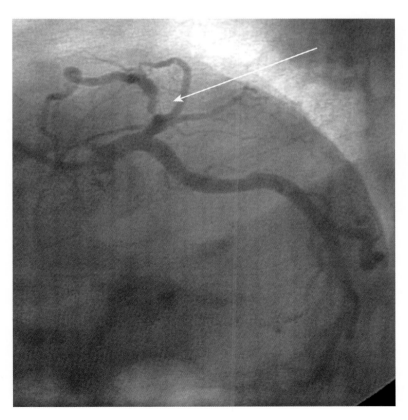

FIGURE 1-5. This figure depicts the second recurrence of in-stent restenosis at the proximal edge of the sirolimus-eluting stent within the proximal left anterior descending artery (*arrow*).

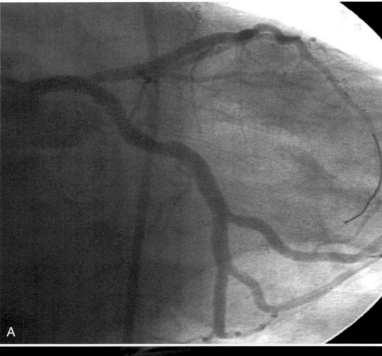

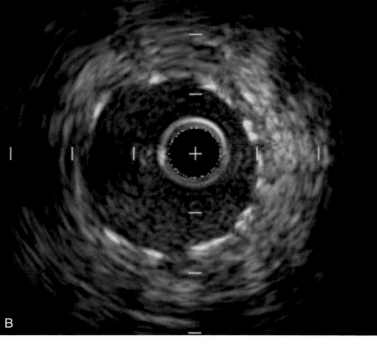

FIGURE 1-6. The second episode of restenosis was treated with a zotarolimus-eluting stent, and the angiographic result *(A)* and representative intravascular ultrasound image *(B)* after receiving a 3 mm diameter by 30 mm long zotarolimus-eluting stent.

CARDIAC CATHETERIZATION

Coronary angiography again demonstrated severe narrowing of the entire stented segment of the proximal left anterior descending artery (Figure 1-7 and Video 1-5), consistent with diffuse in-stent restenosis.

POSTPROCEDURAL COURSE

After discussing the options of repeat percutaneous coronary intervention versus coronary bypass surgery, the patient chose surgical revascularization. He underwent an uncomplicated "off-pump" procedure consisting of a left internal mammary artery graft placed to the mid-portion of the left anterior descending coronary artery. He recovered uneventfully and has had no recurrence of angina 12 months after surgery.

DISCUSSION

This case exemplifies several of the challenges facing a physician managing a patient with recurrent angina after successful stent placement.

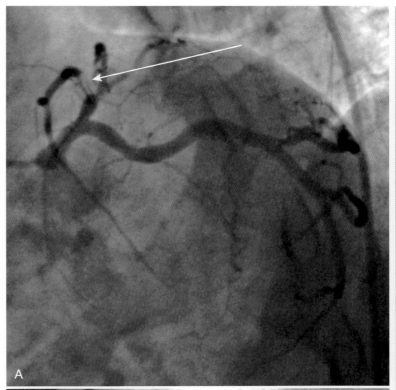

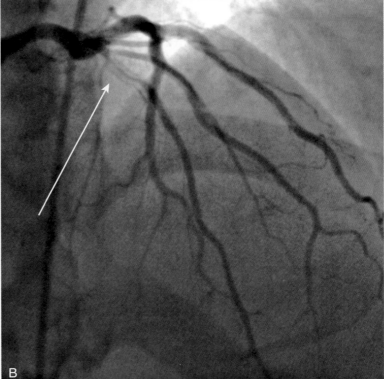

FIGURE 1-7. The third recurrence of in-stent restenosis is shown in the left anterior oblique projection with caudal angulation (*arrow*) *(A)*, and the right anterior oblique projection (*arrow*) *(B)*. There is diffuse in-stent restenosis.

Coronary stents reduced the rate of restenosis compared to balloon angioplasty[1,2]; however, restenosis rates following stent placement remained unacceptably high with 15% to 20% of patients undergoing target vessel revascularization procedures within 9 months of stent implantation. Certain patient subsets, including diabetics and patients with long lesions in small caliber arteries, had rates of restenosis approaching 50% with bare-metal stents. Drug-eluting stents dramatically reduced clinical restenosis rates to about 5% to 10% in all subsets and have become the standard of care for prevention of in-stent restenosis.[3,4]

The mechanism of restenosis after balloon angioplasty is due to elastic recoil and negative vessel remodeling (or vessel shrinkage), while intimal proliferation is the principal mechanism causing in-stent restenosis. The important patient factors associated with bare-metal stent restenosis include diabetes mellitus, female gender, early recurrence, and chronic renal failure. The angiographic and lesion characteristics consistently associated with bare-metal stent restenosis include small vessel diameter, long lesion and stent length, complex lesion subsets (particularly bifurcation and ostial stenoses and chronic total occlusion), and in-stent restenosis lesions. Small final luminal diameter after stenting is also a factor, with optimal outcomes associated with a minimal cross-sectional area greater than 7.0 mm^2 by intravascular ultrasound.[5]

Optimal treatment of in-stent restenosis of a bare-metal stent depends on whether the intimal proliferation is focal (less than 10 mm long) or diffuse (more than 10 mm long and typically involving the entire stent length). Focal in-stent restenosis can be successfully treated with balloon angioplasty with low rates of recurrence; intravascular ultrasound can assist the operator in determining whether stent underexpansion led to the episode of restenosis and can be used to assess the result after angioplasty. Diffuse in-stent restenosis is more problematic, with high rates of recurrence with most conventional therapies including balloon angioplasty, rotational atherectomy, and repeat bare-metal stenting. Local delivery of gamma or beta radiation via brachytherapy devices reduces restenosis, but is cumbersome and has been mostly abandoned. Currently, the treatment of choice for bare-metal stent restenosis is the use of drug-eluting stents.[6]

Although uncommon, restenosis of a drug-eluting stent can be particularly stubborn to manage and is associated with high rates of subsequent recurrence, as is demonstrated in the case presented here. Among drug-eluting stents, there is no clear difference in rates of restenosis between stent types, although there appears to be greater late lumen loss with paclitaxel-eluting stents compared to sirolimus-eluting stents.[7] Intimal proliferation remains the dominant mechanism for drug-eluting stent restenosis; however, many of the episodes occur at the stent edges, and most are focal in-stent restenosis. Presumed causes include stent underexpansion, stent fracture, nonuniform drug deposition or polymer disruption during insertion of the stent, and drug resistance. Predictors are essentially the same as for bare-metal restenosis and include stent length, diabetes, post-procedure minimal luminal diameter, and complex lesion morphology.

Treatment of restenosis within a drug-eluting stent is challenging, with a high rate of recurrent restenosis. Regardless of the percutaneous treatment chosen, almost a third of patients will require target vessel revascularization at 1 year. Options for treatment include balloon angioplasty, restenting with either the same or a different type of drug-eluting stent, bypass surgery, or medical management. There have also been small studies suggesting benefit with brachytherapy or drug-coated balloon angioplasty. There are no large randomized trials comparing different treatments for restenosis of a drug-eluting stent. In patients such as the one presented here, with multiple recurrences of diffuse restenosis, the likelihood of enduring success from another intervention is low, leading to the decision to recommend bypass surgery.

KEY CONCEPTS

1. Drug-eluting stents have significantly reduced the rate of target lesion revascularization due to restenosis. Drug-eluting stents are the treatment of choice for in-stent restenosis of a bare-metal stent.
2. Treatment of restenosis within a drug-eluting stent is challenging, with a high rate of recurrent stenosis. Options for treatment include balloon angioplasty, restenting with either the same or a different type of drug eluting stent, bypass surgery, or medical management.
3. Patients with multiple recurrences of restenosis who are at high risk of repeat revascularization despite treatment should be considered for bypass surgery.

Selected References

1. Fischman DL, Leon MB, Baim DS, Schatz RA, Savage MP, Penn I, Detre K, Veltri L, Ricci D, Nobuyoshi M, Cleman M, Heuser R, Almond D, Teirstein PS, Fish RD, Colombo A, Brinker J, Moses J, Shaknovich A, Hirshfeld J, Bailey S, Ellis S, Rake R, Goldberg S: A randomized comparison of coronary-stent placement and balloon angioplasty in the treatment of coronary artery disease, N Engl J Med 331:496–501, 1994.
2. Serruys PW, DeJaegere P, Kiemeneij F, Macaya C, Rutsch W, Heyndrickx G, Emanuelsson H, Marco J, Legrand V, Materne P, Belardi J, Sigwart U, Colombo A, Goy JJ, Van Den Heuvel P, Delcan J, Morel M: A comparison of balloon expandable-stent implantation with balloon angioplasty in patients with coronary artery disease, N Engl J Med 331:489–495, 1994.
3. Weisz G, Martin B, Leon MB, Holmes DR, Kereiakes DJ, Popma JJ, Teirstein PS, Cohen SA, Wang H, Cutlip DE, Moses JW: Five-year follow-up after sirolimus-eluting stent implantation results of the SIRIUS (sirolimus-eluting stent in de-novo native coronary lesions) trial, J Am Coll Cardiol 53:1488–1497, 2009.
4. Stone GW, Ellis SG, Cannon L, et al: Comparison of a polymer-based paclitaxel-eluting stent with a bare-metal stent in patients with complex coronary artery disease: a randomized controlled trial, JAMA 294:1215–1223, 2005.
5. Hong MK, Park SW, Mintz GS, Lee NH, Lee CW, Kim JJ, Park SJ: Intravascular ultrasonic predictors of angiographic restenosis after long coronary stenting, Am J Cardiol 85:441–445, 2000.
6. Kastrati A, Mehilli J, von Beckerath N, Dibra A, Hausleiter J, Pache J, Schuhlen H, Schmitt C, Dirschinger J, Schomig A, for the ISAR-DESIRE Study Investigators: Sirolimus-eluting stent or paclitaxel-eluting stent vs. balloon angioplasty for prevention of recurrences in patients with coronary in-stent restenosis: A randomized controlled trial, JAMA 293:165–171, 2005.
7. Cosgrave J, Melzi G, Corbett S, Biondi-Zoccai GGL, Agostoni P, Babic R, Airoldi F, Chieffo A, Sangiorgi GM, Montorfano M, Michev I, Carlino M, Colombo A: Comparable clinical outcomes with paclitaxel- and sirolimus-eluting stents in unrestricted contemporary practice, J Am Coll Cardiol 49:2320–2328, 2007.

LAD-Diagonal Bifurcation Lesion

M. Ayoub Mirza, MD, and Michael Ragosta, MD, FACC, FSCAI

CASE PRESENTATION

A 55-year-old woman with diabetes and hypertension presented to the emergency room with sudden onset of chest pain. She had undergone catheterization 5 years earlier, at which time she was found to have nonobstructive coronary disease involving the left anterior descending artery. Initial and subsequent electrocardiograms and serial biomarkers remained normal with no evidence of acute infarction. Diagnosed with unstable angina, she was treated with aspirin, clopidogrel, and low-molecular-weight heparin, and was referred for cardiac catheterization the next day.

CARDIAC CATHETERIZATION

Cardiac catheterization revealed a complex 90% stenosis of the left anterior descending (LAD) artery at the bifurcation of a first diagonal branch (D1). The stenosis extended proximal and distal to the D1 branch; in addition, the D1 branch had an 80% stenosis at the ostium (Figures 2-1, 2-2 and Videos 2-1, 2-2, 2-3). No other significant lesions were observed (Figure 2-3), and left ventricular function was preserved.

The physician chose to treat the artery percutaneously. Using bivalirudin as the procedural anticoagulant, a 6F Judkins left guide coronary catheter with 4 cm curve (JL4) was used to engage the left coronary artery. A 180 cm long,

0.014" floppy-tipped guidewire was advanced into the LAD and the lesion directly stented using a 2.5 mm diameter, 25 mm long sirolimus-eluting stent. This resulted in an excellent angiographic result in the LAD (Figure 2-4 and Video 2-4). A second floppy-tipped guidewire was positioned in the first diagonal branch, passing through the LAD stent. The diagonal stenosis was first dilated with a 2.5 mm diameter by 15 mm long compliant balloon (Figure 2-5) but this produced a suboptimal result at the ostium (Figure 2-6 and Video 2-5). Thus, a 2.5 mm diameter by 18 mm long sirolimus-eluting stent was positioned at the ostium and deployed (Figure 2-7). The final angiographic result is shown in Figure 2-8 and Video 2-6.

POSTPROCEDURAL COURSE

Following the procedure, the patient remained symptom-free and was discharged home the next day on dual antiplatelet therapy (aspirin and clopidogrel) indefinitely. She remained free of cardiac symptoms or events 4 years after the intervention.

DISCUSSION

Atherosclerotic lesions involve the bifurcation of a major side branch in up to 15% of percutaneous coronary interventions, creating significant challenges to the operator.

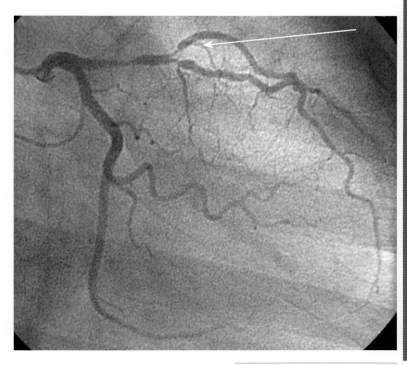

FIGURE 2-1. This is a right anterior oblique angiogram with caudal angulation of the left coronary artery demonstrating a complex lesion in the proximal segment of the left anterior descending artery involving a large diagonal side branch (*arrow*).

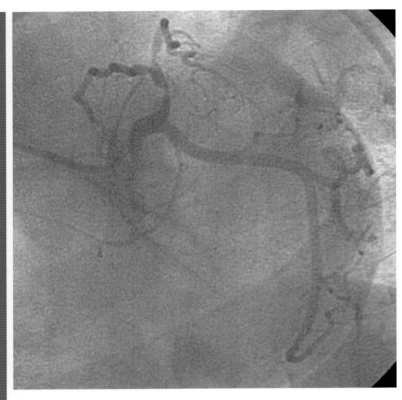

FIGURE 2-2. This is a left anterior oblique view with caudal angulation showing the complex bifurcation disease. This view may be helpful to determine if there is disease involving the ostium of a diagonal side branch, as other views sometimes overlap the diagonal ostium.

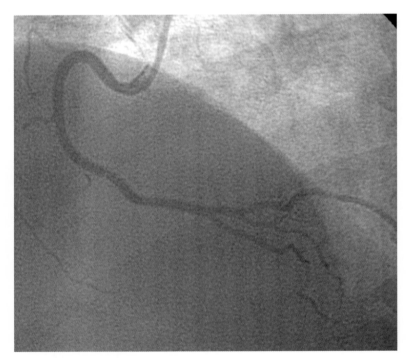

FIGURE 2-3. The right coronary artery was normal.

Compared to nonbifurcation lesions, bifurcation lesions are associated with a higher risk of ischemic complications including periprocedural infarction, primarily due to loss of the side branch. Bifurcation lesions are also associated with a higher risk of stent thrombosis and restenosis, particularly if more than one stent is incorporated into the bifurcation.[1,2]

Lesions classified as "bifurcation" vary greatly, depending on the location of the atherosclerotic plaque relative to the side branch, the angle at which the side branch originates from the parent vessel, and both the caliber and area of myocardium supplied by the side-branch vessel. The heterogeneous nature of bifurcation lesions complicates their management; few studies control for these important

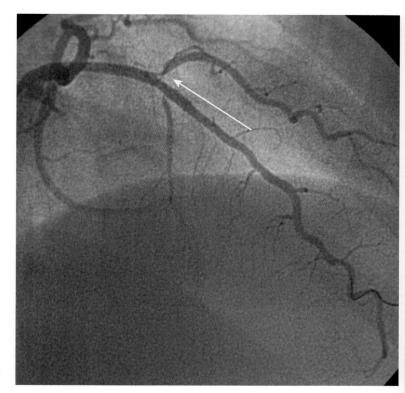

FIGURE 2-4. After stenting the main vessel, there remains significant narrowing in the diagonal side branch (*arrow*).

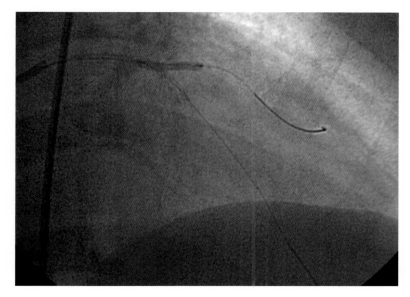

FIGURE 2-5. A guidewire was placed through the stent struts into the diagonal branch and balloon angioplasty of the diagonal was performed.

factors, and both the likelihood of success and the risk of complications are highly dependent on these variables.

Several classification schemes have been described.[3] The Medina classification system (Figure 2-9) uses the number 1 to describe the presence of greater than a 50% stenosis in each of the following three segments in this order: proximal main vessel, distal main vessel, and side branch. Thus, a bifurcation lesion consisting of greater than 50% narrowing of the proximal main vessel and distal main vessel, but sparing the side branch, would be described as 1,1,0.

The risk and outcome of an intervention in the setting of a bifurcation stenosis depends on the lesion morphology and the size of the side branch. Disease involving both sides of the bifurcation as well as the ostium of the side branch (Medina Classification 1,1,1) is associated with the highest risk for side branch occlusion, due to redistribution of atherosclerotic plaque (or plaque "shift").[4] The loss of a major side branch may result in serious sequelae including periprocedural myocardial infarction and its associated complications.

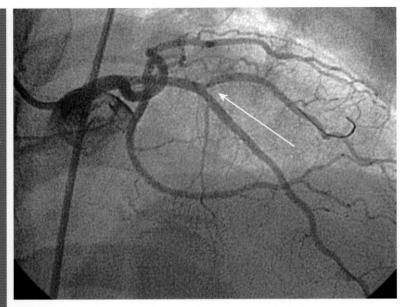

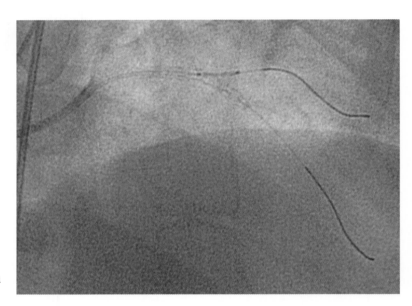

FIGURE 2-6. After balloon angioplasty of the side branch, there remains a suboptimal result at the ostium (*arrow*).

FIGURE 2-7. A stent was positioned at the side branch in a "V" configuration.

A variety of techniques have been proposed to treat bifurcation lesions. Placement of two wires, one in the main artery and a second in the side branch, prior to angioplasty is a standard approach and can help maintain patency after balloon angioplasty. However, in the event of closure after stenting, this wire cannot be used for balloon angioplasty or stenting of the side branch because it lies trapped behind the stent in the main artery. This second wire may maintain patency, however, allowing the operator to identify the location of the side branch ostium and guiding the placement of another guidewire through the stent struts. Debulking techniques using either directional or rotational ather-ectomy, the use of "kissing" balloons, and a variety of side branch stent configurations ("V," "Y," "T," and

"crush stent" configurations) have been developed and advocated by their proponents to prevent loss of the side branch in bifurcation lesions. The optimal treatment of any given bifurcation lesion may incorporate one or more of these techniques; however, recent randomized controlled trials suggest that bifurcation lesions can first be managed with a simple approach of stenting only the main vessel with provisional stenting of the side branch performed only if an unacceptable result is obtained.[5,6] When this strategy is adopted, a second stent is necessary in the side branch in only one third of cases.[6] The case presented here represented a true bifurcation lesion with disease on both sides of the side branch and significant disease involving the side branch ostium. After stenting the

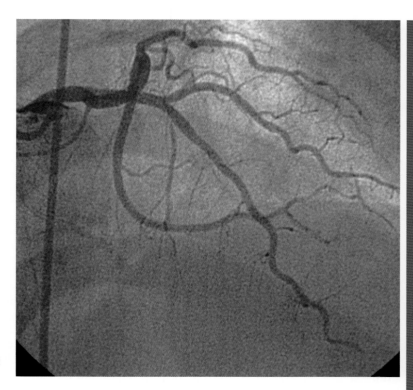

FIGURE 2-8. This is the final angiographic result after stent placement in the side branch ostium.

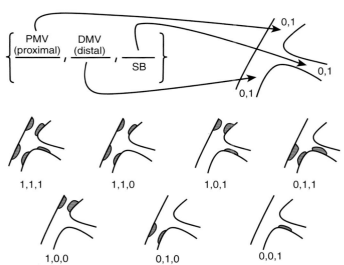

FIGURE 2-9. Medina classification system for coronary bifurcations (from reference 3). PMV = proximal main vessel, DMV = distal main vessel, SB = side branch.

parent vessel, the side branch remained patent but significantly narrowed and balloon angioplasty led to a suboptimal result, leading to placement of the stent in a "V" configuration and an excellent angiographic and long-term clinical result.

KEY CONCEPTS

1. Percutaneous intervention of coronary bifurcation lesions is associated with increased risk of periprocedural infarction from side branch closure and a higher rate of stent thrombosis and restenosis.

2. Careful review of the angiogram is important to characterize the bifurcation and assist in planning the appropriate intervention.

3. A simple strategy of stenting only the main vessel and provisional stenting of the side branch appears to represent the optimal management for most bifurcation lesions.

Selected References

1. Al Suwaidi J, Yeh W, Cohen HA, Detre KM, Williams DO, Holmes DR Jr: Immediate and one year outcome in patients with coronary bifurcation lesions in the modern era (NHLBI dynamic registry), *Am J Cardiol* 87:1139–1144, 2001.

2. Yamashita T, Nishida T, Adamian MG, Briguori C, Vaghetti M, Corvaja N, Albiero R, Finci L, DiMario C, Tobis JM, Colombo A: Bifurcation lesions: two stents versus one stent: immediate and follow-up results, *J Am Coll Cardiol* 35:1145–1151, 2000.

3. Louvard Y, Thomas M, Dzavik V, Hildick-Smith D, Galassi AR, Pan M, Burzotta F, Zelizko M, Dudek D, Ludamn P, Sheiban I, Lassen JF, Darremont O, Kastrati A, Ludwig J, Iakovou I, Brunel P, Lansky A, Meerkin D, Legrand V, Medina A, Lefevre T: Classification of coronary artery bifurcation lesions and treatments: time for a consensus! *Catheter Cardiovasc Interv* 71:175–183, 2008.

4. Aliabadi D, Tillis FV, Bowers TR, Benjuly KH, Safian RD, Goldstein JA, Grines CL, O'Neill WW: Incidence and angiographic predictors of side branch occlusion following high-pressure intracoronary stenting, *Am J Cardiol* 80:994–997, 1997.

5. Steigen TK, Maeng M, Wiseth R, et al: Nordic PCI Study Group Randomized study on simple versus complex stenting of coronary artery bifurcation lesions: the Nordic Bifurcation Study, *Circulation* 114:1955–1961, 2006.

6. Colombo A, Bramucci E, Sacca S, Violini R, Lettieri C, Zanini R, Sheiban I, Paloscia L, Grube E, Schofer J, Bolognese L, Orlandi M, Niccoli G, Latib A, Airoldi F: Randomized study of the crush technique versus provisional side-branch stenting in true coronary bifurcations. The CACTUS (Coronary Bifurcations: Application of the Crushing Technique Using Sirolimus Eluting Stents) Study, *Circulation* 119:71–78, 2009.

Extensive Coronary Calcification

M. Ayoub Mirza, MD, and Michael Ragosta, MD, FACC, FSCAI

CASE PRESENTATION

Three years following placement of a bare-metal stent in the right coronary artery, an otherwise active and healthy 85-year-old woman presented with the acute onset of sharp, stabbing anterior precordial chest pain radiating to the back. The pain was unrelieved by sublingual nitroglycerin and she presented to the hospital. Her only medications were aspirin 81 mg daily and atenolol 50 mg daily. Physical examination revealed a heart rate of 67 and a blood pressure of 110/54 mmHg and the remaining exam was unremarkable. In the emergency room, an electrocardiogram revealed nonspecific T wave inversion in lead III and initial cardiac biomarkers were not elevated. Because of the atypical nature of her chest pain and the absence of objective evidence of ischemia, she first underwent a CT angiogram of the chest to determine if her symptoms were due to an acute aortic dissection. This study showed no evidence of dissection but demonstrated extensive coronary and aortic calcification (Figure 3-1). She was admitted to a telemetry unit with a diagnosis of unstable angina, treated with enoxaparin, and underwent cardiac catheterization the next day.

CARDIAC CATHETERIZATION

Fluoroscopy confirmed the extensive coronary calcification in both the right and left coronary trees seen by CT scan (Figure 3-2). Despite heavy calcification, there was no significant luminal obstruction present in the left coronary artery on angiography. The right coronary artery, however, contained a complex, high-grade stenosis in the proximal segment, with extensive calcification (Figure 3-3 and Video 3-1).

Because of the extensive calcification, the operator planned to treat the artery by first performing rotational atherectomy followed by balloon angioplasty and stenting. After placing a temporary transvenous pacemaker, procedural anticoagulation was accomplished with a double bolus followed by an infusion of eptifibatide, along with a bolus of unfractionated heparin, to achieve an activated clotting time of greater than 200 seconds. A 6 French extra backup right coronary guide catheter was selectively engaged and a floppy RotaWire passed into the distal vessel. The operator used a 1.5 mm atherectomy burr, platformed to 160,000 rotations per minute. After three 30-second runs, the burr passed through the proximal lesion without deceleration and a satisfactory angiographic result was observed (Figure 3-4). The burr was removed from the guide catheter and a 2.5 mm diameter by 15 mm long compliant balloon fully expanded at only 6 atmospheres pressure. A 2.5 mm diameter by 15 mm long bare-metal stent was deployed at 15 atmospheres with an excellent angiographic result (Figure 3-5 and Video 3-2); intravascular ultrasound confirmed full stent deployment at the stent site.

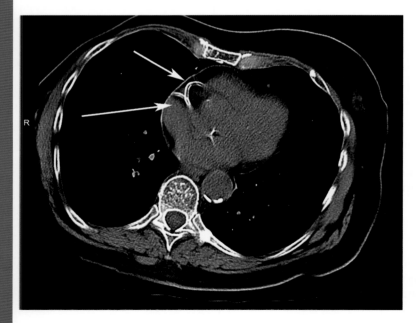

FIGURE 3-1. This is a representative image of a noncontrast CT of the chest demonstrating the extensive coronary calcification present (*arrows*).

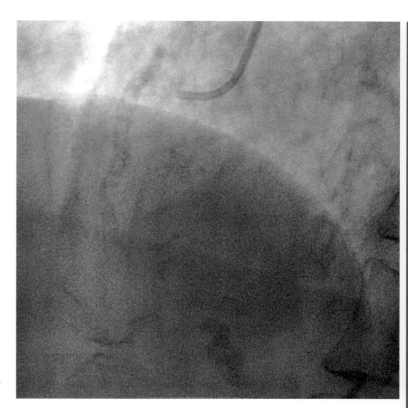

FIGURE 3-2. This is a fluoroscopic image of the right coronary artery showing the heavy calcification present.

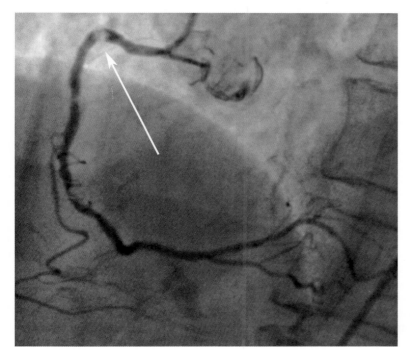

FIGURE 3-3. This is a left anterior oblique angiogram of the right coronary artery demonstrating the severe stenosis of the proximal segment of the right coronary artery within the heavily calcified area (*arrow*).

POSTPROCEDURAL COURSE

She was observed overnight and discharged the next morning with no complications. At follow-up 1 year later, she remained active and free of angina.

DISCUSSION

Calcified coronary lesions offer substantial challenges to the interventional cardiologist. The noncompliant nature of these lesions often leads to difficulty passing balloons

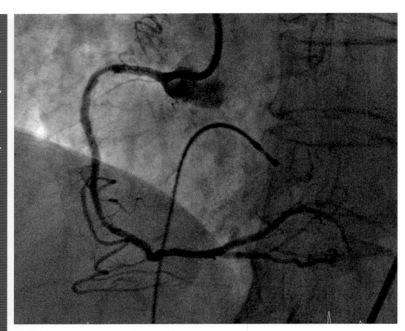

FIGURE 3-4. This is the angiographic result after rotational atherectomy with a 1.5 mm burr.

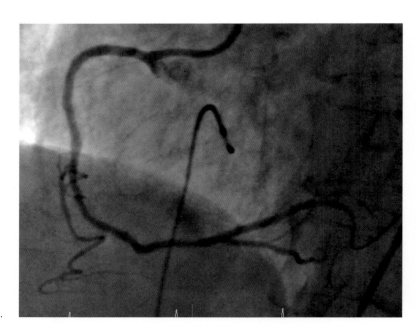

FIGURE 3-5. This is the final angiographic result after stenting.

and stents, and typically requires the use of aggressive guide catheters to provide the back-up necessary to deliver these devices to the lesion. Once a balloon is delivered to the stenosis, the rigid lesion usually responds poorly to balloon angioplasty, leaving a significant residual stenosis, and is associated with a substantial risk of dissection. This can be a serious problem if the coronary calcification subsequently thwarts the operator's ability to deliver a stent. Furthermore, if a stent is successfully delivered, the rigid lesion may prevent full stent expansion, leading to a higher risk of stent thrombosis and restenosis, or, in an effort to fully expand the stent, the operator may resort to balloon inflation using higher and higher pressures, which may cause vessel perforation or extensive edge dissections.

Procedural success in the presence of heavy coronary calcification may be facilitated by first debulking the lesion with rotational atherectomy (RA). Rotational atherectomy involves the use of a diamond-coated burr rotating at high speed to ablate the inelastic tissue of the plaque while preserving elastic tissue of the vessel wall. Ablation of even a small amount of calcified plaque often changes lesion compliance enough to render it more amenable to intervention. Pre-stenting athero-ablation in calcified lesions results in a better acute angiographic result, a larger lumen, and a more favorable clinical outcome compared to either stenting alone or rotational atherectomy alone.[1]

Rotational atherectomy adds complexity to the procedure. Similar to other atheroablative techniques, it is associated with higher complication rates, including periprocedural myocardial infarction, perforation, dissection, and slow- or no-reflow phenomenon. The use of adjunctive platelet glycoprotein IIb-IIIa inhibitors along with heparin helps reduce the risk of no-reflow, and temporary pacemakers are often placed during right coronary interventions because of the heart block and bradycardia associated with rotational atherectomy in this vessel. Marked tortuosity and the presence of a dissection or visible thrombus increase the risk of rotational atherectomy and represent relative contraindications to this procedure.

The decision to first perform rotational atherectomy in a patient such as the one shown here is an important one. While many cases of extensive coronary calcification are successfully treated with balloon angioplasty and stenting, their response is highly unpredictable. A strategy of first attempting balloon angioplasty may be regretted when the operator struggles to dilate the lesion, creates an extensive dissection with a significant residual stenosis, and is then unable to pass a stent. Rotational atherectomy at this point is not possible because of the risk of extending the dissection. Preballoon RA might have prevented this scenario. Interestingly, success does not typically require aggressive atherectomy. Use of a single small-diameter burr such as the one used in this case (1.5 mm) is usually adequate to remove enough luminal calcium to facilitate balloon inflation and stent deployment. In fact, a strategy of aggressive rotational atherectomy (burr to artery ratio > 0.7) offers no advantage over modest atherectomy (burr to artery ratio < 0.7).[2]

KEY CONCEPTS

1. Heavy coronary calcification offers significant challenges to the operator and is associated with a high risk and a lower procedural success rate.
2. Used as an adjunct, prelesion preparation with rotational atherectomy may facilitate balloon angioplasty and stent deployment in the presence of heavy coronary calcification.
3. Rotational atherectomy adds complexity to the procedure, and is associated with a higher risk of periprocedural myocardial infarction, perforation, and no-reflow phenomenon. Adjunctive use of platelet glycoprotein IIb/IIIa inhibitors is recommended to reduce the risk of no-reflow, and a prophylactic pacemaker placement is typically employed for rotational atherectomy of right coronary lesions.

Selected References

1. Hoffmann R, Mintz GS, Kent KM, Pichard AD, Satler LF, Popma JJ, Hong MK, Laird JR, Leon MB: Comparative early and nine-month results of rotational atherectomy, stents, and the combination of both for calcified lesions in large coronary arteries, *Am J Cardiol* 81:552–557, 1998.
2. Whitlow PL, Bass TA, Kipperman RM, Sharaf BL, Ho KKL, Cutlip DE, Zhang Y, Kuntz RE, Williams DO, Lasorda DM, Moses JW, Cowley MJ, Ecclesotn DS, Horrigan DM, Bersin RM, Ramee SR, Feldman T: Results of the study to determine rotablator and transluminal angioplasty strategy (STRATAS), *Am J Cardiol* 87:699–705, 2001.

Coronary Aneurysm

Michael Ragosta, MD, FACC, FSCAI

CASE PRESENTATION

A 68-year-old man with long-standing diabetes mellitus, morbid obesity, prior tobacco abuse, dyslipidemia, and obstructive sleep apnea presents with a several month history of atypical chest pain. Pain involves the left anterior chest wall, occurs sporadically both at rest and with exertion, and may last from a few minutes to several hours before relenting. A noninvasive evaluation performed by his primary care physician revealed inferior ischemia. He was referred for coronary angiography. Of note, he has an impressive family history of aortic aneurysm, with his father, brother, paternal uncles, and several cousins all having aneurysms of the aorta.

CARDIAC CATHETERIZATION

Ventriculography revealed normal left ventricular function. The left coronary artery was angiographically normal. Right coronary angiography, however, demonstrated a large focal aneurysm of the proximal coronary artery, measuring nearly 10 mm in diameter, with a moderate stenosis in the midsegment of the vessel (Figure 4-1 and Videos 4-1, 4-2).

Following the diagnostic cardiac catheterization, the various treatment options were discussed in detail, including medical therapy, surgery, and percutaneous treatment using a covered stent. After much discussion, the patient chose to undergo treatment with a covered stent. After loading with 300 mg of clopidogrel, the patient returned to the cardiac catheterization laboratory for this procedure. Bivalirudin was used as the procedural anticoagulant. The operator engaged the right coronary artery with an 8 French right Judkins guide and positioned an extra-support 0.014" guidewire distally. A 5.0 mm diameter, 22 mm long polytetrafluoroethylene (PTFE) covered stent (Atrium iCast, Atrium Medical Corporation) was centered over the aneurysm (Figure 4-2) and deployed. The angiogram obtained after stent deployment showed a small residual leak into the aneurysm sac at the proximal end of the stent (Figure 4-3 and Video 4-3). The operator proceeded with placement of a 4.0 mm diameter by 15 mm long bare-metal stent at the moderate stenosis in the midsegment of the vessel (Figure 4-4), resulting in an excellent angiographic result at this site; however, there remained a small leak into the aneurysm (Video 4-4). A second covered stent (5.0 mm diameter by 16 mm long) was used to cover this small residual leak (Figure 4-5). This resulted in complete exclusion of the aneurysm from the coronary circulation (Figure 4-6 and Videos 4-5, 4-6).

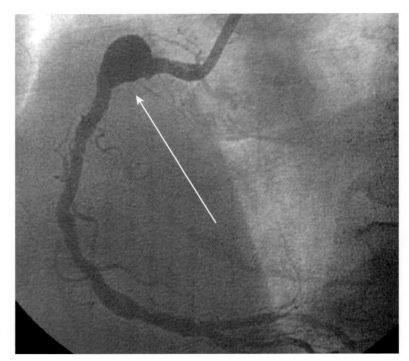

FIGURE 4-1. This is a left anterior oblique angiogram of the right coronary artery. A large aneurysm is seen in the proximal segment (*arrow*) and moderate narrowing is observed in the midsegment.

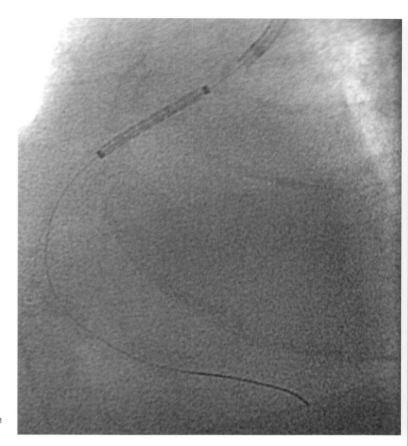

FIGURE 4-2. The covered stent was centered across the neck of the aneurysm.

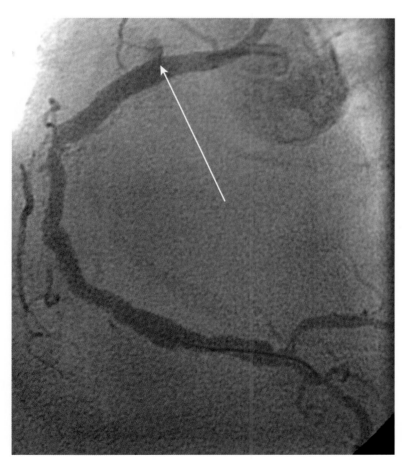

FIGURE 4-3. Angiography obtained after the stent was placed showed a small, persistent leak in the aneurysm sac at the proximal end of the stent (*arrow*).

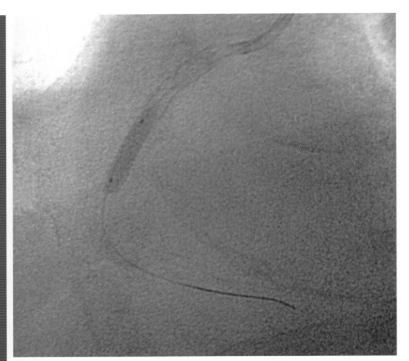

FIGURE 4-4. The moderate stenosis in the midsegment was treated with a bare-metal stent.

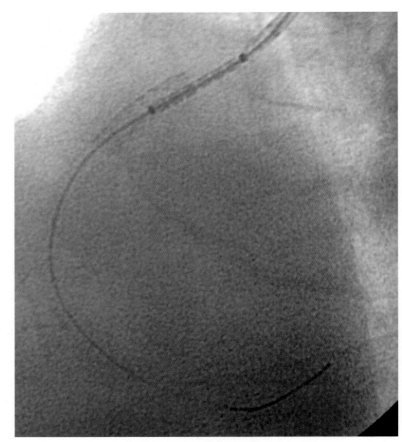

FIGURE 4-5. An additional covered stent was used to cover the persistent leak.

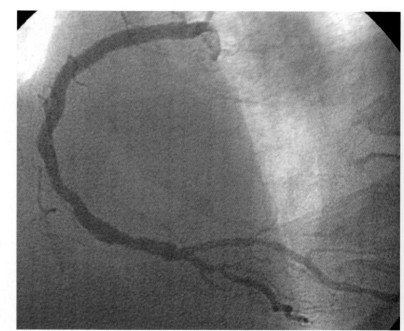

FIGURE 4-6. This is the final angiographic result, demonstrating complete exclusion of the aneurysm sac.

POSTPROCEDURAL COURSE

He was discharged the following day and prescribed clopidogrel and aspirin indefinitely. He remained event free 1 year later.

DISCUSSION

Coronary aneurysms represent abnormal dilatation of the coronary artery and are typically defined by the presence of an enlarged segment greater than 1.5 times the diameter of a normal adjacent segment.[1-3] Coronary aneurysms are not common. They are observed in between 1.5% and 5% of patients undergoing coronary angiography.[1] Similar to this case, they more commonly affect the right coronary artery; the left anterior descending artery is next most commonly involved, followed by the circumflex artery. Multiple aneurysms are frequently observed, but aneurysms of the left main stem are very rare.

By far, the most common cause is atherosclerotic degeneration, accounting for at least 50% of aneurysms. Kawasaki disease is the most common cause worldwide and is the most common nonatherosclerotic cause. Other etiologies are rare and include infection, polyarteritis nodosa, Takayasu arteritis, and connective tissue disorders (Marfan and Ehlers-Danlos syndromes). Coronary aneurysms may also arise iatrogenically from deep vessel injury induced by balloon angioplasty, coronary stenting, or coronary atherectomy procedures. Recently, they have been observed after drug-eluting stent placement.[4]

Many coronary aneurysms are asymptomatic and found incidentally on coronary angiography; however, they may be responsible for symptoms including angina and myocardial infarction. Myocardial infarction can arise from distal embolization or from in-situ thrombosis.[5] Fortunately, rupture of a coronary artery aneurysm is an exceedingly rare occurrence and is only a concern when there is massive enlargement.

There is no consensus regarding the optimal therapy for coronary aneurysms. Most physicians base their therapeutic decision on the size of the aneurysm, the presence of coexisting obstructive lesions, and evidence of ischemia or infarction. Medical therapy with antiplatelet agents and possibly warfarin might reduce the chance of embolization or thrombosis. Surgery is reserved for very large aneurysms involving multiple segments or extending over a long segment. As demonstrated in this case, covered stents are effective at excluding the aneurysm from the coronary circulation but their large bulky nature may result in technical difficulties with delivery.[6] They are also not specifically approved for this indication.

KEY CONCEPTS

1. Coronary aneurysms represent abnormal dilatation of a segment of the coronary artery at least 1.5 times the normal segment and are most commonly caused by atherosclerosis.
2. Many are asymptomatic and cause no significant problems.
3. Potential complications include rupture (very rare) and ischemia from embolic events or thrombosis.
4. There is no consensus regarding optimal therapy. Anticoagulants, surgery, and use of a covered stent to exclude the aneurysm have all been used effectively.

Selected References

1. Chrissoheris MP, Donohue TJ, Young RSK, Ghantous A: Coronary artery aneurysms, *Cardiol Rev* 16:116–123, 2008.
2. Syed M, Lesch M: Coronary artery aneurysm: A review, *Prog Cardiovasc Dis* 40:77–84, 1997.
3. Robinson FC: Aneurysms of the coronary arteries, *Am Heart J* 109:129–135, 1985.
4. Aoki J, Kirtane A, Leon MB, Dangas G: Coronary artery aneurysms after drug-eluting stent implantation, *JACC Cardiovasc Interv* 1:14–21, 2008.
5. von Rotz F, Niederhauser U, Straumann E, Kurz D, Bertel O, Turina MI: Myocardial infarction caused by a large coronary artery aneurysm, *Ann Thorac Surg* 69:1568–1569, 2000.
6. Szalat A, Durst R, Cohen A, Lotan C: Use of polytetrafluoroethylene-covered stent for treatment of coronary artery aneurysm, *Catheter Cardiovasc Interv* 66:203–208, 2005.

Nondilatable Lesion

Michael Ragosta, MD, FACC, FSCAI

CASE PRESENTATION

A 58-year-old man, with a history of documented coronary artery disease found by catheterization 4 years earlier, remained asymptomatic on medical therapy until he presented to his cardiologist with a 6-week history of dyspnea and chest tightness occurring with minimal exertion. Medical therapy consisted of simvastatin, niacin, aspirin, metoprolol, and long-acting nitrates. His past history is also remarkable for diet-controlled diabetes mellitus, hypertension, dyslipidemia, and hypothyroidism. He actively smokes tobacco. The physical exam, electrocardiogram, and routine laboratory evaluations were all normal. Diagnosed with crescendo angina pectoris, he was referred for cardiac catheterization.

CARDIAC CATHETERIZATION

Ventriculography revealed normal left ventricular function. Coronary angiographic findings included a codominant circulation, with a diffusely diseased but small right coronary artery (Figure 5-1) and moderate distal disease in the left circumflex and obtuse marginal branches (Figures 5-2, 5-3). The proximal segment of the left anterior descending artery contained moderate disease (Figure 5-2 and Video 5-1) that in some views appeared nonobstructive (Figures 5-2, 5-3) but in other views appeared more concerning (Figure 5-4 and Video 5-2). Much of the disease present on this study appeared similar to the appearance on angiography 4 years earlier, leaving the operator at a loss for the dramatic change in symptoms.

The concerning symptoms, along with an ambiguous lesion in the proximal left anterior descending artery, prompted the operator to measure fractional flow reserve of this vessel (Figure 5-5). After a 6 French guide catheter was inserted, a pressure wire was advanced past the lesion and hyperemia induced with 100 µg of intracoronary adenosine; fractional flow reserve measured 0.69. Thus, the angiographically-moderate disease represented a flow-limiting lesion, and the operator decided to treat the lesion percutaneously. Following the administration of intravenous heparin and eptifibatide, the procedure

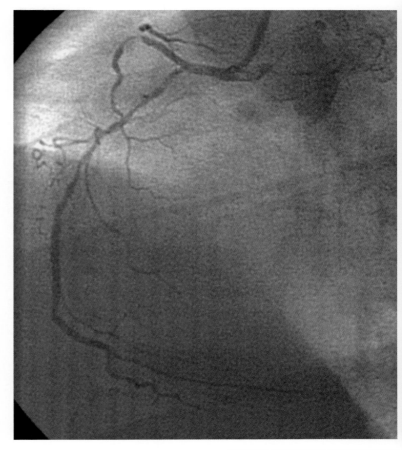

FIGURE 5-1. A small, diffusely-diseased right coronary artery is present but is unchanged from a prior angiogram.

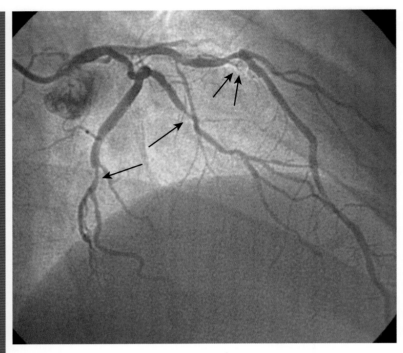

FIGURE 5-2. This view shows the moderate distal disease in the left circumflex and obtuse marginal artery (*arrows*); there is also moderate disease in the left anterior descending artery (*double arrow*).

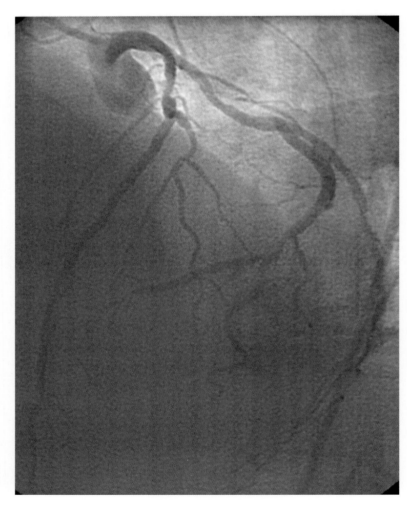

FIGURE 5-3. In this left anterior oblique view of the left coronary artery with cranial angulation, the disease in the left anterior descending artery does not appear significant.

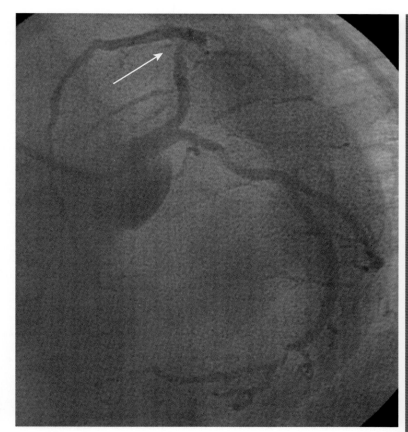

FIGURE 5-4. This left anterior oblique view with caudal angulation suggests a significant lesion in the left anterior descending artery (*arrow*).

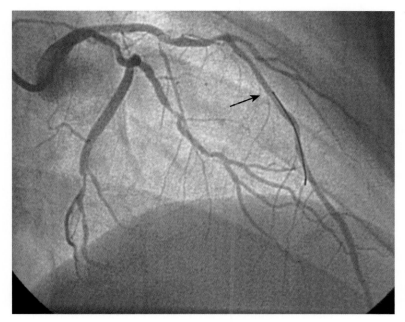

FIGURE 5-5. Pressure wire measurement of the left anterior descending artery. The arrow depicts the location of the transducer.

began with balloon predilatation, using a 2.5 mm by 20 mm long compliant balloon. At nominal inflation pressure, a significant waist remained in the compliant balloon (Figure 5-6 and Video 5-3). Switching to a 2.5 mm by 10 mm noncompliant balloon inflated to 18 atmospheres failed to fully expand the balloon (Figure 5-7). Although these balloon inflations did not improve the luminal appearance, there was no evidence of dissection or perforation (Figure 5-8 and Video 5-4).

Faced with a rigid and undilatable lesion, the operator chose to perform rotational atherectomy with a 1.5 mm burr. Three 30-second runs at 160,000 rpm successfully allowed the burr to pass the diseased area without deceleration (Video 5-5). Following this, a 2.5 mm by

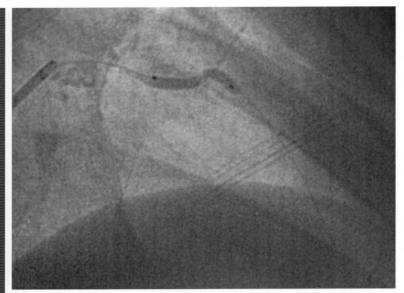

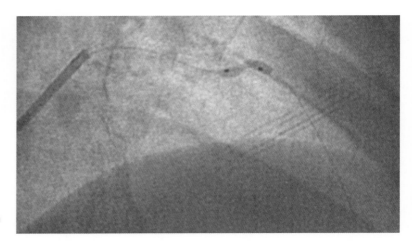

FIGURE 5-6. A compliant balloon failed to fully expand in the lesion.

FIGURE 5-7. A noncompliant balloon inflated to high pressures failed to fully expand in the lesion.

20 mm long compliant balloon fully inflated at nominal pressure (Figure 5-9). Two, everolimus-eluting stents (2.5 mm diameter by 23 mm long and 2.5 mm by 18 mm long) easily crossed and expanded fully at 16 atmospheres of pressure, resulting in an excellent final angiographic appearance (Figure 5-10 and Videos 5-6, 5-7).

POSTPROCEDURAL COURSE

After an uneventful overnight period of observation, he was discharged the next morning on his usual medications, along with clopidogrel for at least 1 year. He remained free of angina at follow-up 1 year later.

DISCUSSION

This case provides two valuable lessons to a budding interventional cardiologist. First, it is an excellent example of one of the important limitations of coronary angiography. The hemodynamic significance of many lesions of only moderate severity may be very difficult to assess by angiography alone, potentially leading to a wrong decision.[1] Although the patient presented with a convincing history of crescendo angina pectoris, on first glance, the angiogram did not reveal an obvious culprit lesion. In fact, the angiogram appeared very similar to one he had 4 years earlier. Despite careful review of the angiogram and multiple angiographic views, the operator was unable to decide if the disease in the left anterior descending artery represented a significant lesion. This is the ideal time to consider further assessment of the artery by either intravascular ultrasound or fractional flow reserve. In this case, fractional flow reserve confirmed the hemodynamic significance of the disease and led to a revascularization decision that successfully eliminated the patient's symptoms.

Once percutaneous intervention was chosen, the rigid nature of the lesion surprised the operator, as this was not expected given the minimal extent of calcium noted by fluoroscopy. When a compliant balloon fails to fully expand at nominal inflation pressures, the operator risks coronary dissection by further increasing inflation pressure. This is due to the fact that a compliant balloon will grow significantly both in diameter and length under increasing pressure. The increasing pressure and enlarging balloon diameter is not transmitted to the offending

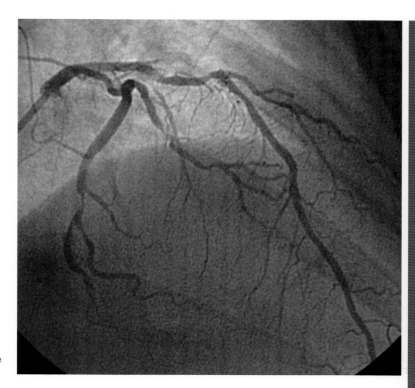

FIGURE 5-8. Angiographic appearance after high pressure balloon inflation.

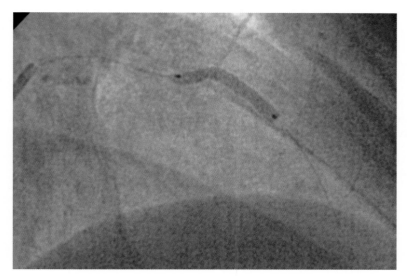

FIGURE 5-9. After rotational atherectomy, a compliant balloon could be fully expanded at nominal inflation pressures.

site, but instead to the softer adjacent sites, often resulting in dissection or perforation. In this case, the operator wisely chose to try a noncompliant balloon, capable of exerting high pressures without significantly changing the balloon size. However, this strategy also failed, with continued underexpansion of the balloon despite very high pressures.

At this point, a decision was made to use rotational atherectomy. It is important to carefully review the angiogram after balloon dilatation in such cases, as the presence of a significant dissection precludes the use of rotational atherectomy. If present, the dissection should be allowed to heal for a few weeks before attempting this strategy. As shown in this case, even minimal debulking with rotational atherectomy led to success; more aggressive debulking was not necessary. Likely,

a small area of luminal calcium prevented balloon expansion. Removal of this component of the plaque allowed full balloon inflation and successful intervention.

This case also provides an example of a potential risk of direct stenting (i.e., without balloon predilatation). Some operators choose this tactic in an effort to save time and reduce equipment cost. However, in this case, this approach would have resulted in an underexpanded and poorly-deployed stent. When this occurs, options are limited, which might have led to aggressive balloon inflations at very high pressures in a desperate effort to expand the stent, potentially causing a perforation or dissection in adjacent segments. Failure to fully expand the stent, in spite of these measures, often leads to an adverse outcome, including stent thrombosis or restenosis.[2,3]

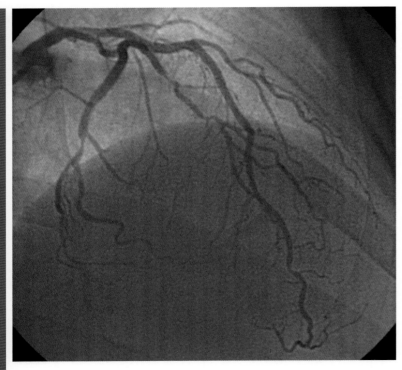

FIGURE 5-10. Final angiographic result after successful stenting.

KEY CONCEPTS

1. Inability to expand a balloon indicates a rigid lesion. Aggressive attempts at balloon dilatation may lead to dissection or perforation.
2. Deployment of a stent should not be attempted when a balloon cannot be fully inflated because of the potential for underexpansion of the stent and subsequent stent thrombosis.
3. Rotational atherectomy can facilitate successful percutaneous intervention of rigid, nondilatable lesions.

Selected References

1. Fischer JJ, Samady H, McPherson JA, Sarembock IJ, Powers ER, Gimple LW, Ragosta M: Comparison between visual assessment and quantitative angiography versus fractional flow reserve for native coronary narrowings of moderate severity, *Am J Cardiol* 90:210–215, 2002.
2. Fujii K, Carlier SG, Mintz GS, Yang YM, Moussa I, Weisz G, Dangas G, Mehran R, Lansky AJ, Kreps EM, Collins M, Stone GW, Moses JW, Leon MB: Stent underexpansion and residual reference segment stenosis are related to stent thrombosis after sirolimus-eluting stent implantation: an intravascular ultrasound study, *J Am Coll Cardiol* 45:995–998, 2005.
3. Fujii K, Mintz GS, Kobayashi Y, Carlier SG, Takebayashi H, Yasuda T, Moussa I, Dangas G, Mehran R, Lansky AJ, Reyes A, Kreps E, Collins M, Colombo A, Stone GW, Teirstein PS, Leon MB, Moses JW: Contribution of stent underexpansion to recurrence after sirolimus-eluting stent implantation for in-stent restenosis, *Circulation* 109:1085–1088, 2004.

High-Risk, Hemodynamically Supported PCI

Angela M. Taylor, MD, MS

CASE PRESENTATION

A fairly active 83-year-old man, with a past medical history notable for previous inferior infarction and ischemic cardiomyopathy, presented with a non-ST elevation myocardial infarction and congestive heart failure. His presenting electrocardiogram revealed an old left bundle branch block. Pertinent laboratory values revealed a brain natriuretic peptide (BNP) of 1473 pg/mL and a peak troponin of 2.28 ng/mL. Cardiac catheterization was performed during his initial hospitalization and revealed a severe mid-right coronary artery stenosis in a diffusely diseased, heavily calcified artery (Figure 6-1 and Video 6-1). The left coronary system was also heavily calcified and demonstrated a moderate-to-severe left main stenosis; a completely occluded circumflex with left to left collateralization (Figure 6-2 and Video 6-2); and a nearly occluded, severely diseased, ostial left anterior descending artery (LAD) (Figure 6-3 and Video 6-3). The LAD also provided collateral flow to the distal RCA territory. A cardiac MRI was subsequently performed to evaluate left ventricular function and myocardial viability. This demonstrated severely reduced left ventricular function (ejection fraction of 12.7%) and viability in the LAD territory. Transmural infarct was present in the inferolateral wall, representing the myocardium supplied by the right coronary and circumflex arteries. He was also noted to have a left ventricular thrombus and a 6 by 9 mm filling defect in the descending thoracic aorta that likely represented atheroma. Based on these findings, he was denied surgical revascularization. Thus, he was managed medically and was discharged on optimal medical therapy including a beta blocker, an ACE inhibitor, a nitrate, a diuretic, aspirin, clopidogrel, and a statin. However, within a 2-week period following discharge, he had two separate admissions for rest chest pain, heart failure, and recurrent non-ST elevation myocardial infarctions. Following the second admission, the decision was made to attempt high-risk percutaneous revascularization of the LAD.

CARDIAC CATHETERIZATION

Repeat angiography at the time of intervention was unchanged. Severe three-vessel disease with left main involvement, heavily calcified coronary arteries, significant collateralization of the RCA from the LAD, and a severely reduced ejection fraction, together placed the patient at significantly high risk for percutaneous intervention. Thus, the operator chose to employ a Tandem-Heart for hemodynamic support during the procedure.

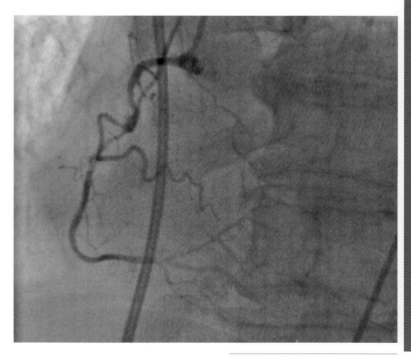

FIGURE 6-1. Severe stenosis in a diffusely diseased, heavily calcified right coronary artery.

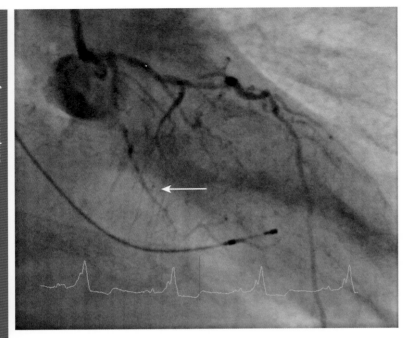

FIGURE 6-2. The left coronary artery system shows an occluded circumflex artery with left to left collaterals (*arrow*) (RAO caudal).

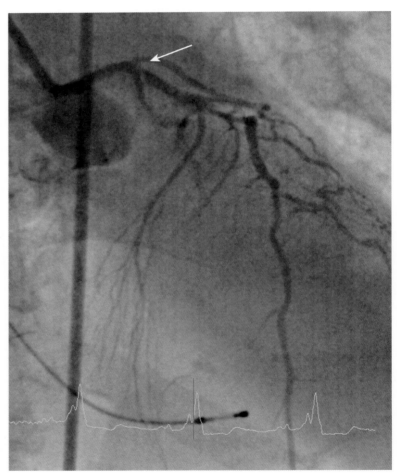

FIGURE 6-3. There is a severe ostial stenosis (*arrow*) in a heavily calcified LAD and a moderate left main stenosis (RAO cranial).

Prior to insertion, the left internal iliac was imaged to assure that the artery was of proper size and was without significant disease burden, to allow passage of the large arterial cannula required for the procedure (Figure 6-4 and Video 6-4). The artery measured 7.7 mm in minimum diameter and thus the operator inserted a 17 French cannula in the left external iliac percutaneously through the left common femoral artery. A transseptal puncture was performed; baseline hemodynamics showed a marked elevation of the left atrial

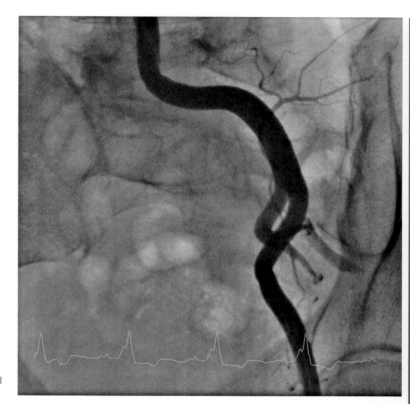

FIGURE 6-4. Angiography of the iliac system showing minimal vascular disease with a minimum artery diameter of 7.7 mm.

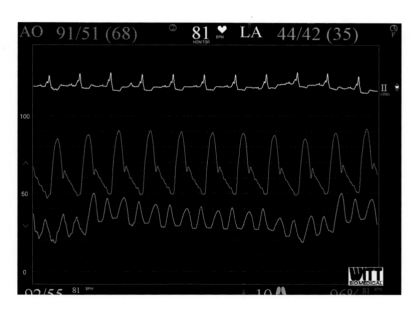

FIGURE 6-5. Baseline hemodynamics showing a marked elevation of the left atrial pressure but preserved arterial pressure.

pressure and preserved arterial pressure (Figure 6-5). The transseptal sheath was exchanged for a 21 French cannula placed via the right femoral vein into the left atrium (Figure 6-6). Unfractionated heparin was used for anticoagulation following the transseptal puncture and ACT was maintained greater than 350 seconds. The arterial and venous cannulae were attached to the extracorporeal centrifugal pump and the system was purged of air. The pump was initiated and maintained at 6500 rpm with resultant flows of 4.5 L/minute. An 8 French sheath was then placed in the right femoral artery, through which the coronary intervention was performed. A temporary pacemaker

was first placed prophylactically via the left femoral vein. Because of the heavy calcification of the proximal LAD, the lesion was debulked using rotational atherectomy with a 1.25 mm burr followed by a 1.5 mm burr. Sequential balloon dilation was performed following successful atherectomy with a 1.5 mm diameter by 15 mm long, a 2.0 mm diameter by 20 mm long, and a 2.5 mm diameter by 20 mm long series of compliant balloons. There was complete inflation of the 2.5 mm balloon along the entire course of the LAD that would require stenting, and the postballoon result appeared suitable for stenting (Figure 6-7 and Video 6-5). Subsequently, a 2.5 mm

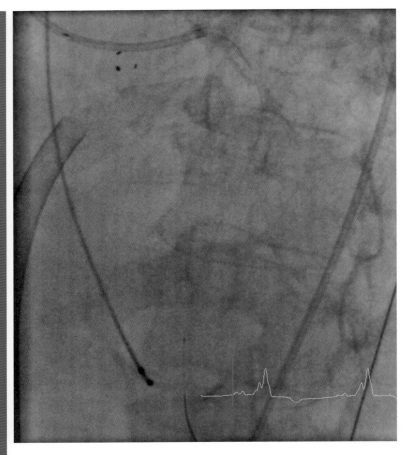

FIGURE 6-6. The transseptal placement of the left atrial cannula of the TandemHeart.

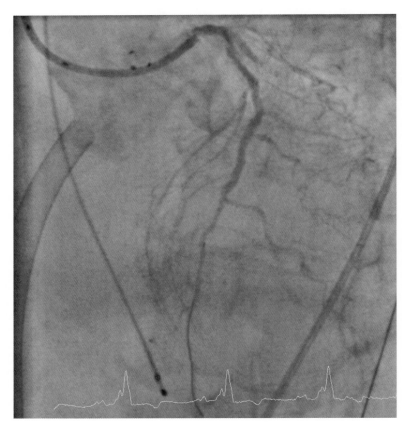

FIGURE 6-7. The LAO cranial projection showing the left main and LAD after rotational atherectomy and balloon angioplasty.

diameter by 28 mm long everolimus-eluting stent was deployed in the LAD and a 2.75 mm diameter by 23 mm long everolimus-eluting stent deployed in the left main. The operator postdilated the left main and LAD stents with a 3.0 mm diameter by 15 mm long semicompliant balloon. The final angiogram demonstrated excellent stent apposition and a widely patent lumen (Figure 6-8, Videos 6-6 and 6-7). Importantly, the patient maintained a normal mean arterial blood pressure of 70 mmHg during the entire procedure while on hemodynamic support (Figure 6-9). The TandemHeart was weaned and removed immediately following the procedure, with hemostasis achieved by manual compression.

POSTPROCEDURAL COURSE

Following the procedure, the patient was monitored and was discharged the next morning with no complications. He was maintained on all of his previous medications with the exception of furosemide, as he had developed contrast nephropathy with a creatinine of 1.7 mg/dL and had mild hypotension at the time of discharge.

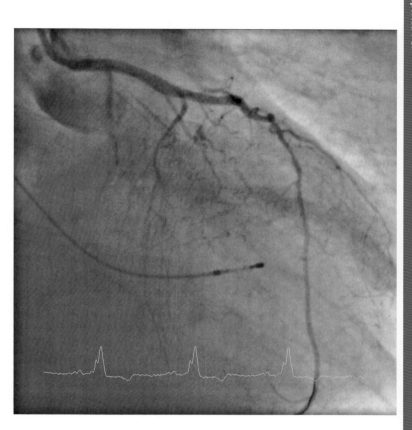

FIGURE 6-8. The RAO caudal projection showing the left main and LAD after stenting and postdilation.

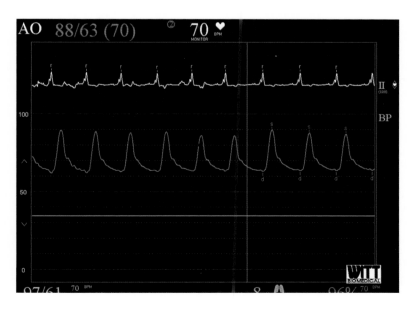

FIGURE 6-9. Intraprocedural hemodynamics while on support showing excellent maintanence of mean arterial pressure at 70 mmHg.

Two days after the procedure, the patient returned to a local hospital with pulmonary edema at which time his furosemide was resumed; he had no further episodes of heart failure. His creatinine had also returned to his previous baseline of 1.0 mg/dL. At 1 month follow-up, he was doing well with no further episodes of angina or heart failure.

DISCUSSION

Clinical goals of cardiac support during high-risk percutaneous coronary intervention (PCI) include maintaining stable hemodynamics for sufficient end-organ perfusion and allowing adequate time for balloon inflation and stent placement. Several support devices are available to support high-risk interventions, including intraaortic balloon pump and percutaneous left ventricular assist devices such as the TandemHeart and Impella. Considerable thought should be given to the requirements and the level of support provided by each device prior to choosing a particular device or beginning a high risk PCI.

The intraaortic balloon pump (IABP) is inserted percutaneously via the femoral artery and advanced in the aorta to the level of the tracheal bifurcation. Most devices require an 8 or 9 French sheath, but can be placed sheathless if a smaller arteriotomy is desired. Balloon volumes range from 30 to 50 cc (average is 40 cc) and are chosen depending on the size of the patient. The balloon inflates during diastole and deflates during systole, augmenting diastolic pressures and reducing afterload. Hemodynamic effects of the IABP include mild increases in cardiac output and stroke volume, decreases in aortic systolic pressure, increases in aortic diastolic and mean pressures, and increases in coronary flow. While the IABP is a useful adjunct to PCI, it is dependent on a fairly stable intrinsic rhythm and cardiac output. It provides the least hemodynamic support of the devices available. Use is contraindicated in the presence of significant aortic regurgitation, aortic dissection, right to left shunts, and severe peripheral vascular disease or tortuosity.[1]

The Impella assist device is inserted percutaneously via the femoral artery into the left ventricle, much in the same way that a left ventricular pigtail catheter is placed. A 13 French sheath requires at least a 5 mm diameter iliofemoral arterial system. Iliac imaging is strongly recommended prior to placement of the device to assure proper vessel size and absence of significant tortuosity. The device functions by removing blood directly from the left ventricle and delivering it to the aorta at the level of the coronary arteries. The Impella provides 2.5 L/min of flow, thus augmenting cardiac output but not providing full support. Hemodynamic effects include direct ventricular unloading, decreased myocardial work and wall tension, increased cardiac output and mean arterial pressure, and increased coronary flow. A 5.0 L/min device, which can provide full left ventricular support, is available, but must be inserted surgically directly into the aorta. The Impella device is contraindicated in patients with severe peripheral vascular disease or tortuosity, mechanical prosthetic aortic valves, significant aortic stenosis, or in the presence of left ventricular thrombus.[2]

The TandemHeart requires percutaneous placement of a 15 to 17 Fr arterial sheath and a transseptally placed 21 Fr venous sheath. The arterial sheath is placed via the femoral artery and advanced into the iliac artery where retrograde arterial flow is delivered. The iliofemoral system should measure at least 6 mm for safe insertion. Due to the large arterial cannula size, iliofemoral imaging is mandatory prior to placement of the device to assure proper vessel size and absence of significant tortuosity or disease. Oxygenated blood is withdrawn from the left atrium via the 21 French cannula placed transseptally via the right femoral vein, and delivered in a retrograde fashion to the artery cannula via a rotary pump. The TandemHeart functions as a percutaneous left ventricular assist device and can provide full cardiac support, up to 4.5 L/min. It is useful for support of high-risk PCI when hemodynamic collapse is likely, such as left main PCI or PCI of a main artery in the setting of severe left ventricular dysfunction. The TandemHeart requires full systemic anticoagulation similar to the extent needed for cardiopulmonary bypass. Hemodynamic effects include increases in cardiac output and mean arterial pressure and decreases in pulmonary capillary wedge pressure. It is contraindicated in the presence of severe peripheral vascular disease, an inferior vena cava filter, left atrial thrombus, and in cases where anticoagulation is contraindicated or transseptal puncture cannot be performed safely.[3]

In the case presented here, TandemHeart was chosen, since the operator anticipated the need for full hemodynamic support based on his profound left ventricular dysfunction and severe disease in the only remaining artery. Furthermore, the presence of left ventricular thrombus precluded the use of Impella. The device clearly resulted in hemodynamic stability despite a prolonged, complex intervention.

KEY CONCEPTS

In the setting of high-risk PCI:
1. Several ventricular support devices are available, including the intraaortic balloon pump, the Impella, and the TandemHeart. The device should be chosen based on the level of support needed and specific patient characteristics, particularly the status of the iliofemoral vessels.
2. The intraaortic balloon pump provides the least support, while the TandemHeart provides maximum and full cardiac support. The percutaneous Impella provides an intermediate level of support.
3. The intraaortic balloon pump requires an 8 French sheath and at least a 4 mm diameter femoral artery. The Impella requires a 13 French sheath and at least a 5 mm diameter femoral artery. The TandemHeart requires a 17 to 19 French sheath and at least a 6 mm diameter femoral artery.
4. All support devices are contraindicated in patients with severe peripheral vascular disease or severe arterial tortuosity. This should be taken into account before committing to a complex intervention in a high-risk patient.

Selected References

1. Brodie BR, Stuckey TD, Hansen C, Muncy D: Intra-aortic balloon counterpulsation before primary percutaneous transluminal coronary angioplasty reduces catheterization laboratory events in high-risk patients with acute myocardial infarction, *Am J Cardiol* 84:18–23, 1999.
2. Dixon SR, Henriques JPS, Mauri L, Sjauw K, Civitello A, Kar B, Loyalka P, Resnic FS, Teirstein P, Makkar R, Palacios IF, Collins M, Moses J, Benali K, O'Neill WW: A prospective feasibility trial investigating the use of the Impella 2.5 system in patients undergoing high-risk percutaneous coronary intervention (PROTECT I), *JACC Cardiovasc Interv* 2(2):91–96, 2009.
3. Aragon J, Lee MS, Kar S, Makkar RR: Percutaneous left ventricular assist device: "TandemHeart" for high risk coronary intervention, *Catheter Cardiovasc Interv* 65(3):346–352, 2005.

Saphenous Vein Graft Disease

Michael Ragosta, MD, FACC, FSCAI

CASE PRESENTATION

This case involves a 72-year-old man with a history of prior inferior infarction and coronary bypass surgery 16 years earlier, consisting of a left internal mammary artery graft to the left anterior descending (LAD) and a saphenous vein graft to a large ramus intermedius. Past medical history also includes chronic atrial fibrillation, hypertension, insulin-requiring diabetes, tobacco abuse, and hyperlipidemia.

He had known left ventricular dysfunction with an ejection fraction of 40%, but had remained asymptomatic since his bypass operation until 2 to 3 weeks before presentation, when he noted progressive shortness of breath with any exertion associated with chest tightness. He developed rest dyspnea and then became unable to lie flat without developing a sense of suffocating. He presented to the emergency room and was promptly admitted with a diagnosis of congestive heart failure and unstable angina. His electrocardiogram showed nonspecific abnormalities that were unchanged from prior ECGs, and serial troponin assays remained in the normal range. However, an echocardiogram showed deterioration in his left ventricular

function with an ejection fraction of 15% to 20%. He subsequently underwent cardiac catheterization, which found a chronically-occluded right coronary artery and a patent left internal mammary to the LAD with large collateral vessels to the right coronary (Figure 7-1 and Video 7-1). The native proximal LAD and circumflex arteries were completely occluded. The saphenous vein graft to the ramus had a very severe stenosis located in the proximal segment near the aortic anastomosis (Figures 7-2, 7-3 and Videos 7-2, 7-3). He was referred for percutaneous coronary intervention of the saphenous vein graft.

CARDIAC CATHETERIZATION

The night prior to the procedure, the patient received a loading dose of 600 mg clopidogrel and, after obtaining arterial access, the operator administered bivalirudin as the procedural anticoagulant. A 6 French Judkins right 4.0 guide catheter was engaged in the saphenous vein graft. To achieve distal embolic protection, the operator advanced a filter wire past the

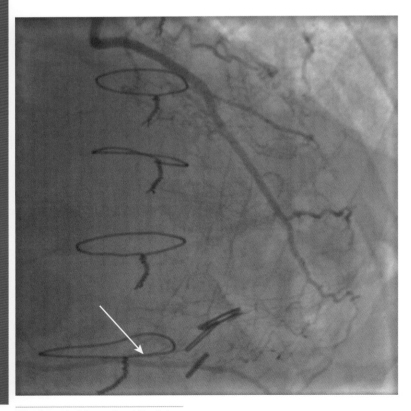

FIGURE 7-1. This is an angiogram of the left internal mammary graft to the left anterior descending artery. There is a large collateral vessel to the right coronary artery (*arrow*).

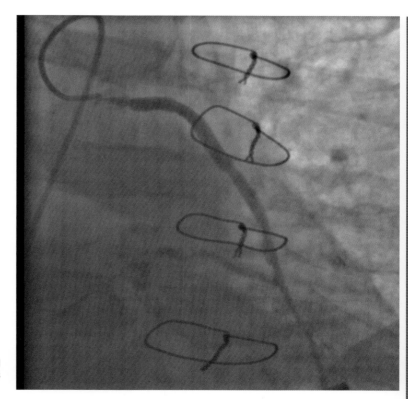

FIGURE 7-2. A severe stenosis was seen in the proximal segment of the saphenous vein graft to the ramus intermedius (right anterior oblique projection).

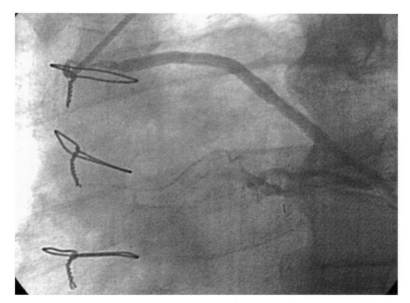

FIGURE 7-3. A severe stenosis was seen in the proximal segment of the saphenous vein graft to the ramus intermedius (left anterior oblique projection).

stenosis and positioned the filter in the distal portion of the vein graft (Figure 7-4). The lesion in the proximal vein graft was first treated with a 3.0 mm diameter by 20 mm long compliant balloon and then with a 4.0 mm diameter by 23 mm long bare-metal stent. The stent was postdilated with a 4.5 mm diameter noncompliant balloon to high atmospheres. The filter wire was retrieved and angiography showed normal flow in the ramus with no evidence of distal embolization and an excellent luminal result. The final angiographic results are shown in Figure 7-5 and Video 7-4.

POSTPROCEDURAL COURSE

He had no postprocedure complications and was discharged the next morning on lisinopril, atenolol, furosemide, rosuvastatin, aspirin, clopidogrel, and insulin. At follow-up visits 6 weeks and 3 months later, he remained free of chest pain, orthopnea, or significant dyspnea on exertion. Repeat echocardiography found no change in his severe left ventricular dysfunction, and his physician planned to refer him for an implantable defibrillator. However, 4 months after the intervention, he

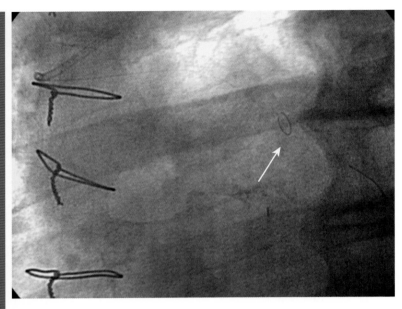

FIGURE 7-4. Distal embolic protection was accomplished with a filter wire positioned in the vein graft (*arrow*).

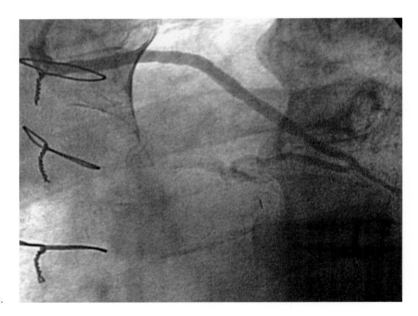

FIGURE 7-5. Final angiographic result after stenting.

experienced recurrent chest tightness and presented to the emergency room after a prolonged episode. He became pain-free after nitroglycerin administration, and his troponin peaked at 4.0 ng/mL. Repeat catheterization showed no change in the left internal mammary to the LAD, but severe focal in-stent restenosis was seen in the saphenous vein graft to the ramus (Figure 7-6 and Video 7-5). Again, a distal embolic protection device was placed and intervention performed first with a 3.5 mm balloon (Figure 7-7). A sirolimus-eluting stent (3.5 mm diameter by 18 mm long, postdilated with a 4.0 mm noncompliant balloon) was deployed within the stent (Figure 7-8 and Video 7-6). There were no complications, and, after an overnight observation, he was discharged the next morning. He remained symptom-free at follow-up visits 3 and 9 months after this second intervention.

DISCUSSION

Saphenous vein grafts are subject to accelerated atherosclerosis. This phenomenon limits the long-term efficacy of coronary bypass surgery, as more than half of saphenous vein grafts are either occluded or have severe disease 10 years after surgery.[1] Graft failure occurring very early after bypass surgery (i.e., within a month) is due to thrombotic occlusion of the graft and is often due to technical issues related to graft harvest, graft quality, or the nature of the distal vessel. Beyond the first month, lesions developing within the first year of coronary bypass surgery are typically caused by intimal proliferation, and are usually located at the aorto-ostium or distal anastomosis. After 1 year, lesions are due to more typical atherosclerosis; however, these lesions

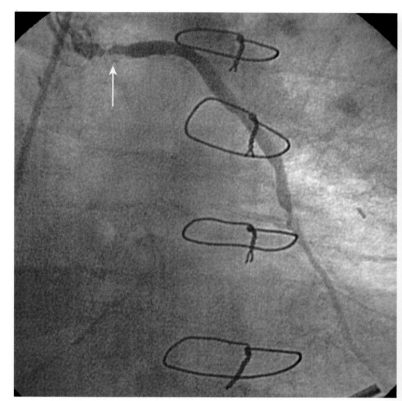

FIGURE 7-6. Four months after stenting, the patient developed recurrent symptoms and severe in-stent restenosis was observed in the vein graft (*arrow*).

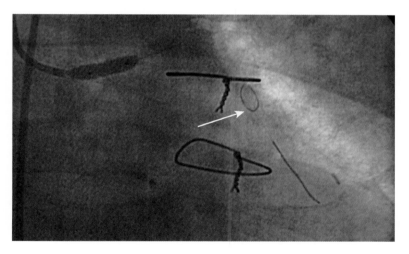

FIGURE 7-7. Balloon angioplasty was performed on the restenotic lesion. A distal embolic protection device was used (*arrow*).

behave differently than those that affect native coronary arteries. Once atherosclerosis begins, saphenous vein graft lesions tend to rapidly progress. More importantly, unlike lesions in native coronary arteries, lesions in saphenous vein grafts are friable and prone to distal embolization when treated percutaneously. This later feature is the primary reason contributing to the high risk of saphenous vein graft interventions.

Atheroembolism occurring after saphenous vein graft interventions may have very serious consequences. Macroembolization may occlude distal branches but, more commonly, extensive embolization of small particles causes microcirculatory obstruction and "no-reflow" or "slow-flow." These events may lead to sizeable

periprocedural myocardial infarctions and, depending on the size of the vascular territory involved and the status of left ventricular function, may result in serious morbidity and increased mortality.

Various methods to improve the safety and efficacy of saphenous vein graft interventions have been tried. Atherectomy devices and covered stents are associated with an increased risk of distal embolization and have essentially been abandoned for this indication. In contrast to other high-risk lesions, the glycoprotein IIb/IIIa receptor antagonists have not shown any benefit in this subgroup.[2] The only approach that has shown significant benefit in reducing the risk of distal embolization and periprocedural myocardial infarction in saphenous

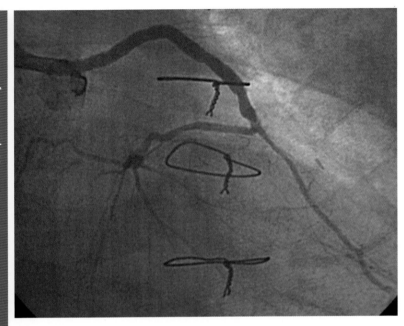

FIGURE 7-8. Final angiographic result after placement of a drug-eluting stent.

vein graft interventions is the use of distal embolic protection devices.[3-5] The first generation device consisted of distal balloon occlusion during intervention, followed by aspiration of the embolic material.[3] This technique has mostly been replaced by the use of distal filters, such as that used in the present case. Proximal protection is also possible, in the event that disease involves the distal segment of the graft and a filter cannot be placed beyond the lesion.[5] All these devices have reduced the risk of periprocedural MI and the incidence of no-reflow and should be routinely used when performing an intervention on an atherosclerotic lesion within a vein graft. As noted above, lesions occurring at the anastomosis within the first year after bypass surgery are usually due to intimal proliferation and do not have the tendency to embolize. Similarly, although a distal protection device was used during treatment of the restenotic lesion present in this case, restenosis lesions have a very low likelihood of distal embolization and a distal protection device may not be necessary.[6]

For the initial intervention, a bare-metal stent was used. Unfortunately, despite the fact that the stent was postdilated to 4.5 mm diameter, the patient developed in-stent restenosis and required an additional revascularization procedure. The routine use of drug-eluting stents to treat saphenous vein graft lesions and reduce rates of restenosis is controversial. One randomized, controlled trial found a lower rate of target lesion revascularization at 6 months in patients treated with sirolimus-eluting stents compared to patients treated with bare-metal stents (5.3% vs. 27%).[6] However, this effect disappeared during long-term follow-up, and, in fact, there was an unexpected higher mortality seen in the drug-eluting stent group.[7] Additional studies did not show an increase in mortality among patients treated with drug-eluting stents but did not find any benefit over bare-metal stents.[8,9] The most recent randomized trial comparing paclitaxel-eluting stents to bare metal stents found a similar mortality but lower rates of angiographic restenosis and target vessel failure in patients treated with drug-eluting stents.[10] Thus, it is unclear whether drug-eluting stents should be routinely used in this population. As done in this case, many operators planning to use large-diameter stents employ bare-metal stents initially and reserve the use of drug-eluting stents for restenotic lesions.

Even with the use of distal protection, the rate of periprocedural myocardial infarction is higher than for native coronary arteries, particularly if the vein graft is extensively diseased (also known as a "degenerated" vein graft). Furthermore, some vein graft lesions are surprisingly rigid and it may be difficult to fully expand a stent. Clearly, saphenous vein graft lesions represent high-risk lesions and are likely to continue to challenge the interventional cardiologist.

KEY CONCEPTS

1. Accelerated atherosclerosis of saphenous vein grafts limits the long-term efficacy of coronary bypass surgery.
2. Percutaneous treatment of saphenous vein grafts is associated with a high risk of distal embolization and periprocedural myocardial infarction.
3. Distal embolic protection devices improve the safety of percutaneous intervention of atherosclerotic lesions in saphenous vein grafts.
4. The role of drug-eluting stents in reducing rates of restenosis is unclear.

Selected References

1. Motwani JG, Topol EJ: Aortocoronary saphenous vein graft disease: Pathogenesis, predisposition, and prevention, *Circulation* 97:916–931, 1998.

2. Roffi M, Mukherjee D, Chew DP, Bhatt DL, Cho L, Robbins MA, Ziada KM, Brennan DM, Ellis SG, Topol EJ: Lack of benefit from intravenous platelet glycoprotein IIb/IIIa receptor inhibition as adjunctive treatment for percutaneous interventions of aortocoronary bypass grafts. A pooled analysis of five randomized clinical trials, *Circulation* 106:3063–3067, 2002.

3. Baim DS, Wahr D, George B, et al: on behalf of the Saphenous vein graft Angioplasty Free of Emboli Randomized (SAFER) Trial Investigators: Randomized trial of a distal embolic protection device during percutaneous intervention of saphenous vein aorto-coronary bypass grafts, *Circulation* 105:1285–1290, 2002.

4. Stone GW, Rogers C, Hermiller J, et al: for the FilterWire EX Randomized Evaluation (FIRE) Investigators: Randomized comparison of distal protection with a filter-based catheter and a balloon occlusion and aspiration system during percutaneous intervention of diseased saphenous vein aorto-coronary bypass grafts, *Circulation* 108:548–553, 2003.

5. Mauri L, Cox D, Hermiller J, Massaro J, Wahr J, Tay SE, Jonas M, Popma JJ, Pavliska J, Wahr D, Rogers C: The PROXIMAL Trial: Proximal protection during saphenous vein graft intervention using the proxis embolic protection system. A randomized, prospective, multicenter clinical trial, *J Am Coll Cardiol* 50: 1442–1449, 2007.

6. Vermeersch P, Agostoni P, Verheye S, Van den Heuvel P, Convens C, Bruining N, Van den Branden F, van Langenhove G: Randomized double-blind comparison of sirolimus-eluting stent versus bare-metal stent implantation in diseased saphenous vein grafts. Six-month angiographic, intravascular ultrasound, and clinical follow-up of the RRISC Trial, *J Am Coll Cardiol* 48: 2423–2431, 2006.

7. Vermeersch P, Agostoni P, Verheye S, Van den Heuvel P, Convens C, Van den Branden F, van Langenhove G: for the DELAYED RRISC (Death and Events at Long-term follow-up AnalYsis: Extended Duration of the Reduction of Restenosis in Saphenous vein grafts with Cypher stent) Investigators: Increased late mortality after sirolimus-eluting stents versus bare-metal stents in diseased saphenous vein grafts. Results from the randomized DELAYED RRISC Trial, *J Am Coll Cardiol* 50:261–267, 2007.

8. Okabe T, Lindsay J, Buch AN, Steinberg DH, Roy P, Slottow TLS, Smith K, Torguson R, Xue Z, Satler LF, Kent KM, Pichard AD, Weissman NJ, Waksman R: Drug-eluting stents verus bare-metal stents for narrowing in saphenous vein grafts, *Am J Cardiol* 102:530–534, 2008.

9. Vignali L, Saia F, Manari A, Santarelli A, Rubboli A, Varani E, Piovaccari G, Menozzi A, Percoco G, Benassi A, Rusticali G, Marzaroli P, Guastaroba P, Grilli R, Maresta A, Marzocchi A: Long-term outcomes with drug-eluting stents verus bare metal stents in the treatment of saphenous vein graft disease (Results from the REgistro Regionale AngiopLastiche Emilia-Romagna Registry), *Am J Cardiol* 101:947–952, 2008.

10. Brilakis ES, Lichenwalter C, de Lemos JA, et al: A randomized controlled trial of a paclitaxel-eluting stent versus a similar bare-metal stent in saphenous vein graft lesions. The SOS (Stenting of Saphenous Vein Grafts) Trial, *J Am Coll Cardiol* 53:919–928, 2009.

STEMI Intervention and Stent Thrombosis

Lawrence W. Gimple, MD, FACC, FSCAI

CASE PRESENTATION

A 45-year-old man presented to the emergency department with severe substernal chest pain of 2.5 hours duration. In the emergency department, the initial ECG showed sinus rhythm at a rate of 71 bpm with ST segment elevation in leads II, III, aVF, and V4 to V6. A "STEMI-Alert" was initiated to facilitate rapid coordination of reperfusion therapy.

The patient had a past history of atypical chest pain, hyperlipidemia, and gout. He worked as a self-employed artist; he denied tobacco abuse but smoked marijuana daily. He took no prescription medications. His physical examination was unremarkable, and laboratory studies found an initial troponin of 0.03 ng/mL, normal blood count and renal function, and marked lipid abnormalities (HDL 48 and LDL 213 mg/dL). Initial treatment began in the emergency room with aspirin (325 mg), clopidogrel (600 mg), and unfractionated heparin intravenous bolus (60 U/kg). He was referred for an emergency catheterization.

CARDIAC CATHETERIZATION

An ACT was measured and additional heparin administered to achieve an ACT between 250 and 300 seconds. Based on the ECG, the right coronary artery was the suspected infarct artery and was engaged first using a 6 French JR4 guiding catheter. Right coronary angiography revealed occlusion of the distal vessel, with retained contrast at the occlusion site (Figure 8-1 and Video 8-1). Eptifibatide was administered (two boluses, each of 180 mcg per kg, and an infusion of 2.0 mcg/kg per minute for 14 hours). The operator crossed the occlusion with a 0.014 inch floppy-tipped guidewire and TIMI-3 flow was restored after balloon dilatation with a 2.5 mm diameter by 15 mm long, compliant balloon. Following this, a 3.0 mm diameter by 23 mm long bare-metal stent was selected based on visual determination of the proximal and distal reference segments (Figure 8-2 and Video 8-2). A bare-metal stent was selected due to uncertainty about future medication compliance. The stent was positioned across the narrowed arterial segment and deployed at

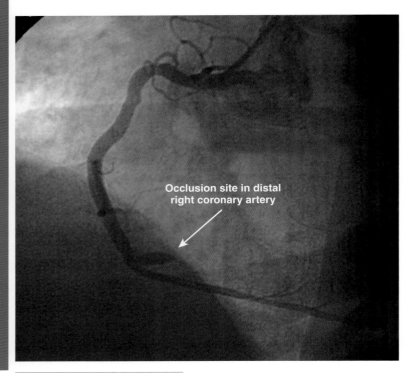

FIGURE 8-1. Initial angiogram of the right coronary artery in the LAO cranial view showing the acute occlusion of the distal right coronary.

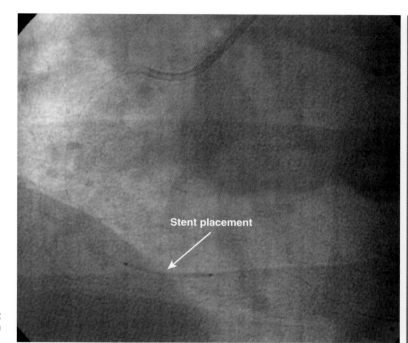

FIGURE 8-2. Placement of a bare-metal stent in the right coronary artery in the LAO cranial view following balloon angioplasty.

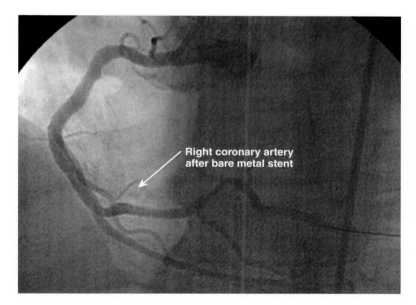

FIGURE 8-3. Final image of the right coronary artery in the LAO cranial view showing an excellent angiographic result in the distal right coronary artery. The more distal lesion was not significant in additional views.

14 atmospheres of pressure. The operator achieved a satisfactory angiographic result (Figure 8-3 and Video 8-3); intravascular ultrasound was not used.

Following stenting of the right coronary artery, the left coronary, imaged in standard views, showed minimal coronary atherosclerosis. A biplane left ventriculogram showed inferior and inferolateral hypokinesis with a preserved global ejection fraction estimated at 55%. The patient remained hemodynamically stable throughout the procedure. The vascular access sheath was removed with manual compression after 4 hours when the ACT was measured at less than 180 secs but while the eptifibatide infusion was continuing. He was treated during "off hours" with a door-to-balloon time of 64 minutes.

POSTPROCEDURAL COURSE

The patient recovered uneventfully, with his troponin level rising to 69 ng/mL. He was enrolled in cardiac rehabilitation and counseled regarding lifestyle modification, diet, weight loss, physical activity, and smoking (tobacco and marijuana) avoidance. He was discharged on the third hospital day and prescribed full-dose aspirin, clopidogrel, simvastatin, ezetimibe, lisinopril, and metoprolol. The importance of medical compliance, especially with aspirin and clopidogrel, was emphasized to the patient.

Three months later, the patient again presented to the emergency department after suffering chest pains for 5 hours. The initial ECG demonstrated 3 to 4 mm ST elevations in leads 2, 3, and aVF with Q waves in those leads.

The patient had not kept his previous medical follow-up appointments and admitted to stopping all of his medications after running out of prescriptions 3 weeks prior to the current presentation. Again, he was promptly treated in the emergency department with aspirin (325 mg), clopidogrel (600 mg), and unfractionated heparin (60 U/kg) and brought emergently to the cardiac catheterization laboratory. Right coronary angiography confirmed the suspected occlusion at the site of the previously-placed bare-metal stent (Figure 8-4 and Video 8-4). Adjunctive pharmacology consisted of therapeutic levels of unfractionated heparin along with eptifibatide double bolus and infusion. The operator crossed the occluded stent with a conventional, 0.014 inch floppy-tipped guidewire, taking great care to avoid passing the wire behind stent struts. Similar to the first event, TIMI-3 flow was promptly restored after balloon dilatation with a

2.5 diameter by 15 mm long, compliant balloon (Figure 8-5 and Video 8-5). The operator chose to further expand the stent with a 3.0 mm diameter by 20 mm long, noncompliant balloon inflated to 18 atmospheres of pressure. Angiography confirmed the lack of any distal embolization and an acceptable angiographic result (Figure 8-6). Hemostasis was achieved with a closure device and the patient was transferred to the coronary care unit. Again, the patient was treated during "off hours" with a door-to-balloon time of 74 minutes.

The patient remained asymptomatic throughout the admission. The serum troponin peaked at 6.6 ng/mL. The patient was advised to continue taking clopidogrel indefinitely for his late stent thrombosis. His medications were reinitiated as before and he was again strongly advised regarding lifestyle, medication, compliance, and follow-up.

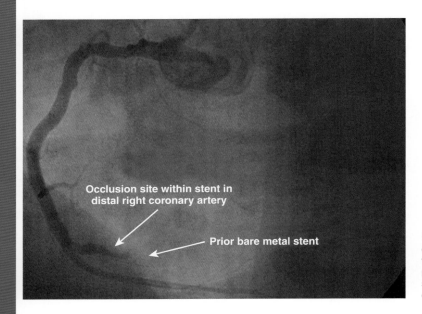

Occlusion site within stent in distal right coronary artery

Prior bare metal stent

FIGURE 8-4. Angiogram of the right coronary artery obtained during the second admission showing the acute occlusion of the distal right coronary at the site of the prior bare-metal stent placed 3 months earlier (late stent thrombosis). The occlusion site is clearly within the prior stent. The patient had stopped all of his medications due to cost and noncompliance.

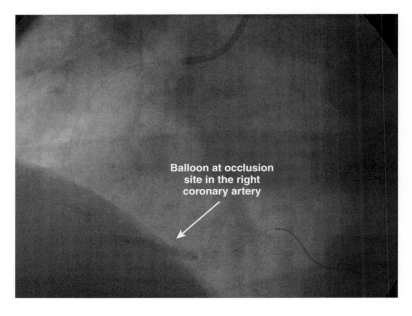

Balloon at occlusion site in the right coronary artery

FIGURE 8-5. After careful wire placement in the distal right coronary artery, a balloon is inflated within the prior stent.

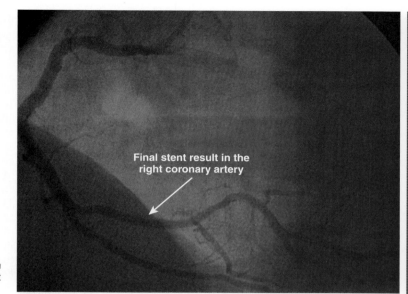

Final stent result in the right coronary artery

FIGURE 8-6. Final angiogram of the right coronary artery in the LAO cranial view following repeat balloon angioplasty at high pressure for late stent thrombosis.

DISCUSSION

This patient presented initially with an acute ST-segment elevation myocardial infarction with chest pain of 2.5 hours duration. Consistent with modern practice, he was rapidly evaluated according to a prespecified protocol that activated the cardiac catheterization laboratory staff and an interventionalist for rapid reperfusion therapy with direct PCI. The goal of therapy is to achieve a "door-to-balloon time" of less than 90 minutes; in the present case, this was accomplished in 64 minutes. The patient was first treated in the emergency department according to prespecified protocols with aspirin 325 mg, clopidogrel 600 mg load, and unfractionated heparin (60 U/kg). The exact protocols vary between institutions. In our catheterization laboratory, we visualized the presumed infarct-related artery first using a guiding catheter, with the intent to treat rapidly with PCI if there was no doubt about the clinical story and infarct artery. Other laboratories might choose to image the noninfarct artery first to have a complete definition of the coronary anatomy. The advantage of the former approach is speed to reperfusion. The advantage of the latter is more complete information prior to a specific therapy being initiated. There is no consensus regarding this strategy.

The approach to PCI reperfusion has been a rapidly evolving field. There is increasingly compelling data to suggest that thrombus extraction with a simple aspiration catheter improves clinical outcomes prior to stenting for acute ST-elevation MI.[1] This was not done in our laboratory at the time this case occurred but has currently become the preferred approach, when technically feasible. Similarly the optimal adjunctive pharmacologic therapy is in a state of evolution. In this case, unfractionated heparin and eptifibatide were used, but other heparins and GP IIb/IIIa inhibitors are also appropriate. The HORIZON trial has established the role of bivalirudin without routine GP IIb/IIIa inhibitors in such cases.[2] Although early stent thrombosis was increased with bivalirudin, this was not significant at later time points and the reduction in bleeding with bivalirudin was associated with decreased mortality at 1 year in patients with STEMI. In a separate publication, the HORIZON's investigators also established the role of drug-eluting stents in ST-elevation MI and showed significantly reduced angiographic evidence of restenosis and recurrent ischemia necessitating repeat revascularization procedures with no safety concerns apparent at 1 year with drug-eluting stents.[3] The challenge of such cases is to establish the bleeding risk and patient compliance issues during the "fast-forward" environment of an acute PCI. In this case, there were concerns raised regarding compliance with medications and a bare-metal stent was selected.

This patient did well for 2 months, but then became noncompliant with his follow-up and stopped taking all his medications, including aspirin and clopidogrel. Predictably, he developed late stent thrombosis within 3 weeks. The role of aspirin and clopidogrel (dual antiplatelet therapy) in the prevention of late stent thrombosis is well established. Clopidogrel has replaced ticlopidine as the ADP-receptor blocker of choice due to its improved safety profile. However, there is a defined incidence of clopidogrel resistance which results from multiple factors including its complex pharmacology and need for conversion from a pro-drug to its active form. Stent thrombosis has been associated with clopidogrel resistance as measured by platelet aggregation studies and with bedside platelet monitoring. Newer agents such as prasugrel (Triton TIMI 38) and ticagrelor (PLATO) may have improved efficacy against stent thrombosis.[4]

Stent thrombosis complicates approximately 2% of coronary interventional procedures and is associated with significant morbidity and mortality and a high risk of myocardial infarction. Certain situations are known to have increased risk of stent thrombosis including unstable angina, diabetes mellitus, low ejection fraction, renal failure, small vessel diameter, long lesions (with multiple stents), bifurcation lesions, downstream poorly-functioning myocardium, residual uncovered dissection, poor distal runoff, and suboptimal final postprocedure lumen.

Proper stent deployment with optimal sizing and avoidance of malapposition are important technical factors in avoiding stent thrombosis. Intravascular ultrasound may be helpful in defining risk factors for stent thrombosis, including improper sizing, stent malapposition, and edge dissections. Whether the "on label" use of drug-eluting stents treated with dual antiplatelet therapy results in increased late and very late thrombosis compared with bare-metal stents remains uncertain.[5]

In this case, the late stent thrombosis was treated with high-pressure balloon angioplasty alone. There is increasing evidence that placement of additional stents can result in still greater increases in recurrent stent thrombosis, so additional stents are typically avoided in these cases unless specifically indicated due to dissection or unacceptable angiographic result. Whether intravascular ultrasound can more precisely define therapy and diminish repeat episodes of stent thrombosis remains unproven.

In research trials, stent thrombosis is often classified using the ARC definition as definite, probable, or possible; and as early (0 to 30 days), late (31 to 360 days), or very late (over 360 days). The definition of definite stent thrombosis requires the presence of an acute coronary syndrome with angiographic or autopsy evidence of thrombus or occlusion. Probable stent thrombosis includes unexplained deaths within 30 days after the procedure, or acute myocardial infarction involving the target-vessel territory without angiographic confirmation. Possible stent thrombosis also includes all unexplained deaths occurring at least 30 days after the procedure. Intervening target lesion revascularization is defined as any repeated percutaneous revascularization of the stented segment, including the 5-mm proximal and distal margins that preceded stent thrombosis.

KEY CONCEPTS

1. Stent thrombosis complicates up to 2% of coronary interventions and is associated with increased morbidity and mortality. Several specific patient and lesion characteristics predispose to this event.
2. The use of high-pressure balloon inflations and dual antiplatelet therapy has reduced the incidence of stent thrombosis. Stent thrombosis remains a significant clinical challenge with the widening use of both bare-metal and drug eluting stents for "off label indications." The optimal duration of dual antiplatelet therapy is unclear. Current guidelines recommend daily aspirin (162 to 325 mg daily) for at least 1 month after bare-metal stent implantation, and 3 to 6 months after drug-eluting stent placement, after which daily long-term aspirin should be continued indefinitely at a dose of 75 to 162 mg. Clopidogrel should be loaded with 600 mg and continued for at least 12 months for patients receiving a drug-eluting stent. Patients receiving a bare-metal stent should continue clopidogrel for at least 1 month and ideally for up to 12 months, especially for acute coronary syndromes.
3. Thrombus extraction using an aspiration catheter has been shown to improve outcomes in patients with acute ST-elevation MI, but has not been specifically studied for acute stent thrombosis with MI.
4. Most cases of acute stent thrombosis can be treated with balloon angioplasty alone, with repeat stenting reserved for cases where a dissection or other mechanical cause of stent thrombosis can be identified.

Selected References

1. Svilaas T, Vlaar PJ, van der Horst IC, Diercks GFH, de Smet BJGL, van den Heuvel AFM, Anthonio RL, Jessurun GA, Tan ES, Suurmeijer AJH, Zijlstra F: Thrombus aspiration during primary percutaneous coronary intervention, *N Engl J Med* 358:557–567, 2008.
2. Stone GW, Witzenbichler B, Guagliumi G, Peruga JZ, Brodie BR, Dudek D, Kornowski R, Hartmann F, Gersh BJ, Pocock SJ, Dangas G, Wong SC, Kirtane AJ, Parise H, Mehran R: the HORIZONS-AMI Trial Investigators: Bivalirudin during primary PCI in acute myocardial infarction, *N Engl J Med* 358:2218–2230, 2008.
3. Stone GW, Lansky AJ, Pocock SJ, Gersh BJ, Dangas G, Wong SC, Witzenbichler B, Guagliumi G, Peruga JZ, Brodie BR, Dudek D, Mockel MO, Andrzej K, Alison PH, Mehran R: the HORIZONS-AMI Trial Investigators: Paclitaxel-eluting stents versus bare-metal stents in acute myocardial infarction, *N Engl J Med* 360:1946–1959, 2009.
4. Wallentin L, Becker RC, Budaj A, Cannon CP, Emanuelsson H, Held C, Horrow J, Husted S, James S, Katus H, Mahaffey KW, Scirica BM, Skene A, Steg PG, Storey RF, Harrington RA: the PLATO Investigators: Ticagrelor versus clopidogrel in patients with acute coronary syndromes, *N Engl J Med* 361:1045–1057, 2009.
5. Marroquin OC, Selzer F, Mulukutla SR, Williams DO, Vlachos HA, Wilensky RL, Tanguay JF, Holper EM, Abbott JD, Lee JS, Smith C, Anderson WD, Kelsey SF, Kip KE: A comparison of bare-metal and drug-eluting stents for off-label indications, *N Engl J Med* 358:342–352, 2008.

Unprotected Left Main Coronary Intervention

Michael Ragosta, MD, FACC, FSCAI

CASE PRESENTATION

An unfortunate 54-year-old man experienced numerous complications from paraplegia as a result of a gunshot wound at age 18. He has a neurogenic bladder with an indwelling catheter, and underwent resection of the left proximal femur following hip disarticulation. He has had multiple debridement and surgical procedures on chronic sacral decubitus ulcers. The most recent surgery, performed 2 weeks earlier, consisted of a gluteal flap.

While recuperating from this surgery, he developed a left facial droop and left arm weakness and also reported profound dyspnea but no chest pain. The neurologic symptoms resolved after a few hours but dyspnea continued. An electrocardiogram found lateral lead ST depressions and serial troponins were elevated, peaking at 17.54 ng/mL. Echocardiography uncovered severely reduced left ventricular function and a chest X-ray revealed congestive heart failure. He was diagnosed with a non-ST segment elevation myocardial infarction and heart failure; the transient ischemic attack was thought possibly due to a cardiac embolism. Although cardiac catheterization was indicated, the plastic surgeons advised against lying on his back side because pressure on the graft might jeopardize the viability of the gluteal flap. His extensive past medical history is also notable for prior myocardial infarction, diabetes mellitus, dyslipidemia, nephrolithiasis, and depression.

He was treated medically with aspirin, clopidogrel, beta blockers, and nitrates, and ultimately became stable with no further cardiac or neurologic symptoms. Surgery recommended that he continue to avoid lying on his back side for at least 2 more weeks. His physician decided to postpone catheterization for about 4 weeks to allow his decubitus graft to heal. However, 2 weeks later, he developed acute-onset shortness of breath and was admitted with pulmonary edema. He was referred for cardiac catheterization.

CARDIAC CATHETERIZATION

Obtaining arterial access proved challenging as his longstanding paraplegia resulted in substantial lower extremity atrophy and contracture at the hip. The femoral pulses were barely palpable; however, the right femoral artery was finally accessed successfully using ultrasound guidance, and angiography showed a small, diseased external iliac (Figure 9-1). The right coronary

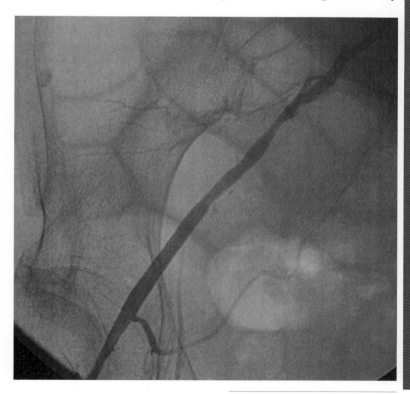

FIGURE 9-1. The femoral and external iliac vessels were very small and diffusely diseased.

artery was without significant disease (Figure 9-2). Upon engagement of the left coronary artery, the operator observed pressure damping and ventricularization. The left main stem was severely diseased at the ostium (Figures 9-3, 9-4 and Videos 9-1, 9-2). In addition, there was significant obstructive disease noted in the proximal left anterior descending (LAD) and circumflex (LCX) arteries.

A cardiac surgeon reviewed his medical history and deemed him a very poor surgical candidate because of his substantial comorbidities. After discussion about the options of continuing medical therapy versus a high-risk percutaneous coronary intervention, the patient agreed to proceed with a stenting procedure of the left main stem as well as the LCX and LAD lesions, primarily because he clearly failed a course of medical therapy.

The operator inserted an 8 French sheath in the right femoral artery and procedural anticoagulation was achieved with bivalirudin; he had already been on clopidogrel therapy. An 8 French, left Judkins guide catheter was engaged and floppy-tipped guidewires passed into the LAD and LCX. The lesions in the LAD and LCX were

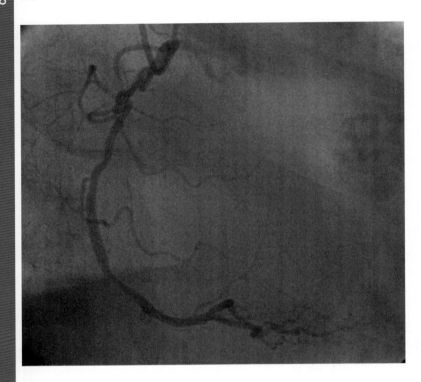

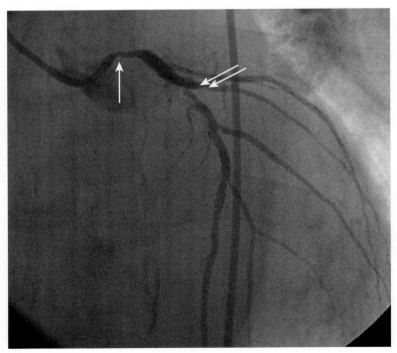

FIGURE 9-2. There was moderate atherosclerotic disease in the right coronary artery.

FIGURE 9-3. The ostium of the left main stem was severely narrowed (*arrow*) and there was a high grade lesion of the proximal LAD (*double arrow*).

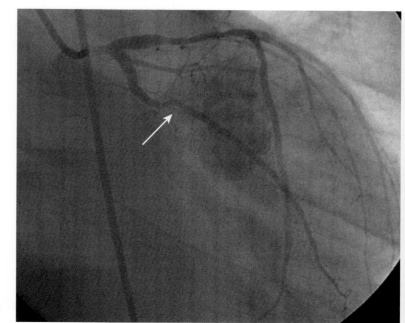

FIGURE 9-4. There was also severe disease of the circumflex artery (*arrow*).

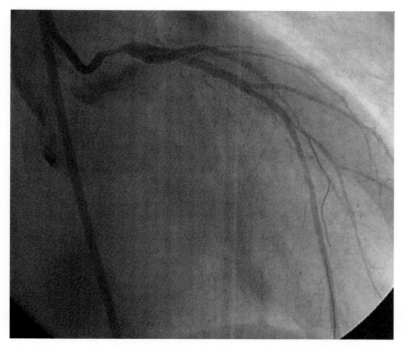

FIGURE 9-5. The LAD and LCX were stented first, with an excellent angiographic result.

treated successfully with balloon dilatation followed by placement of paclitaxel-eluting stents (Figure 9-5).

In order to protect the circumflex artery, the operator chose to use a modified "crush stent" technique to treat the left main stem lesion. Two stents were positioned in the left main/LAD and LCX: a 3.0 mm diameter by 20 mm long paclitaxel-eluting stent in the left main into the LAD, and a 3.0 mm diameter by 12 mm long paclitaxel-eluting stent in the circumflex (Figure 9-6). The left circumflex stent was deployed first (Figure 9-7); following this, the stent catheter and wire was removed from the circumflex artery and the left main stent deployed (Figure 9-8). The operator re-crossed the circumflex stent with another 0.014 inch guidewire and simultaneously

inflated two 3.0 mm diameter noncompliant balloons ("kissing balloons") to high pressure (Figure 9-9). A 3.5 mm noncompliant balloon was used to postdilate the left main stem. The final angiographic result was excellent (Figures 9-10, 9-11 and Videos 9-3, 9-4). Intravascular ultrasound was used to assess stent deployment and showed excellent stent apposition and a widely patent lumen (Figure 9-12).

POSTPROCEDURAL COURSE

He recovered uneventfully and was discharged 2 days later on aspirin, clopidogrel, simvastatin, and metoprolol. In follow-up 3 months later, he reported no symptoms of

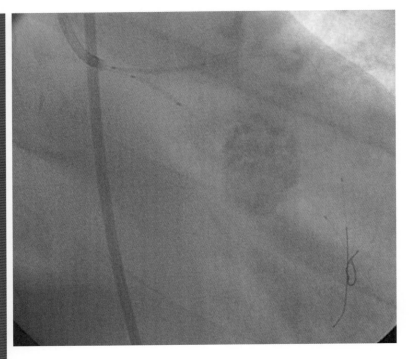

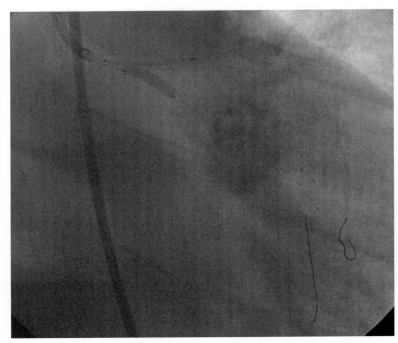

FIGURE 9-6. The initial step in managing the left main lesion is shown here. An 8 French guide catheter is engaged in the left main, and stents are positioned in the left main into the LAD and in the circumflex artery with the distal end of the circumflex stent at the ostium.

FIGURE 9-7. The LCX stent is deployed first.

chest pain, dyspnea, or recurrent heart failure. Unfortunately, he continued to be limited due to his chronic sacral decubitus ulcer and experienced new areas of skin breakdown in another sacral location. He was again seen 18 months after the coronary intervention and remained symptom-free and without cardiac events.

DISCUSSION

Left main stem disease is traditionally treated with bypass surgery, and this mode of revascularization is generally accepted as the standard of care for this high-risk subgroup. Percutaneous intervention of unprotected left main stem disease (i.e., without a patent bypass graft to one or more branches of the left coronary artery) has generally been reserved for patients too unstable for bypass or, as in this case, for patients who are not surgical candidates. However, there is a growing interest in and experience of treating this disease with stents instead of bypass surgery. Numerous registries and nonrandomized comparative trials have shown feasibility, relative safety, and efficacy of left main stenting using both bare-metal and drug-eluting stents.[1] These data suggest that left main stenting can be done, but do not answer

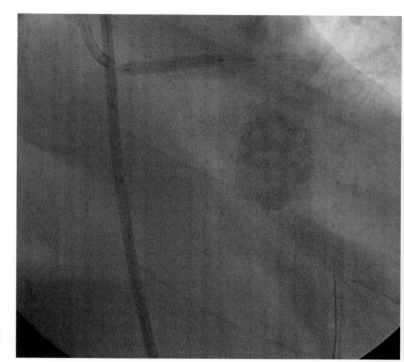

FIGURE 9-8. After deploying the LCX stent, the stent catheter and guidewire were removed from the LCX and the left main/LAD stent deployed.

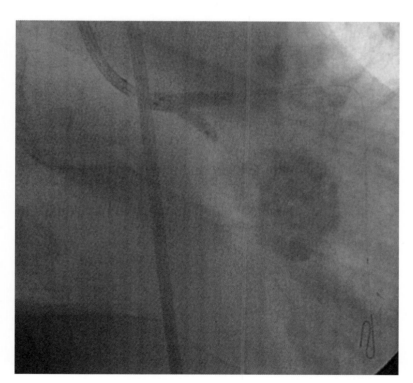

FIGURE 9-9. Final kissing balloons performed with noncompliant balloons.

the question of whether it should be done. Only randomized, controlled trials comparing left main PCI to bypass surgery can answer that question, and PCI would need to show equivalence to bypass surgery in order to gain a Class I recommendation.

Left main stem stenting is a high-risk lesion subset for several reasons. First, the left main stem supplies a very large vascular territory and there is the potential for cardiovascular collapse with ischemia, particularly if the left coronary is dominant, the right coronary is occluded, or left ventricular function is reduced. Patients with left main coronary disease often have other disease requiring revascularization; isolated involvement of the left main stem occurs in only 9% of patients with left main stem disease.[2] Often, this other disease is extensive or not amenable to percutaneous approaches, thus favoring surgical revascularization. Furthermore, left main stem disease involves the bifurcation in more than

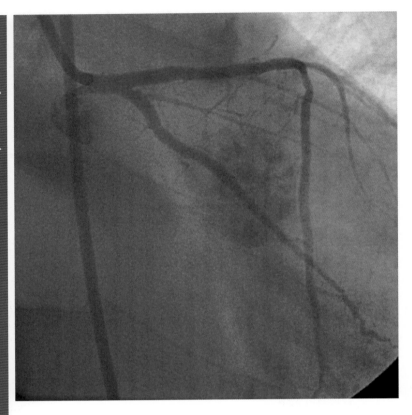

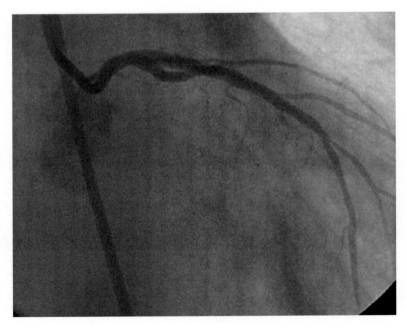

FIGURE 9-10. Final angiographic result in the RAO caudal projection.

FIGURE 9-11. Final angiographic result in the RAO cranial projection.

half the cases, introducing additional complexity and risk. Finally, the occurrence of either restenosis or stent thrombosis may be fatal events in patients with left main stents.

Several randomized controlled trials comparing bypass surgery to drug-eluting stents for treatment of left main disease are in progress or have been reported. A small series of 105 patients randomized to PCI versus surgery found similar anginal status at 12 months, but better left ventricular ejection fraction, shorter length of stay, and lower rate of adverse events at 12-month follow-up in the group randomized to stenting.[3] The SYNTAX trial was a much larger randomized controlled trial that included patients with three-vessel or left main disease and compared stenting to bypass surgery.[4] In the subgroup of patients with left main disease, patients treated with stents had similar rates of death and MI as patients treated with bypass surgery. Similar to the multivessel PCI versus CABG trials, patients treated with stents had a significantly higher rate of repeat revascularization.

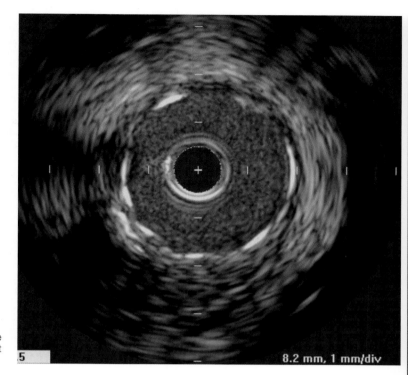

FIGURE 9-12. Representative intravascular ultrasound image of the left main stem after stenting, showing excellent stent deployment.

In the SYNTAX trial, the patients treated with bypass surgery had a higher rate of stroke.

Based on the SYNTAX trial, the most recently revised guidelines changed the classification of left main stenting from Class III to Class IIb, with several important caveats.[5] Patients considered for left main stenting must have lesions suitable for PCI. Complex bifurcations and patients with multivessel disease are better served with surgery. Furthermore, the guidelines suggest that only experienced operators, backed-up by surgeons and competent support staff, should consider PCI of left main lesions.

There are several other issues and concerns relating to left main stenting. Regarding the choice of drug-eluting stent, based on the ISAR LEFT MAIN study, there does not appear to be a difference in outcomes in patients with left main disease treated with paclitaxel-eluting compared to sirolimus-eluting stents.[6] Late stent thrombosis is a concern in this subgroup, as thrombosis of a left main stent would likely prove fatal. In the ISAR LEFT MAIN trial, no late thrombosis was seen beyond 30 days, alleviating this worry in this population. There is also uncertainty about how best to follow these patients after stenting. Many practitioners have advocated the performance of routine coronary angiography at 6 to 9 months; however, the most recent guidelines do not recommend this practice.

Selection of patients is clearly important in deciding on the optimal method of revascularization in this subgroup. In patients undergoing left main PCI, the most significant predictor of a major adverse event and repeat revascularization is bifurcation involvement.[7] Treatment of bifurcation disease remains challenging, but nonbifurcation left main PCI has very favorable outcomes. The SYNTAX score can help choose the optimal revascularization strategy in patients with complex CAD including left main stem disease.[8] This score takes into account disease complexity and the presence of additional disease; the higher the SYNTAX score, the better the outcome with CABG compared to PCI.

KEY CONCEPTS

1. Isolated left main disease is rare. Left main stem disease involves the bifurcation in more than half the cases and is often accompanied by multivessel disease.
2. Left main stem stenting represents a high-risk subgroup because of the extent of myocardium supplied and the often complex nature of the disease; however, it is safe and feasible in properly-selected patients.
3. Left main PCI is a potential revascularization option, particularly in nonbifurcation disease and in poor surgical candidates.

Selected References

1. Taggart DP, Kaul S, Boden WE, Ferguson TB, Guyton RA, Mack MJ, Sargeant PT, Shemin RJ, Smith PK, Yusuf S: Revascularization for unprotected left main stem coronary artery stenosis: Stenting or surgery, *J Am Coll Cardiol* 51:885–892, 2008.
2. Ragosta M, Dee S, Sarembock IJ, Lipson LC, Gimple LW, Powers ER: Prevalence of unfavorable angiographic characteristics for percutaneous intervention in patients with unprotected left main coronary artery disease, *Catheter Cardiovasc Interv* 67: 357–362, 2006.
3. Buszman PE, Kiesz SR, Andrzej Bochenek AJ, et al: Acute and late outcomes of unprotected left main stenting in comparison with surgical revascularization, *J Am Coll Cardiol* 51:538–545, 2008.
4. Serruys PW, Morice MC, Kappetein AP, et al: Percutaneous coronary intervention versus coronary-artery bypass grafting for severe coronary artery disease, *N Engl J Med* 360:961–972, 2009.

5. Kushner FG, Hand M, Smith SC, et al: Focused Updates: ACC/AHA guidelines for the management of patients with ST-elevation myocardial infarction (updating the 2004 guideline and 2007 focused update) and ACC/AHA/SCAI guidelines on percutaneous coronary intervention (updating the 2005 guideline and 2007 focused update): A report of the American College of Cardiology Foundation/American Heart Association Task Force on Practice Guidelines, *J Am Coll Cardiol* 54:2205–2241, 2009.

6. Mehilli J, Kastrati A, Byrne RA, Bruskina O, Iijima R, Schulz S, Pache J, Seyfarth M, Maßberg S, Laugwitz KL, Dirschinger J, Schömig A, and ISAR-LEFT-MAIN (Intracoronary Stenting and Angiographic Results: Drug-Eluting Stents for Unprotected Coronary Left Main Lesions) Study Investigators: Paclitaxel-versus sirolimus-eluting stents for unprotected left main coronary artery disease, *J Am Coll Cardiol* 53:1760–1768, 2009.

7. Biondi-Zoccai GGL, Lotrionte M, Moretti C, et al: A collaborative systematic review and meta-analysis on 1278 patients undergoing percutaneous drug-eluting stenting for unprotected left main coronary artery disease, *Am Heart J* 155:274–283, 2008.

8. Sianos G, Morel MA, Kappetein AP, Morice MC, Colombo A, Dawkins K, van den Brand M, Van Dyck N, Russell ME, Mohr FW, Serruys PW: The SYNTAX Score: an angiographic tool grading the complexity of coronary artery disease, *Euro Intervention* 1:219, 2005.

PCI of an Ostial Right Coronary Artery Lesion

Michael Ragosta, MD, FACC, FSCAI

CASE PRESENTATION

A healthy and active 83-year-old woman without prior cardiac history presented with 1 week of intermittent chest pain, culminating in a prolonged episode of severe rest pain prompting hospital admission. In the emergency department, her initial electrocardiogram showed inferior T-wave changes, and she quickly became pain-free with nitrates, aspirin, a beta blocker, and unfractionated heparin. Subsequent serial troponin values peaked at 3.9 ng/mL. She was diagnosed with a non-ST segment elevation myocardial infarction. Her past medical history is notable only for hypertension, hyperlipidemia, and degenerative joint disease, and she lives independently. Her physical examination was unremarkable and her laboratory studies were notable only for a serum creatinine of 1.3 mg/dL. She was referred for cardiac catheterization.

CARDIAC CATHETERIZATION

Coronary angiography found no significant obstructive disease in the left coronary artery (Figure 10-1) but a severe ostial stenosis of the right coronary artery, with extensive calcification (Figure 10-2 and Video 10-1).

Based on the angiogram, her physician decided to proceed with a percutaneous approach and, anticipating great difficulty because of the ostial location and the degree of calcification observed, the operator planned to debulk the lesion with rotational atherectomy.

Femoral venous access was obtained and a temporary pacemaker wire positioned in the right ventricular apex. The operator then engaged an 8 French right Judkins guide catheter with side holes and administered eptifibatide as a double bolus plus infusion along with unfractionated heparin to achieve an activated clotting time (ACT) greater than 200 seconds. A floppy-tipped rotational atherectomy guidewire was positioned distally in the right coronary artery. Rotational atherectomy was accomplished first with a 1.5 mm burr, followed by a 2.0 mm burr. The angiographic result after rotational atherectomy is shown in Figure 10-3 and Video 10-2. The operator removed the rotational atherectomy guidewire and positioned a conventional 0.014 inch floppy-tipped guidewire distally in the right coronary artery. The lesion was dilated with a 3.0 mm diameter by 20 mm long compliant balloon and a 3.5 mm diameter by 23 mm long sirolimus-eluting stent positioned to cover the ostium (Figure 10-4 and Video 10-3) and postdilated with a 4.0 mm diameter by 9 mm long noncompliant

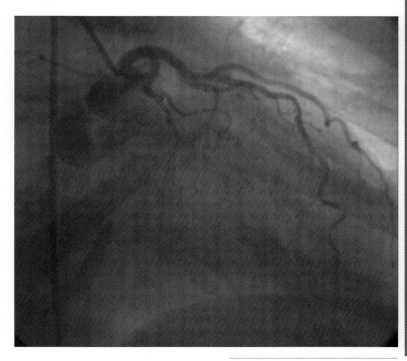

FIGURE 10-1. This is the left coronary angiogram; there were no significant obstructive lesions noted.

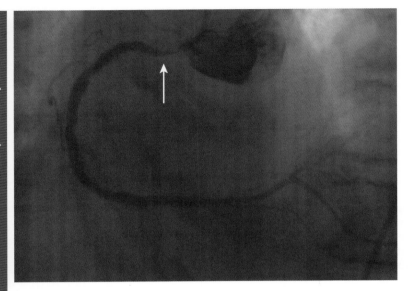

FIGURE 10-2. The ostium of the right coronary artery was severely narrowed with heavy calcification noted around the ostium (*arrow*).

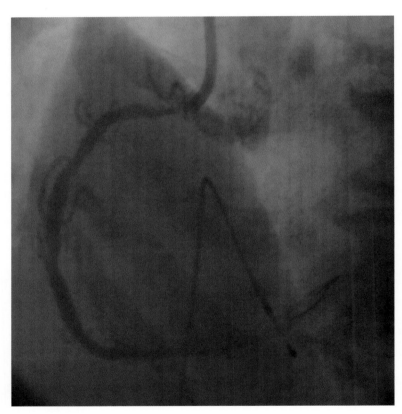

FIGURE 10-3. This is the angiographic result after rotational atherectomy with a 2.0 mm burr.

balloon to high pressures. The final angiographic images satisfied the operator, although mild narrowing remained at the ostium (Figure 10-5 and Video 10-4); intravascular ultrasound was not performed and the procedure was terminated.

POSTPROCEDURAL COURSE

The pacing electrode was withdrawn and the femoral sheaths removed using manual pressure when the ACT fell below 180 seconds. After an uncomplicated overnight stay, she was discharged the next morning on clopidogrel, aspirin, atenolol, atorvastatin, and lisinopril.

She remained symptom-free for 5 months, and then developed recurrent severe chest pain similar to her initial symptoms. She was again admitted to the hospital, but this time, serial troponins were negative. Repeat cardiac catheterization revealed severe, in-stent restenosis of the ostium of the right coronary artery (Figure 10-6 and Video 10-5). Her physician decided to treat this lesion percutaneously with a cutting balloon. Using bivalirudin as the procedural anticoagulant, the operator dilated the stenosis with a 3.5 mm diameter cutting balloon

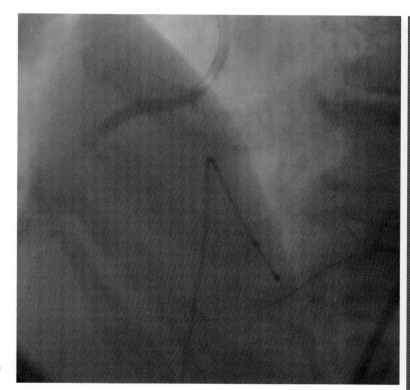

FIGURE 10-4. This figure demonstrates the position of the stent relative to the right coronary ostium.

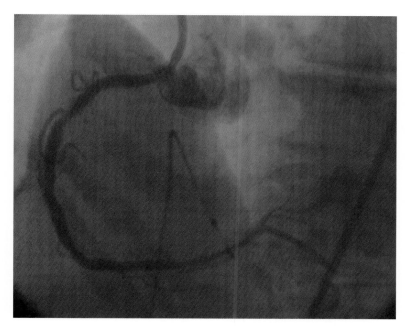

FIGURE 10-5. Final angiographic results after stenting the right coronary ostial lesion.

followed by a 4.0 mm noncompliant balloon to high pressures. Although the angiographic result appeared acceptable (Figure 10-7), there remained a gentle narrowing of the ostium. Intravascular ultrasound was performed and demonstrated excellent stent expansion distally (Figure 10-8), but the ostium remained deformed with a 7 mm^2 minimal lumen area, despite aggressive balloon dilatation (Figure 10-9). In order to treat this apparent recoil, the operator placed a 4.5 mm diameter by 13 mm long bare-metal stent and expanded it to high pressures

(Figure 10-10). The angiographic result appeared much improved (Figure 10-11 and Video 10-6); importantly, the post-stent intravascular ultrasound images showed wide expansion of the stent at the ostium (Figure 10-12).

She had an uncomplicated course following the procedure and enjoyed resolution of her symptoms. Unfortunately, 3 months later she again developed recurrent severe angina. When another catheterization confirmed recurrent, severe in-stent restenosis at the ostium, she was referred for a single-vessel bypass operation.

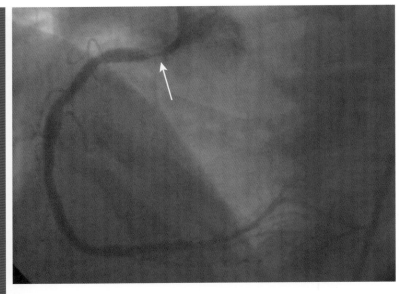

FIGURE 10-6. Angiogram obtained after the patient developed recurrent chest pain, showing severe in-stent restenosis (*arrow*).

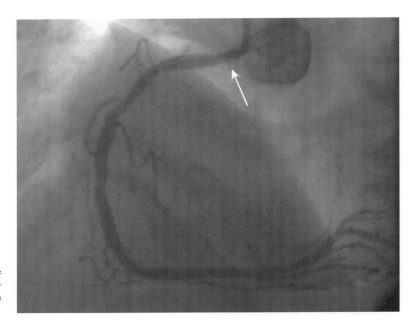

FIGURE 10-7. Angiographic result obtained after treatment of the in-stent restenosis lesion with a cutting balloon and further high pressure dilatation with a noncompliant balloon. There remains mild narrowing of the ostium (*arrow*).

She recovered uneventfully from this surgery and has remained asymptomatic during follow-up.

DISCUSSION

Coronary artery disease is classified as "aorto-ostial" when it involves the left main or right coronary ostium, or "branch-ostial" when it involves the ostium of a large side branch such as a diagonal or obtuse marginal artery. Aorto-ostial disease is relatively uncommon; observed in less than 1% of patients with coronary artery disease. In addition to atherosclerotic heart disease, it is also seen in association with prior therapeutic chest irradiation, diseases of the aorta such as syphilitic aortitis and Takayasu arteritis, and with calcific aortic valve stenosis.

Percutaneous treatment of aorto-ostial disease presents several important technical challenges. First, the operator may find it difficult to accurately image the ostium by angiography, a critically important component of the procedure in order to ensure that the true ostium is covered by the stent. The true ostium is often obscured by the guide catheter, or from reflux of contrast in the aorta or by the sinuses themselves, making it very difficult for the operator to be confident in the placement of the stent. Second, aorto-ostial lesions are often calcified and rigid and subject to greater amounts of elastic recoil because the lesion involves the aortic wall and not just the coronary artery. Finally, there are often significant technical challenges associated with the choice of a satisfactory guide catheter. The operator needs to engage the artery with a guide that will allow adequate angiographic

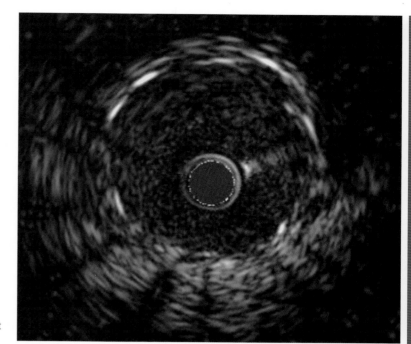

FIGURE 10-8. Distal to the ostium, the right coronary stent appears well-expanded.

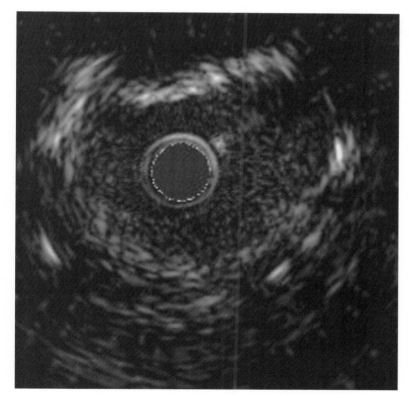

FIGURE 10-9. At the ostium, there is deformity and under-expansion of the stent.

imaging and provide support for device delivery, but also allow the operator the ability to gently disengage the guide when positioning the stent at the ostium without resulting in the guidewire and stent catheter flying out of the coronary artery. The use of an extra-supportive guidewire may help stabilize the system, particularly with right coronary ostial lesions.

The acute technical success for percutaneous interventions of aorto-ostial lesions is very high, but restenosis rates are higher as compared to similar lesions that do not involve the ostium.[1] As demonstrated in this case, there is a high restenosis rate for right coronary artery ostial lesions as compared to left main stem ostial lesions; the mechanism, by intravascular ultrasound studies, appears to be stent recoil as well as neointimal formation.[2]

Some operators advocate pre-stenting rotational atherectomy or cutting balloon angioplasty to reduce the

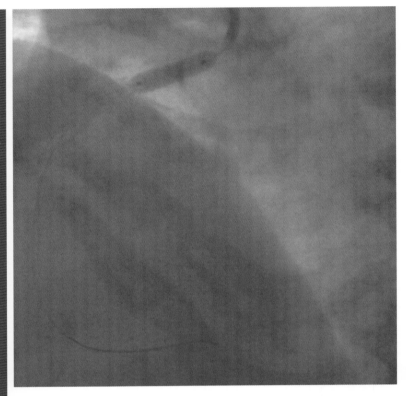

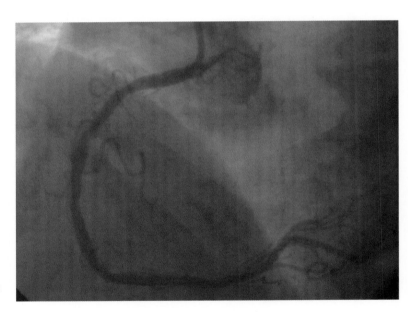

FIGURE 10-10. Bare-metal stent deployment at the ostium.

FIGURE 10-11. The angiographic appearance is much improved after repeat stenting of the ostium.

elastic recoil component, theoretically improving the long-term results for ostial lesions.[3] Currently, there are little data and no randomized controlled data to support this strategy for the treatment of aorto-ostial lesions. This strategy did not appear effective in this case.

Similar to other lesion subsets, drug-eluting stents reduce the rate of restenosis for aorto-ostial lesions as compared to bare-metal stents.[4,5] However, as shown in this case, restenosis remains a significant problem.

Several important technical tricks may improve the operator's success. Incomplete coverage of the ostium is the most commonly encountered mistake during treatment of these challenging lesions. This is often due to the previously mentioned difficulty in accurately imaging the true ostium by angiography. In addition, if the operator "overshoots," causing an excessive length of the stent to protrude into the aorta, it may create difficulties with re-engagement later on. One trick to ensure coverage of the ostium involves the "stent tail wire" technique in which another 0.014 inch guidewire (the tail anchor wire) is placed alongside the stent catheter and inserted behind the last strut. The stent, along

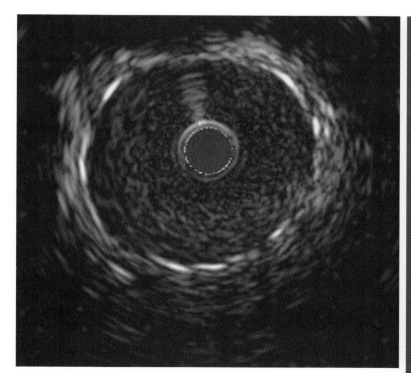

FIGURE 10-12. Following stent placement, the intravascular ultrasound showed improved expansion of the ostium.

with the attached tail anchor wire, is advanced along the guidewire already in place in the coronary artery positioned in the ostium. The tail anchor wire does not enter the coronary artery, but instead straddles the aorto-ostium and helps identify the exact location of the aorto-ostium.[6]

It may not be enough to position the end of the stent flush with the ostium, since the final row of struts may not have adequate strength to resist the force of recoil, leading some experienced operators to state, "When you think you have covered the ostium, pull the stent back a bit further." As noted above, however, the risk of this maneuver is to have an excessive amount of stent outside the coronary artery.

Intravascular ultrasound is helpful to assure that the stent has completely covered the ostium and that it has been fully expanded, and, in the opinion of the author, should be a part of all interventions involving aorto-ostial lesions. In the event that the ultrasound reveals excessive recoil resistant to repeat balloon inflations, a second stent may be necessary to provide adequate radial strength against the aorto-ostial wall.

KEY CONCEPTS

1. Aorto-ostial lesions are uncommon and provide important technical challenges to the operator including: a) difficulty imaging the ostium, b) the presence of calcification and excessive rigidity, c) greater amounts of elastic recoil, d) choice of guide catheter, and e) difficulty ensuring proper position of the stent at the aorto-ostium.
2. Restenosis rates remain high and are due, in part, to the greater amount of elastic recoil present in these lesions.

Selected References

1. Mavromatis M, Ghazzal Z, Veledar E, Diamandopoulos L, Weintraub WS, Douglas JS, Kalynych AM: Comparison of outcomes of percutaneous coronary intervention of ostial versus nonostial narrowing of the major epicardial coronary arteries, *Am J Cardiol* 94:583–587, 2004.
2. Tsunoda T, Nakamura M, Wada M, Ito N, Kitagawa Y, Shiba M, Yajima S, Iijima R, Nakajima R, Yamamoto M, Takagi T, Yoshitama T, Anzai H, Nishida T, Yamaguchi T: Chronic stent recoil plays an important role in restenosis of the right coronary ostium, *Coron Artery Dis* 15:39–44, 2004.
3. Motwani JG, Raymone RE, Franco I, Ellis SG, Whitlow PL: Effectiveness of rotational atherectomy of right coronary artery ostial stenosis, *Am J Cardiol* 85:563–567, 2000.
4. Iakovou I, Ge L, Michev I, Sangiorgi GM, Montorfano M, Airoldi F, Chieffo A, Stankovic G, Vitrella G, Carlino M, Corvaja N, Briguori C, Colombo A: Clinical and angiographic outcome after sirolimus-eluting stent implantation in aorto-ostial lesions, *J Am Coll Cardiol* 44:967–971, 2004.
5. Park DW, Hong MK, Suh IW, Hwang ES, Lee SW, Jeong YH, Kim YH, Lee CW, Kim JJ, Park SW, Park SJ: Results and predictors of angiographic restenosis and long-term adverse cardiac events after drug-eluting stent implantation for aorto-ostial coronary artery disease, *Am J Cardiol* 99:760–765, 2007.
6. Kern MJ, Ouellette D, Frianeza T: A new technique to anchor stents for exact placement in ostial stenoses: The stent tail wire or Szabo technique, *Catheter Cardiovasc Interv* 68:901–906, 2006.

Chronic Total Occlusion Intervention

Michael Ragosta, MD, FACC, FSCAI

CASE PRESENTATION

A 49-year-old man with numerous atherosclerotic risk factors was referred for cardiac catheterization because of exertional angina and an abnormal stress test. He has no prior cardiac history, but is being treated for hyperlipidemia and hypertension with atorvastatin and carvedilol. He also takes a baby aspirin each day. He smokes more than one pack of cigarettes per day and also has a strong family history for premature coronary disease. Beginning at least 6 months earlier, he noted the gradual development of anginal chest pain with exertion. He happened to report this symptom to his primary care physician during a routine physical examination, prompting his physician to order a nuclear perfusion exercise stress test. During this test, he achieved 7 METS of exercise and had to stop because of chest pain. The perfusion images showed exercise-induced ischemia of the entire anterior wall and apex, and he was referred to a cardiologist for catheterization.

CARDIAC CATHETERIZATION

The left ventriculogram was normal, with an ejection fraction of 60% and no segmental wall motion abnormalities. A severe stenosis was noted in the right coronary artery (Figure 11-1). There was also a prominent collateral vessel to the left anterior descending (LAD) artery (Figure 11-2 and Video 11-1). As was suspected because of the presence of collateral circulation from the right coronary artery, there was total occlusion of the LAD. The circumflex artery appeared free of significant narrowing (Figures 11-3, 11-4 and Video 11-2). Although the right coronary lesion appeared readily amenable to percutaneous coronary intervention (PCI), the angiographic appearance and clinical history suggested that the LAD occlusion was likely chronic and might not be successfully treated percutaneously. The physician decided to terminate the procedure and discuss therapeutic options in more detail with the patient.

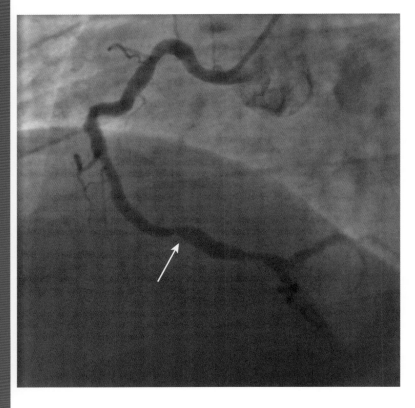

FIGURE 11-1. The right coronary artery was severely narrowed (*arrow*).

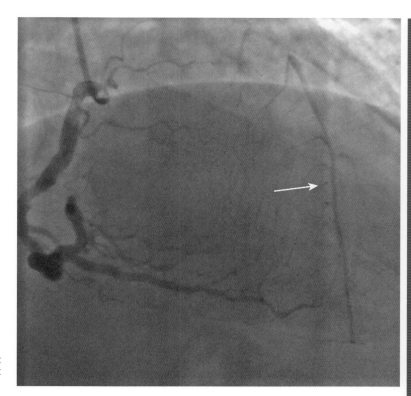

FIGURE 11-2. This right anterior oblique projection of the right coronary artery demonstrates a prominent collateral to the left anterior descending artery (*arrow*) via septal perforators.

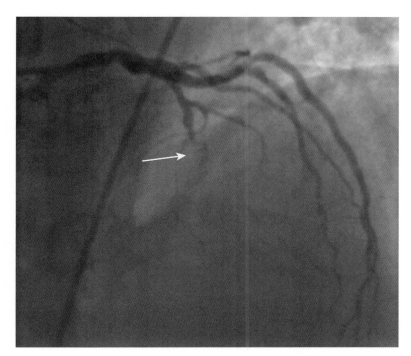

FIGURE 11-3. The left anterior descending artery was completely occluded (*arrow*).

After a lengthy discussion regarding the options of medical therapy, coronary bypass surgery, or an attempt at multivessel coronary intervention, the patient chose a percutaneous approach. The interventional cardiologist explained that if percutaneous intervention of the chronically-occluded LAD proved unsuccessful, then coronary bypass surgery would be necessary.

The patient returned to the cardiac catheterization laboratory. The operator decided to use the prominent collateral to the LAD from the right coronary artery to help guide attempts at crossing the occluded segment. Therefore, two angiographic manifolds were prepared and femoral arterial access obtained from both the right and left femoral arteries. After engaging the right

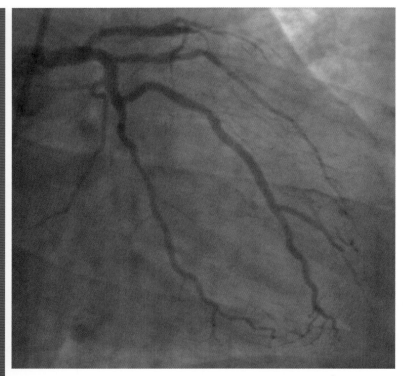

FIGURE 11-4. There was no significant disease in the circumflex artery.

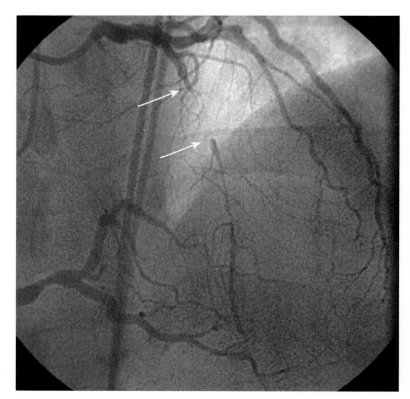

FIGURE 11-5. Simultaneous injection of the right and left coronary arteries shows the extent of the occlusion (*arrows*).

coronary artery with a diagnostic catheter and the left coronary artery with a guide catheter, contrast was injected first in the right coronary artery and then in the left coronary to define the extent of the LAD occlusion (Figure 11-5 and Video 11-3).

Unfractionated heparin was administered as a bolus to achieve a therapeutic activated clotting time; clopidogrel had not been given prior to the procedure in the event that PCI was unsuccessful and bypass surgery was required. The operator chose a tapered tip guidewire specifically designed for chronic total occlusions (Asahi Miracle Bros 3.0) and loaded this wire into a 2.0 mm diameter by 20 mm long "over-the-wire" compliant balloon. In the right anterior oblique projection, the operator advanced the stiff-tipped guidewire through the occluded segment, using occasional injections into the right coronary artery to visualize the collateral. Eventually, it appeared that the wire had advanced all the way through the occlusion (Figure 11-6 and Video 11-4). Angiography of the wire and collateral in the lateral projection, however, demonstrated that the wire tip was parallel to the artery and not in the true lumen of the LAD (Figure 11-7 and Video 11-5). The wire was gently withdrawn and

repositioned, ultimately achieving the distal lumen of the LAD (Figure 11-8 and Video 11-6). The balloon easily advanced through the occlusion but, prior to inflation, the operator removed the guidewire and gently injected contrast through the balloon lumen to confirm location within the true lumen of the distal LAD (Figure 11-9 and Video 11-7). A floppy-tipped, 0.014 inch guidewire was reinserted within the balloon catheter and positioned distally in the LAD, and balloon angioplasty was performed

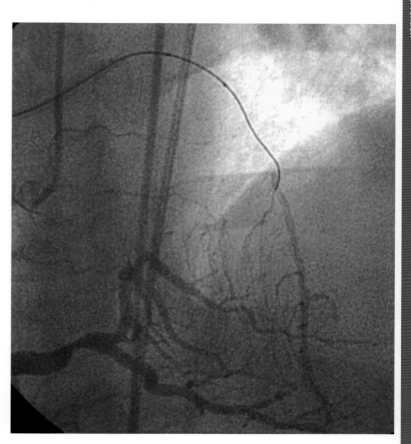

FIGURE 11-6. A stiff-tipped guidewire penetrated the occluded segment and, in this view, the tip appeared to enter the true lumen of the distal left anterior descending artery. The collateral is imaged by injection of the right coronary artery.

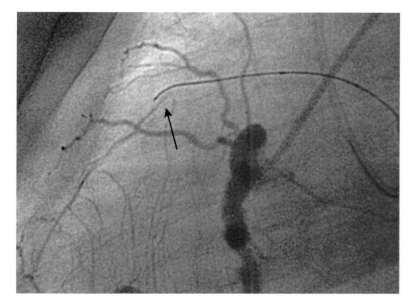

FIGURE 11-7. In the lateral projection, it is apparent that the tip of the guidewire was not within the true lumen of the LAD (arrow). The collateral is imaged by injection of the right coronary artery.

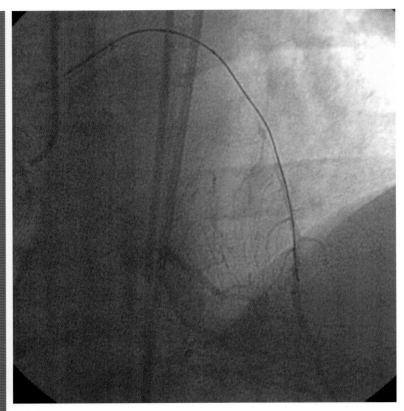

FIGURE 11-8. The guidewire has been repositioned into the true lumen (this was confirmed in the lateral projection, not shown). The collateral is imaged by injection of the right coronary artery.

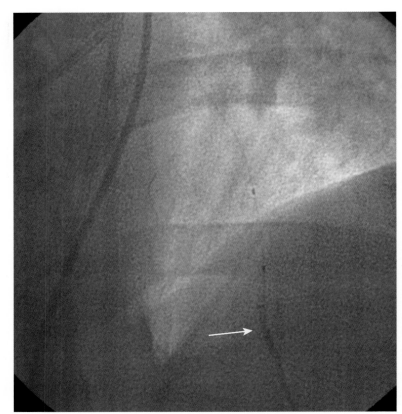

FIGURE 11-9. An injection of contrast via the lumen of the balloon catheter confirmed the location within the true lumen (*arrow*).

with a 2.5 mm compliant balloon followed by placement of two sirolimus-eluting stents (2.5 mm diameter by 28 mm long stent distally and a 2.75 mm diameter by 13 mm long stent proximally). The final angiographic result for the LAD is shown in Figure 11-10 and Videos 11-8, 11-9. Satisfied with the result, the operator chose a 4.0 mm by 15 mm long bare-metal stent for the right coronary artery and postdilated it with a 4.5 mm noncompliant balloon (Figure 11-11). Hemostasis was achieved at the completion of the case by use of a closure device.

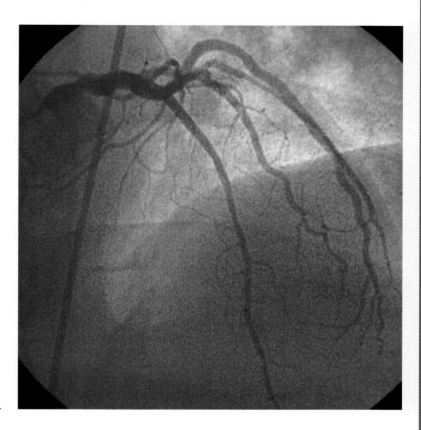

FIGURE 11-10. Angiographic result after stenting the LAD.

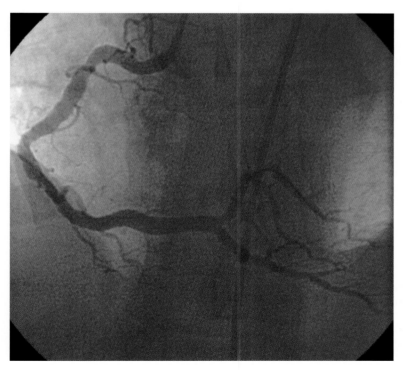

FIGURE 11-11. Following the LAD intervention, the right coronary artery was stented successfully.

POSTPROCEDURAL COURSE

He recovered uneventfully and was discharged the next day on his usual medications, along with clopidogrel indefinitely. At follow-up, 3 months, 12 months, and 19 months later, he remained free of symptoms, although he continued to smoke cigarettes.

DISCUSSION

Chronic total coronary occlusions (CTO) remain one of the most difficult lesion subsets confronting an interventional cardiologist. Defined as a complete occlusion of more than 3 months duration, these lesions are technically challenging and have a lower success rate of approximately 70%, compared to nonoccluded lesions whose success rate typically exceeds 95%.

Chronic total occlusions are fairly common. It is estimated that about one third of patients undergoing angiography for evaluation of coronary disease have at least one chronically occluded artery, with the right coronary artery most commonly involved.[1] However, despite their prevalence, only about 10% of percutaneous coronary interventions (PCI) involve CTOs. In fact, many interventionalists are reluctant to attempt PCI of a chronic occlusion because of the lower success rate, the potential risk of perforation, and the commitment in time and patience required by the operator. For these reasons, the presence of one or more chronically occluded arteries in the setting of multivessel disease is often the justification for choosing coronary bypass surgery instead of multivessel PCI.[2] The case presented here with a chronically occluded LAD and a focal lesion in the RCA is an example of a case where many physicians might have chosen bypass surgery as the initial revascularization strategy instead of a PCI strategy.

Many patients with CTO are asymptomatic and can be treated medically; but, as is present in this case, chronic stable angina is common and most patients manifest ischemia on a stress test.[1] In addition to improvement in anginal symptoms and the freedom from need for coronary bypass surgery, successful PCI of a chronically-occluded coronary artery is also associated with improvement in left ventricular function and improved survival.[3,4] One nonrandomized observational study involving over 2000 patients undergoing PCI for a chronic total occlusion during the 1980-1999 time period observed a success rate of 70% and an in-hospital adverse event rate that was similar between CTO patients (3.8%) and non-CTO patients (3.7%).[4] Ten-year survival was better if the CTO was successfully opened (73.5%), compared to patients with failed CTO treatment (65%).[4] It should be emphasized that, despite these apparent benefits, PCI for a chronic total occlusion is not justified in asymptomatic patients without evidence of ischemia and with normal left ventricular function.[3]

In patients with chronically occluded arteries, the major obstacle to success lies in the inability to pass a guidewire through the occluded segment. Predictors of successful wire passage include: 1) short duration of occlusion; 2) short length of occlusion; 3) tapered entry into the stump; 4) absence of a side branch at the occluded site; and 5) lack of lesion calcification, vessel tortuosity, or ostial location.[5] Numerous techniques, devices, and strategies have been designed to improve procedural success.[5] Advances in guidewire technology, particularly the tapered tip and stiff-tipped guidewires, have helped many operators achieve success for anterograde attempts at crossing the lesion.[3,6] Furthermore, the use of another angiographic catheter to image the collateral vessels originating from another coronary artery, as used in this case, greatly facilitates success and eliminates much of the uncertainty, particularly in the presence of long occlusions. Guide backup is important to allow the operator the ability to push and penetrate the fibrous cap of the occlusion. Loading the guidewire into an over-the-wire balloon allows the operator to advance the balloon close to the occluded site and provides additional backup. In addition, it allows the operator to exchange for a floppy-tipped wire once the occlusion is crossed, preventing the migration of the stiff-tipped wire into a small branch and leading to a distal perforation. If anterograde approaches fail, experts in total occlusion angioplasty have developed numerous retrograde approaches via the collateral vessels to penetrate the distal cap.[3]

The risk of a chronic total occlusion PCI is fairly low and there is usually little or no consequence if the attempt fails. However, there are unique complications associated with a CTO PCI. These include perforation, proximal dissection and loss of side branches proximal to the occlusion, damage to the collateral vessels, and the associated risk of a prolonged procedure including excessive contrast use and radiation exposure. The risk of perforation for CTO PCI is about 0.9% compared to 0.2% in the non-CTO population.[3] To minimize the consequences of a wire perforation complicating an attempt at PCI of CTO, glycoprotein IIb/IIIa inhibitors or direct thrombin inhibitors without antidotes should not be used until the operator is confident that the wire is safely in the distal true lumen. Unfractionated heparin is a wise choice as it can be readily reversed in the event of a wire perforation.

Interestingly, collaterals appear to regress almost immediately after a successful PCI of a CTO.[7,8] Therefore, stent thrombosis occurring after successful PCI for a CTO might result in an acute ST-segment elevation myocardial infarction, as the collaterals previously present can no longer be relied upon for ischemic protection if the artery occludes.

The final challenge relates to maintaining patency and preventing restenosis. Reocclusion rates are as high as 10% to 15% after stenting[9] and restenosis with bare-metal stents approaches 30%.[10] Similar to other lesion subtypes, drug-eluting stents reduce restenosis compared to bare-metal stents in patients undergoing chronic total occlusion PCI,[11] and thus, in the absence of contraindications, drug-eluting stents are preferable in this complex lesion subgroup.

KEY CONCEPTS

1. Chronic total occlusions are present in 30% of patients undergoing angiography for coronary syndromes.
2. PCI of chronic total occlusions is difficult, with a lower success rate than non-chronic occlusions. Failure to cross the occluded segment is the primary cause of failure.
3. PCI of a chronic occlusion can be considered in patients with angina or ischemia on a noninvasive test and anatomy favorable for an attempted PCI.
4. Angiographic features predicting success include a tapered entry, short occlusion, and absence of calcification, angulation, or ostial location.
5. Advances in guidewires and novel techniques improve procedural success.
6. Drug-eluting stents reduce restenosis rates in this subgroup.

Selected References

1. Stone GW, Kandzari DE, Mehran R, Colombo A, et al: Percutaneous recanalization of chronically occluded coronary arteries. A consensus document. Part I, *Circulation* 112:2364–2372, 2005.
2. Christofferson RD, Lehmann KG, Martin GV, Every N, Caldwell JH, Kapadia SR: Effect of chronic total occlusion on treatment strategy, *Am J Cardiol* 95:1088–1091, 2005.
3. Grantham JA, Marso SP, Spertus J, House J, Holmes DR, Rutherford BD: Chronic total occlusion angioplasty in the United States, *J Am Coll Cardiol Interv* 2:479–486, 2009.
4. Suero JA, Marso SP, Jones PG, Laster SB, Huber KC, Giorgi LV, Johnson WL, Rutherford BD: Procedural outcomes and long-term survival among patients undergoing percutaneous coronary intervention of a chronic total occlusion in native coronary arteries: A 20-year experience, *J Am Coll Cardiol* 38:409–414, 2001.
5. Stone GW, Reifart NJ, Moussa I, Hoye A, et al: Percutaneous recanalization of chronically occluded coronary arteries. A consensus document. Part II, *Circulation* 112:2530–2537, 2005.
6. Saito S, Tanaka S, Hiroe Y, Miyashita Y, Takahashi S, Satake S, Tanaka K: Angioplasty for chronic total occlusion by using tapered tip guide wires, *Catheter Cardiovasc Interv* 59:305–311, 2003.
7. Werner GS, Richartz BM, Gastmann O, Ferrari M, Figulla HR: Immediate changes of collateral function after successful recanalization of chronic total coronary occlusions, *Circulation* 102:2959–2965, 2000.
8. Zimarino M, Ausiello A, Contegiacomo G, Riccardi I, Renda G, DiIorio C, Caterina R: Rapid decline of collateral circulation increases susceptibility to myocardial ischemia, *J Am Coll Cardiol* 48:59–65, 2006.
9. Buller CE, Dzavik V, Carere RG, Mancini J, Barbeau G, Lazzam C, Anderson TJ, Knudtson ML, Marquis JF, Suzuki T, Cohen EA, Fox RS, Teo KK: for the TOSCA Investigators: Primary stenting versus ballon angioplasty in occluded coronary arteries. The Total Occlusion Study of Canada (TOSCA), *Circulation* 100:236–242, 1999.
10. Sirnes PA, Gold S, Myreng Y, Mølstad P, Emanuelsson H, Albertsson P, Brekke M, Mangschau A, Endresen K, Kjekshus J: Stenting in chronic coronary occlusion (SICCO): A randomized, controlled trial of adding stent implantation after successful angioplasty, *J Am Coll Cardiol* 28:1444–1451, 1996.
11. Suttorp MJ, Laarman GJ, Rahel BM, et al: Primary stenting of totally occluded native coronary arteries II (PRISON II): A randomized comparison of bare-metal stent implantation with sirolimus-eluting stent implantation for the treatment of total coronary occlusions, *Circulation* 114:921–928, 2006.

Excessive Coronary Tortuosity

Michael Ragosta, MD, FACC, FSCAI

CASE PRESENTATION

A 49-year-old man with no significant past medical history presented to the hospital after a prolonged episode of chest pain associated with nausea and diaphoresis. Initial troponin was only slightly abnormal (0.07 ng/mL) and he was admitted with the diagnosis of a non-ST segment elevation myocardial infarction. He was treated with a beta blocker, nitrates, and low-molecular-weight heparin and referred for cardiac catheterization.

CARDIAC CATHETERIZATION

The culprit lesion involved the right coronary artery. There was a severe stenosis in the midportion of the right coronary artery past an extremely tortuous segment of the artery (Figures 12-1, 12-2, 12-3 and Video 12-1). There was moderate disease in the left anterior descending artery (Figures 12-4, 12-5).

Based on the angiogram and the clinical presentation, the patient's physician decided to proceed with a percutaneous intervention of the right coronary artery. The severe tortuosity of the proximal right coronary concerned the operator and, anticipating difficulty passing wires, balloons, and stents around the tortuous segment, the operator decided to use a supportive guide catheter and engaged the right coronary artery with a 6 French extra-support right guide catheter (Cordis, XBRCA). Procedural anticoagulation was accomplished with a bolus of unfractionated heparin and a double bolus

plus infusion of eptifibatide. The operator crossed the lesion with a floppy-tipped, 0.014 inch guidewire. This wire successfully straightened the proximal tortuosity and allowed passage of a 2.5 mm diameter by 15 mm long compliant balloon (Figure 12-6). The operator chose a 3.0 mm diameter by 18 mm long bare-metal stent. Advancing the stent to the desired segment of the artery proved very difficult. Ultimately, this stent was successfully delivered to the lesion (Figure 12-7 and Video 12-2). The post-stent angiogram revealed a new and concerning lesion proximal to the stent. This segment of the artery straightened substantially with the floppy-tipped guidewire and the physician was unsure if the angiographic appearance represented a "pseudolesion" due to straightening of the tortuous segment by the guidewire or if it represented an injury to the artery from the vigorous attempts at passing the stent. The operator decided to pass another 3.0 mm by 18 mm stent, but was unable to advance it to the desired location (Figure 12-8). After positioning an extra-supportive guidewire (Mailman, Boston Scientific) alongside the first wire, and after deeply inserting the guide catheter, the operator successfully delivered this stent. The angiogram obtained after the second stent was placed showed that the additional wire further straightened the artery (Figure 12-9) creating a prominent pseudolesion. However, in addition to the pseudolesion, there was retention of contrast at the ostium that was concerning for a guide catheter dissection (Video 12-3). A third 3.5 mm diameter by 23 mm long bare-metal stent was placed over

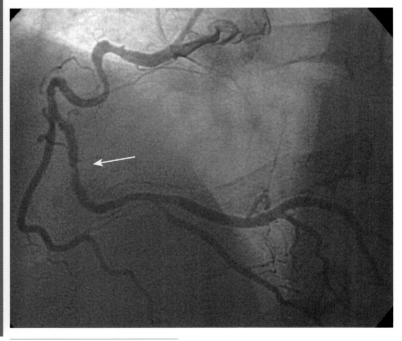

FIGURE 12-1. This is a left anterior oblique projection of the right coronary artery showing a severe stenosis in the midsegment (*arrow*). There is a severely tortuous segment of the artery proximal to the lesion, with moderate atherosclerotic disease.

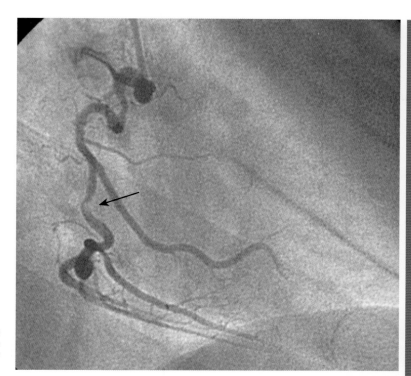

FIGURE 12-2. This is a right anterior oblique projection of the right coronary artery showing the severe stenosis in the midsegment (*arrow*) and marked tortuosity of the artery proximal to the lesion.

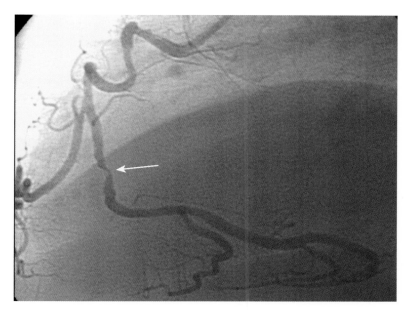

FIGURE 12-3. This is a left lateral projection of the right coronary artery showing a severe stenosis in the midsegment (*arrow*) and marked tortuosity proximal to the lesion.

this segment. The final angiographic result in multiple projections and with the guidewires removed is shown in Figures 12-10, 12-11 and Videos 12-4, 12-5.

POSTPROCEDURAL COURSE

His postprocedural course was uncomplicated, and he was discharged the next morning on clopidogrel, aspirin, atorvastatin, and metoprolol. At follow-up 2 and 8 months after this intervention, he remained free of cardiac events and symptoms but had discontinued his atorvastatin. He remained well until 18 months after the intervention when he developed recurrent angina.

Cardiac catheterization performed at another hospital without open heart surgery backup found wide patency of the right coronary stents but observed a new and severe stenosis of the proximal left anterior descending artery (LAD). He underwent attempted intervention, but the procedure was complicated by abrupt vessel closure. He was transferred emergently to a hospital capable of performing open heart surgery and underwent emergency bypass surgery consisting of a left internal mammary artery to the LAD. He recovered from this and the associated periprocedural infarction. Two years after the initial right coronary stents were placed, he developed recurrent atypical chest pain and underwent

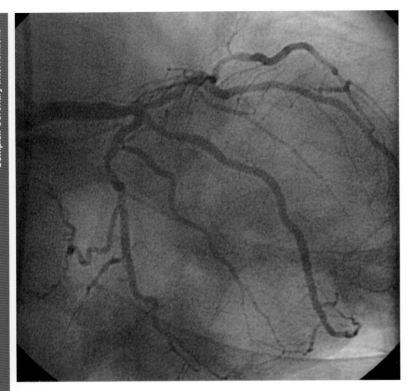

FIGURE 12-4. Representative angiogram of the left coronary artery in the right anterior oblique projection with caudal angulation.

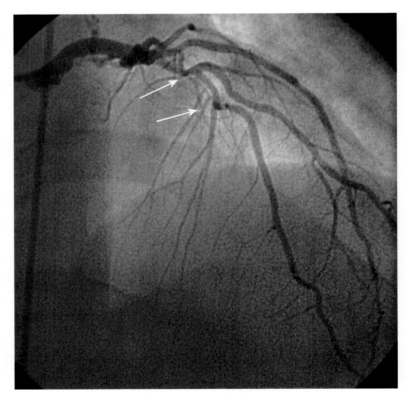

FIGURE 12-5. Representative angiogram of the left coronary artery in the right anterior oblique projection with cranial angulation, showing moderate disease of the left anterior descending artery (*arrows*).

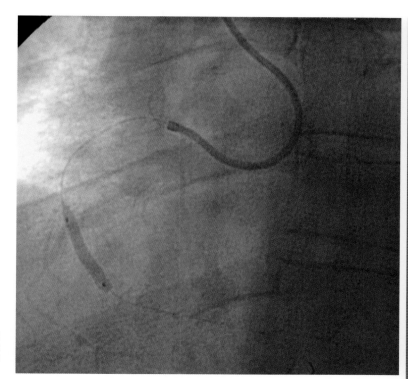

FIGURE 12-6. An extra-support guide catheter is placed in the right coronary artery and balloon angioplasty of the lesion performed. Notice the straightening of the tortuous segment by the guidewire.

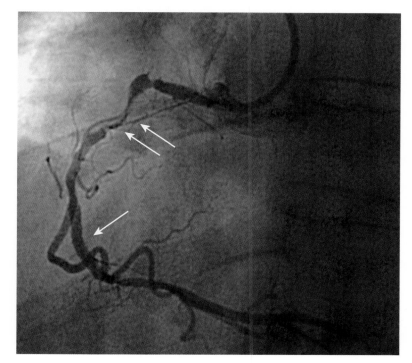

FIGURE 12-7. Following stenting of the mid lesion (*arrow*), there is a suspicious lesion in the tortuous segment (*double arrow*).

another catheterization that again showed wide patency of the previously placed right coronary stents and a patent left internal mammary graft to the LAD.

DISCUSSION

Severe vessel tortuosity has long been identified as a high-risk feature for PCI. This case exemplifies many of the challenges facing the operator treating a tortuous coronary artery.

Marked tortuosity of the coronary arteries is often seen in patients with longstanding hypertension and in elderly individuals. Tortuosity impairs the operator's ability to advance guidewires, balloons, and stents. Even floppy-tipped guidewires are sometimes difficult to position, and the operator may encounter considerable loss of torque control after advancing past one or more sharply angled and tortuous segments. The operator must achieve appropriate guide catheter support before beginning a PCI on a tortuous coronary. This typically

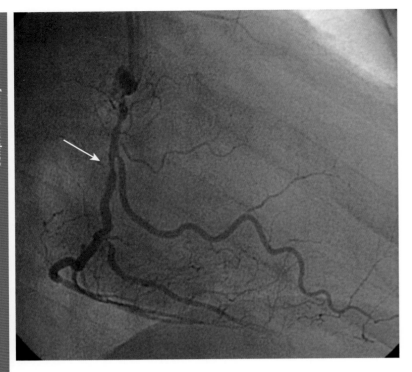

FIGURE 12-8. Right anterior oblique projection obtained after stenting. Resistance to passage of the second stent was encountered proximal to the first stent, at a lesion of moderate severity (*arrow*).

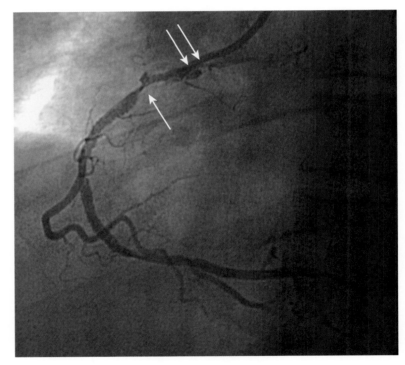

FIGURE 12-9. Placement of the second stent required an additional supportive wire and aggressive engagement of the guide. A pseudolesion is present in the proximal segment (*arrow*). There is also a guide catheter injury at the ostium (*double arrow*).

requires the use of guides with larger bores and aggressive curves. If a high-torque floppy guidewire is not successfully advanced, a hydrophilic wire may prove valuable as this type tends to "float" down the artery and requires less manipulation. Many operators employ extra-supportive wires to help straighten the tortuous curves and help deliver equipment. However, the extra stiffness of their shafts may hinder their delivery. In these cases, many physicians use a floppy-tipped wire as the primary wire and the stiffer, supportive wire

as a second or "buddy" wire.[1] Compliant balloons are usually deliverable despite severe tortuosity. Stents, however, may not pass easily around the curves. Tricks for success include the use of an aggressive guide, employment of extra-supportive guidewires or "buddy" wires[1] and adequate lesion predilatation. In addition, it is often wise to use multiple short stents instead of a single long stent to cover the diseased segment. Finally, drug-eluting stents are sometimes more difficult to pass than the thin-strut, bare-metal stents.

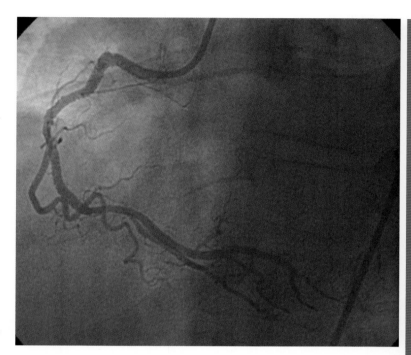

FIGURE 12-10. Final angiogram obtained after removal of the guidewire (left anterior oblique projection).

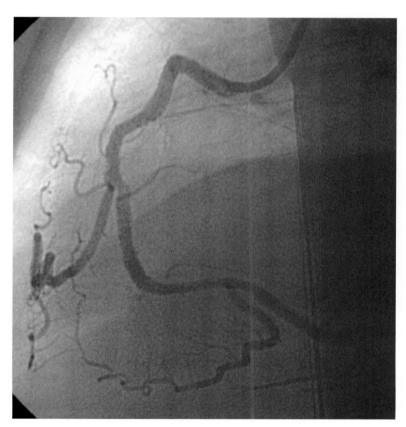

FIGURE 12-11. Final angiogram obtained after removal of the guidewire (left lateral projection).

Marked vessel tortuosity increases the risk of PCI-related complications. Difficulty with wire manipulation may result in intimal injury or vessel dissection. Balloon angioplasty of a tortuous and angulated segment often leads to dissection. This could pose a serious problem if the operator cannot subsequently deliver a stent. Tortuosity is a well-recognized risk factor for coronary perforation from rotational atherectomy.[2] Finally, the use of aggressive guide catheters necessary to provide adequate support may also result in guide-related injury to the proximal coronary as observed in this case.

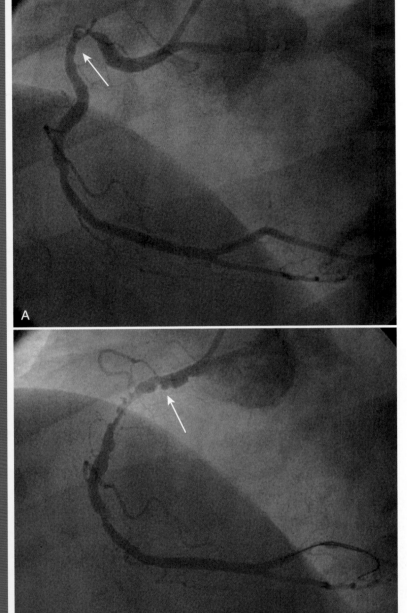

FIGURE 12-12. These images are from another patient and demonstrate the classic angiographic features of a pseudolesion. There is severe angulation of the proximal right coronary artery (A). After placement of a guidewire, the artery straightened and created multiple "new" lesions, characteristic of pseudolesions or the accordion phenomenon (B, arrow).

In the setting of significant vessel tortuosity, guidewires and balloon catheters may straighten the artery and create "pseudolesions."[3-6] This angiographic artifact represents an invagination or crumpling of the redundant segments of the vessel from straightening, and has also been termed "the accordion phenomenon."[6] Characteristically, it appears as the development of a "new" lesion after the guidewire has been placed but appears smooth and beaded (Figure 12-12). The unenlightened PCI operator may misinterpret these artifacts as a dissection, thrombus, or spasm, which often leads to the use of additional (and unnecessary) stents. As displayed in this case, pseudolesions are commonly observed in the right coronary artery, but have also involved the left anterior descending, circumflex arteries, and left internal mammary grafts.

Guidewire removal restores the artery to its original configuration and resolves the pseudolesion. Fearing a dissection, many physicians are reluctant to do this as they are not entirely confident that the angiographic appearance is solely due to straightening artifact. Withdrawal of the guidewire so that just the floppy-tipped portion is across the area of concern is one technique offered to prove that the apparent lesion is an artifact and not a dissection without giving up access to the distal lumen.[7]

KEY CONCEPTS

1. Severe vessel tortuosity creates substantial challenges to the operator, including difficulty passing guidewires, balloons, and stents, and an increased risk of dissection and perforation.
2. Adequate guide support, the use of supportive wires or "buddy" wires, and passage of multiple short stents instead of one long stent increases the chance of success.
3. It is important for PCI operators to recognize the commonly encountered "pseudolesions" due to straightening of the angulated segment, as they resolve with guidewire removal and do not require additional stenting.

Selected References

1. Burzotta F, Trani C, Mazzari MA, Mongiardo R, Rebuzzi AG, Buffon A, Niccoli G, Biondi-Zoccai G, Romagnoli E, Ramazzotti V, Schiavoni G, Crea F: Use of a second buddy wire during percutaneous coronary interventions: a simple solution for some challenging situations, *J Invasive Cardiol* 17:171–174, 2005.
2. Cohen BM, Weber VJ, Relsman M, Casale A, Dorros G: Coronary perforation complicating rotational ablation: the U.S. multicenter experience, *Catheter Cardiovasc Diagn* (Suppl 3):55–59, 1996.
3. Tenaglia AN, Tcheng JE, Phillips HR, Stack RS: Creation of pseudo narrowing during coronary angioplasty, *Am J Cardiol* 67:658–659, 1991.
4. Hays JT, Stein B, Raizner AE: The crumpled coronary: an enigma of arteriographic pseudopathology and its potential for misinterpretation, *Catheter Cardiovasc Diagn* 31:293–300, 1994.
5. Doshi S, Shiu MF: Coronary pseudo-lesions induced in the left anterior descending and right coronary artery by the angioplasty guide-wire, *Int J Cardiol* 68:337–342, 1999.
6. Muller O, Hamilos M, Ntalianis A, Sarno G, DeBruyne B: The accordion phenomenon. Lesson from a movie, *Circulation* 118: e677–e678, 2008.
7. Chalet Y, Chevalier B, el Hadad S, Guyon P, Lancelin B: "Pseudo-narrowing" during right coronary angioplasty: how to diagnose correctly without withdrawing the guidewire, *Catheter Cardiovasc Diagn* 31:37–40, 1994.

Complex Coronary Disease

Michael Ragosta, MD, FACC, FSCAI

CASE PRESENTATION

The onset of severe substernal chest pain awakened a 50-year-old diabetic woman without prior cardiac history from her sleep. The pain waxed and waned all morning until she finally presented to the emergency room 9 hours later. She was found to have an inferior wall ST-segment elevation myocardial infarction and was taken emergently to the cardiac catheterization laboratory. As suspected, based on the electrocardiographic changes, the right coronary artery was completely occluded (Figure 13-1); however, the operator was surprised to find severe and complex disease affecting the left anterior descending (LAD) and diagonal arteries (Figure 13-2 and Video 13-1) and moderate disease in the left circumflex artery (Figure 13-3 and Video 13-2). Lush collaterals filled the distal right coronary artery from the left coronary injections.

With the goal of achieving rapid reperfusion of the infarct-related artery, the operator decided to open the right coronary artery. This was promptly and successfully accomplished with balloon angioplasty followed by deployment of two 4.5 mm diameter bare-metal stents. The operator obtained an excellent luminal result and TIMI-3 flow (Figure 13-4 and Video 13-3).

She recovered uneventfully from the acute infarction. During this hospitalization, a transthoracic echocardiogram showed an ejection fraction of 35% to 40% from an extensive inferoposterior wall motion abnormality. Uncertain about the optimal management of the incidentally-noted disease in the LAD and diagonal branch, her physician carefully considered several options. Surgical revascularization was thought to be unattractive because of the small caliber of the vessel and the presence of diffuse disease distally at the site of the usual graft anastomosis. Percutaneous revascularization would be complex and technically difficult because of the presence of bifurcation disease in the LAD and the small caliber of the LAD and diagonal vessels. In addition, given the recent sizeable inferior infarction and reduced left ventricular function, a PCI-related complication involving the LAD, such as abrupt vessel closure or loss of the diagonal side branch, might lead to serious morbidity and even death. Based on these considerations, her physician decided to pursue aggressive medical therapy as the initial management strategy. Thus, she was discharged on aspirin, clopidogrel, metoprolol, lisinopril, and atorvastatin.

At follow-up 2 months later, she reported significant shortness of breath associated with substernal chest pain

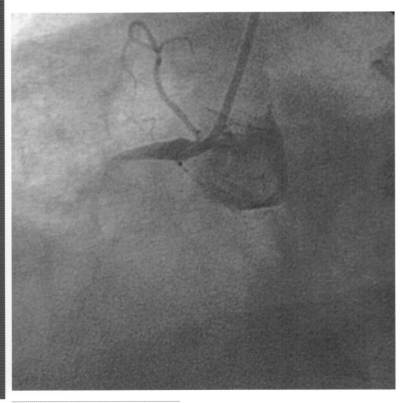

FIGURE 13-1. This is the occluded right coronary and the infarct-related artery.

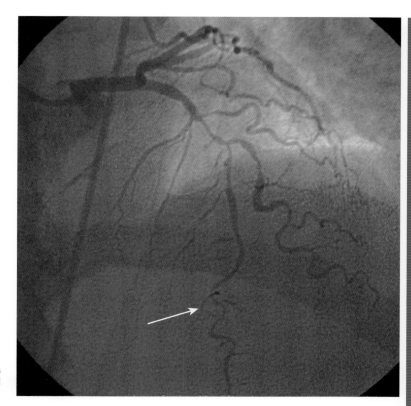

FIGURE 13-2. The left anterior descending artery was severely diseased, with complex disease involving the diagonal and the bifurcation. There is also distal disease present (*arrow*).

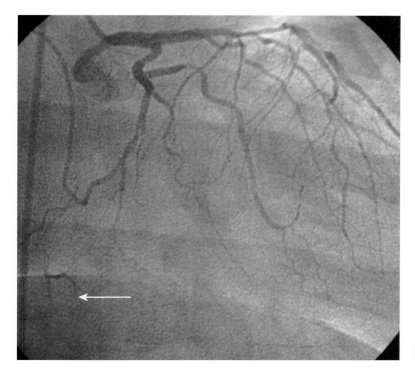

FIGURE 13-3. There is moderate disease of the obtuse marginal artery and collaterals to the right coronary artery (*arrow*).

when walking up the stairs at her home. A repeat echocardiogram showed improvement in left ventricular function with ejection fraction of 45% to 50%. Her physician again weighed the risks and benefits of surgery, percutaneous revascularization of the LAD, or continued medical therapy and referred her for stenting of the LAD.

CARDIAC CATHETERIZATION

She returned to the cardiac catheterization laboratory for an elective complex intervention of the LAD and diagonal. After achieving therapeutic anticoagulation, the operator advanced 0.014 inch floppy-tipped guidewires in both the LAD and diagonal and performed balloon

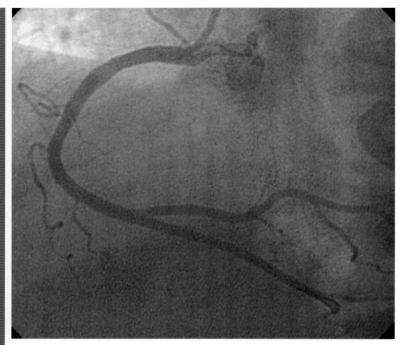

FIGURE 13-4. Angiogram obtained after stenting the right coronary artery.

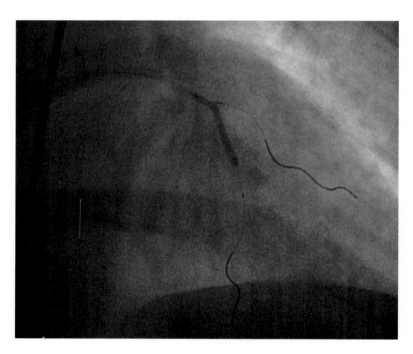

FIGURE 13-5. First, the LAD was treated with balloon angioplasty after a guidewire was positioned in the diagonal branch.

angioplasty in the LAD with a 2.0 mm diameter by 20 mm long compliant balloon (Figure 13-5). The first diagonal was then treated with two everolimus-eluting stents; the first one (2.5 mm diameter by 14 mm long) placed in the mid-diagonal (Figures 13-6, 13-7) and a second one (also 2.5 mm diameter by 14 mm long) placed in the diagonal but extended into the proximal part of the LAD (Figures 13-8, 13-9 and Video 13-4). The operator withdrew the LAD wire to the guide catheter because the wire was trapped behind the latter stent. This guidewire was then repositioned in the distal LAD through the stent struts. Balloon angioplasty was performed and a single 2.5 mm diameter by 18 mm long

everolimus-eluting stent positioned in the LAD using a "T" configuration just distal to the diagonal bifurcation (Figure 13-10). Following the deployment of this stent, the ostium of the diagonal was postdilated with a 2.5 mm diameter noncompliant balloon (Figure 13-11). The final angiographic result, shown in Figure 13-12 and Video 13-5, appeared satisfactory to the operator.

POSTPROCEDURAL COURSE

Her post-PCI course was uncomplicated and she was discharged the following morning. She remained event- and symptom-free at follow-up 15 months later.

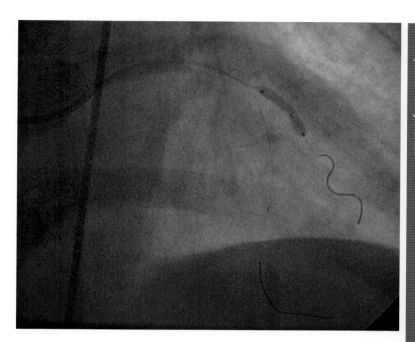

FIGURE 13-6. Next, the operator stented the diagonal branch.

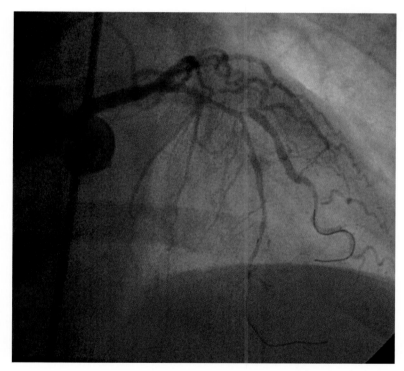

FIGURE 13-7. Angiographic appearance after the first diagonal stent was placed.

DISCUSSION

The complex disease and challenging revascularization decisions evident in this case are familiar to practitioners of interventional cardiology. This patient first presented with an ST-segment elevation myocardial infarction. At that point, the physician's primary focus was to achieve prompt reperfusion of the infarct-related artery; this was successfully accomplished using percutaneous techniques. However, during this procedure, significant obstructive coronary disease was identified in the non-infarct–related arteries. The decision regarding how to best manage this other coexisting disease was not entirely clear to the physician, as each of the various options had limitations, risks, and uncertainty.

First, it was not clear if and when revascularization of this other disease was indicated. Multivessel coronary disease is found in up to 60% of patients undergoing emergent cardiac catheterization for ST-segment elevation myocardial infarction.[1-3] The optimal management of these "bystander" lesions is unclear and controversial. Because of the concern about the risks of intervening upon a non-infarct–related artery when there is acute infarction in another vascular territory, current practice

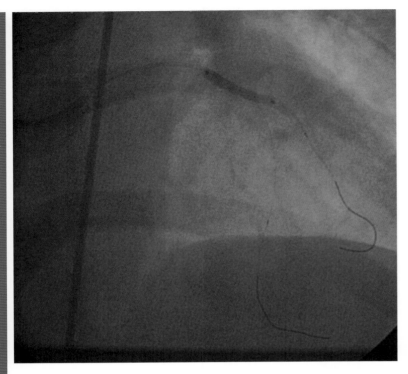

FIGURE 13-8. The proximal end of the diagonal was treated with another stent that extended into the LAD.

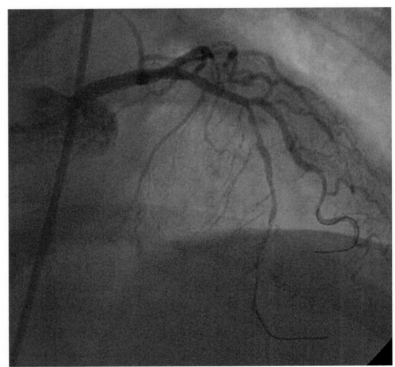

FIGURE 13-9. Angiographic appearance after the second diagonal stent was placed.

guidelines discourage the performance of an intervention on obstructive lesions in the non-infarct–related artery at the time of acute infarct angioplasty. It is not known if these lesions should be treated during the hospital phase while the patient is still recovering from the infarction, in the weeks to months following the event when the infarction has healed, or deferred indefinitely unless there is objective evidence of ischemia. In this case, the complexity of the disease led to the decision

to pursue medical therapy as the initial strategy. During follow-up, her ongoing symptoms despite appropriate medical therapy caused her physicians to recommend revascularization.

Second, once it was determined that the patient needed revascularization, it was not clear how it might best be accomplished. Surgical revascularization might have been the simplest solution, but the small caliber of the patient's arteries as well at the presence of diffuse disease

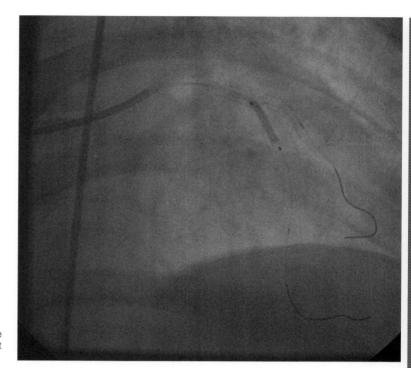

FIGURE 13-10. After repositioning the LAD wire through the stent struts and performing balloon angioplasty, the LAD stent was placed flush to the origin of the diagonal side branch.

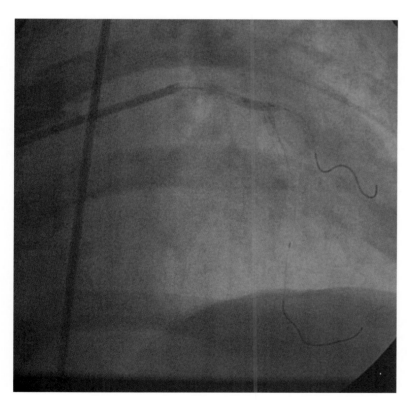

FIGURE 13-11. As a final step, the operator ballooned the origin of the diagonal to ensure proper stent apposition.

located at the usual site of a graft anastomosis discouraged her physicians from pursuing this option. Percutaneous revascularization was also problematic and associated with increased risk because of the presence of bifurcation disease and small-caliber arteries.

Finally, once the option of percutaneous revascularization was chosen, the operator was faced with several crucial technical decisions regarding treatment of the complex disease. The small caliber of the involved arteries (<2.5 mm diameter) is associated with an increased risk of procedural complication and an increased risk for restenosis. Bare-metal stents are superior to balloon angioplasty in small arteries but are associated with at least a 25% restenosis rate[4]; this rate approaches 50% in diabetics. Drug-eluting stents reduce the rate of restenosis in small arteries compared to bare-metal stents.[5,6]

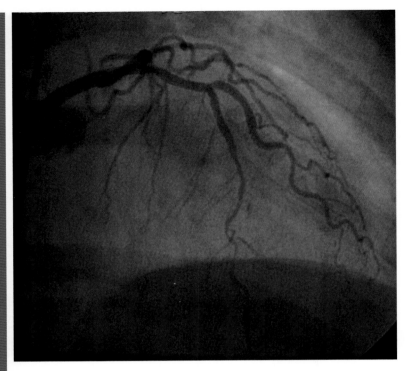

FIGURE 13-12. Final angiographic result after stenting the LAD and diagonal.

In the present case, it was not clear to the operator that the involved arteries were large enough to accommodate a drug-eluting stent; fortunately, 2.5 mm diameter drug-eluting stents were successfully placed without creating distal edge dissections or other complications. Management of the bifurcation represented another significant technical challenge. Because of the diffuse disease in the distal LAD, the operator decided to prioritize the large diagonal branch and considered the LAD the "side branch" vessel. Choosing a relatively simple approach to stenting the bifurcation and avoiding overlapping stents at the bifurcation in this diabetic patient with small-caliber vessels likely contributed to the excellent outcome.

KEY CONCEPTS

1. Multivessel disease is common in patients with acute ST-segment elevation myocardial infarction and the optimal management of this coexisting disease is not clear.
2. Small-caliber arteries are difficult to treat percutaneously. Drug-eluting stents appear to be beneficial at preventing restenosis in this subgroup.

Selected References

1. Muller DW, Topol EJ, Ellis SG, et al: Multivessel coronary artery disease: a key predictor of short-term prognosis after reperfusion therapy for acute myocardial infarction. Thrombolysis and Angioplasty in Myocardial Infarction (TAMI) Study Group, *Am Heart J* 121(4 Pt 1):1042–1049, 1991.
2. Jaski BE, Cohen JD, Trausch J, et al: Outcome of urgent percutaneous transluminal coronary angioplasty in acute myocardial infarction: comparison of single-vessel versus multivessel coronary artery disease, *Am Heart J* 124:1427–1433, 1992.
3. Kahn JK, Rutherford BD, McConahay DR, et al: Results of primary angioplasty for acute myocardial infarction in patients with multivessel coronary artery disease, *J Am Coll Cardiol* 16:1089–1096, 1990.
4. Moreno R, Fernandez C, Alfonso F, Hernandez R, Perez-Vizcayno MJ, Escaned J, Sabate M, Banuelos C, Angiolillo DJ, Azcona L, Macaya C: Coronary stenting versus balloon angioplasty in small vessels: a meta analysis from 11 randomized studies, *J Am Coll Cardiol* 43:1964–1972, 2004.
5. Menozzi A, Solinas E, Ortolani P, Repetto A, Saia F, Piovaccari G, Manari A, Magagnini E, Vignali L, Bonizzoni E, Merlini PA, Cavallini C, Ardissino D: SES-SMART Investigators: Twenty-four months of clinical outcomes of sirolimus-eluting stents for the treatment of small coronary arteries: the long-term SES-SMART clinical study, *Eur Heart J* 30:2095–2101, 2009.
6. Hermiller JB, Fergus T, Pierson W, Su X, Sood P, Sudhir K, Stone GW: Clinical and angiographic comparison of everolimus-eluting and paclitaxel-eluting stents in small coronary arteries: a post hoc analysis of the SPIRIT III randomized trial, *Am Heart J* 158:1005–1010, 2009.

Extensive Coronary Thrombus

Michael Ragosta, MD, FACC, FSCAI

CASE PRESENTATION

After experiencing a 1-month history of intermittent chest discomfort, a 47-year-old man suddenly developed severe left-sided chest pain while loading a truck. The chest pain continued despite stopping to rest and was associated with nausea, diaphoresis, and light-headedness. He drove himself to a hospital without the capacity to perform primary angioplasty. In the emergency room, he was discovered to have an acute ST-segment elevation inferoposterior myocardial infarction, and the emergency room physician administered sublingual nitroglycerin without relief of pain. The patient was within 1 hour of symptom onset and the treating physician decided to reperfuse with thrombolysis rather than delay reperfusion in order to transfer to a hospital with PCI capability. Therefore, while still in the emergency room, the patient received aspirin, clopidogrel, and tenecteplase, along with enoxaparin (30 mg intravenously and 100 mg subcutaneously). Twenty-five minutes after receiving thrombolysis, the patient noted improvement in chest pain. A repeat electrocardiogram confirmed near complete resolution of ST-segment elevation. Unfortunately, approximately 30 minutes later, his chest pain returned, along with marked ST-segment elevation, hypotension, and bradycardia. At this point, the emergency room physician decided to transfer the patient for rescue intervention, to a hospital 60 minutes away by helicopter.

Upon arrival, the patient continued to report chest pain, and there remained persistent ST-segment elevation present on the electrocardiogram. A review of the patient's medical history was relevant only for ongoing tobacco abuse and a family history of premature coronary disease. Physical exam was notable for a heart rate of 69 bpm, a blood pressure of 105/63 mmHg, elevated neck veins, and clear lung fields. Initial troponin I was normal and all other laboratory evaluations were within normal limits. He was taken emergently to the cardiac catheterization laboratory.

CARDIAC CATHETERIZATION

The patient arrived in the cardiac catheterization laboratory approximately 2 hours after receiving thrombolysis. As expected, the right coronary artery was completely occluded (Figure 14-1). There was no significant obstructive disease noted in the left coronary arteries. An additional intravenous bolus of enoxaparin was administered, along with a bolus plus infusion of eptifibatide. The operator inserted a guide catheter and easily passed a 0.014 inch floppy-tipped guidewire to the distal artery. A 2.5 mm by 20 mm long compliant

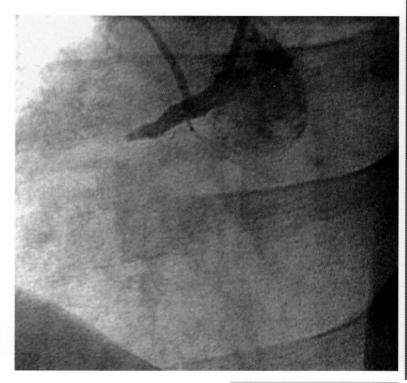

FIGURE 14-1. This is a right coronary angiogram demonstrating complete occlusion of the proximal right coronary artery in a patient with an acute ST-segment elevation inferoposterior myocardial infarction.

balloon inflated at the occlusion site immediately restored TIMI-3 flow, and resulted in resolution of chest pain and ST-segment elevation. However, an extensive filling defect was observed, consistent with a large intra-coronary thrombus (Figure 14-2 and Video 14-1). The operator passed a Pronto extraction catheter over the floppy-tipped guidewire to the distal artery and, using a 30 cc syringe, gently aspirated as the catheter was withdrawn to the guide catheter. A large amount of clot was successfully removed and improved the angiographic appearance of the artery with no evidence of distal embolization (Figure 14-3 and Video 14-2). A 4 mm diameter by 28 mm long bare-metal stent postdilated with a 4.5 mm noncompliant balloon successfully treated

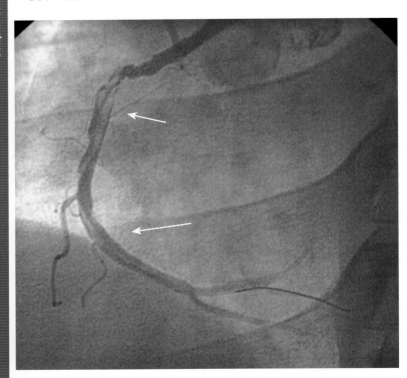

FIGURE 14-2. This angiogram, taken after balloon angioplasty of the proximal segment, shows extensive filling defects consistent with thrombus within the lumen of the artery (*arrows*).

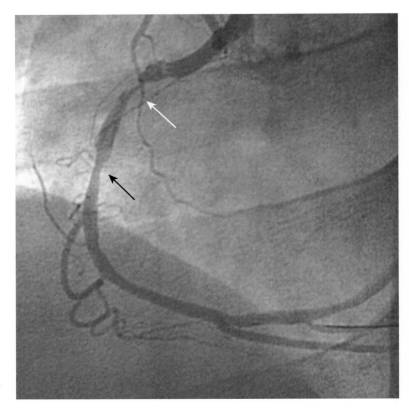

FIGURE 14-3. After aspiration of thrombus, the filling defects are gone. There are residual stenoses present (*arrows*).

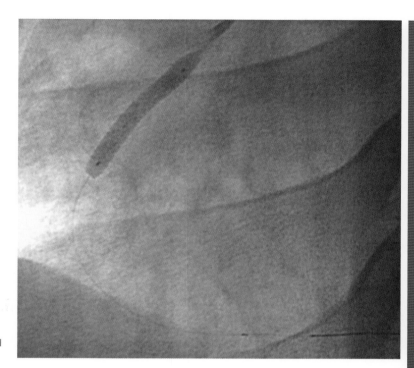

FIGURE 14-4. A bare-metal stent was placed in the proximal artery.

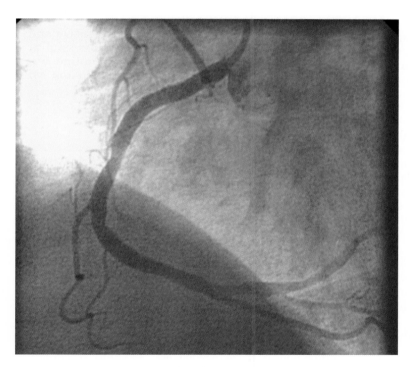

FIGURE 14-5. Final angiographic result after stenting.

the residual stenosis (Figures 14-4, 14-5 and Video 14-3). At the completion of the procedure, the patient had no further chest pain and was transferred to the coronary care unit.

POSTPROCEDURAL COURSE

After a femoral angiogram confirmed puncture of the common femoral artery, the arterial sheaths were removed in the cardiac catheterization laboratory and hemostasis achieved with a closure device. The patient completed a 14-hour course of eptifibatide and remained asymptomatic. Echocardiography showed mildly decreased left ventricular function with inferior hypokinesis. The remainder of his hospital stay was uneventful, and he was discharged 72 hours after admission on aspirin, clopidogrel, metoprolol, lisinopril, and atorvastatin. At follow-up 6 months and again 1 year following the procedure, he remained completely asymptomatic and off cigarettes.

DISCUSSION

Using angiographic criteria, a thrombus is definitely present when a filling defect surrounded by contrast on all sides is observed within the lumen of a coronary artery. Typically, the clot appears to dangle from the distal end of an atherosclerotic plaque of varying severity. A probable thrombus is defined by the presence of a hazy or "washed-out" appearance to the lesion. However, angiography is not very sensitive for thrombus; angioscopy is better at identifying intracoronary clot but is not used clinically. Intravascular ultrasound is not useful because organized thrombus usually appears indistinguishable from a fatty plaque.

Angiographic thrombus is most often encountered in patients undergoing an intervention for acute coronary syndromes. Visible clot often occurs in patients with ST-segment elevation infarction. Similarly, patients undergoing PCI for failed thrombolysis (i.e., rescue angioplasty), as demonstrated in this case, also are likely to have a large thrombus burden. The presence of visible clot is a high-risk feature and is associated with a higher rate of death, myocardial infarction, and abrupt vessel closure,[1] and is also associated with other adverse angiographic outcomes such as failure to achieve TIMI-3 flow post-PCI for acute MI, development of no-reflow phenomenon, and distal embolization.

Adjunctive pharmacology helps reduce the risk of complication from PCI in the setting of visible thrombus. Antiplatelet agents are highly efficacious in this setting and both pretreatment with aspirin and clopidogrel and the adjunctive use of the glycoprotein IIb/IIIa inhibitors are essential for success. Additionally, it is important to achieve an adequate antithrombin effect. If unfractionated heparin is used, the activated clotting time (ACT) should be at least within the therapeutic range (>200 seconds if a glycoprotein IIb/IIIa inhibitor is used); some operators prefer higher levels (250 to 300 seconds) in the presence of a visible clot. Although anecdotal reports abound, the role of intracoronary glycoprotein IIb/IIIa inhibitors or intracoronary lytics has not been well established in a randomized controlled manner.[2] Similarly, although bivalirudin is an effective antithrombin agent for PCI in the setting of acute myocardial infarction (especially if pre-loaded with clopidogrel), the efficacy of this agent without glycoprotein IIb/IIIa inhibitors for PCI in the setting of visible thrombus is unclear.

Numerous mechanical methods have been developed for physical removal of the thrombus. The more complex devices such as the rheolytic thrombectomy device (Angiojet) and an atherectomy-type device (X-Sizer catheter) have not been shown to be beneficial and may be associated with increased risk of adverse outcomes, likely due to distal embolization.[3,4] Aspiration catheters are simply large-bore catheters that use manual aspiration with a syringe to remove clot. They are highly effective at removing clot and employ much simpler techniques and more limited device inventory than the more complex devices. Importantly, aspiration devices have been shown to improve outcomes when used routinely in patients with ST-segment elevation myocardial infarction.[5] Distal protection devices have not shown benefit when applied routinely to patients with STEMI;[6] whether they are helpful in preventing distal embolization in patients with large, visible thrombus such as this case is unclear.

KEY CONCEPTS

1. The lesions associated with acute myocardial infarction are often complex and laden with thrombus.
2. The presence of residual thrombus represents a high-risk lesion and may result in an unsuccessful PCI, failure to achieve TIMI-3 flow, reocclusion, no-reflow phenomenon, or distal embolization.
3. Adjunctive pharmacology with glycoprotein IIb/IIIa inhibitors and antithrombin agents may improve success.
4. While a variety of sophisticated thrombectomy devices have been developed to treat coronary thrombus, they are expensive and associated with poor outcomes, likely due to their propensity to cause distal embolization.
5. Simple aspiration catheters are inexpensive and easy to use and are often highly successful at removing visible thrombus. Their routine use during PCI for acute ST-segment elevation MI appears to improve outcomes.

Selected References

1. Singh M, Reeder GS, Ohman EM, et al: Does the presence of thrombus seen on a coronary angiogram affect the outcome after percutaneous coronary angioplasty? An angiographic trials pool data experience, J Am Coll Cardiol 38:624–630, 2001.
2. Kelly RV, Crouch E, Krumnacher H, Cohen MG, Stouffer GA: Safety of adjunctive intracoronary thrombolytic therapy during complex percutaneous coronary intervention: initial experience with intracoronary tenecteplase, Catheter Cardiovasc Interv 66:327–332, 2005.
3. Kelly RV, Cohen MG, Stouffer GA: Mechanical thrombectomy options in complex percutaneous coronary interventions, Catheter Cardiovasc Interv 68:917–928, 2006.
4. Ali A, Cox D, Dib N, et al: Rheolytic thrombectomy with percutaneous coronary intervention for infarct size reduction in acute myocardial infarction. 30-day results from a multicenter randomized study, J Am Coll Cardiol 48:244–252, 2006.
5. Silva-Orrego P, Colombo P, Bigi R, et al: Thrombus aspiration before primary angioplasty improves myocardial reperfusion in acute myocardial infarction. The DEAR-MI (Dethrombosis to Enhance Acute Reperfusion in Myocardial Infarction) Study, J Am Coll Cardiol 48:1552–1559, 2006.
6. Stone GW, Webb J, Cox DA, et al: Enhanced myocardial efficacy and recovery by aspiration of liberated debris (EMERALD) Investigators: Distal microcirculatory protection during percutaneous coronary intervention in acute ST-segment elevation myocardial infarction: A randomized controlled trial, JAMA 293:1063–1072, 2005.

Transplant Vasculopathy

Michael Ragosta, MD, FACC, FSCAI

CASE PRESENTATION

A 61-year-old man underwent orthotopic heart transplantation 16 years ago for ischemic cardiomyopathy. He now presents for his annual routine right and left heart catheterization, coronary angiogram, and endomyocardial biopsy. A coronary angiogram performed 1 year earlier showed only mild atheromatous disease in the left anterior descending artery without significant luminal narrowing (Figure 15-1). He remains free of all cardiac symptoms including chest pain, dyspnea, exercise intolerance, syncope, or edema. Other pertinent medical history includes peripheral vascular disease treated with an aortobifemoral bypass, hypertension, hyperlipidemia, and mild renal insufficiency with a baseline creatinine of 1.4 mg/dL. Medications include simvastatin, diltiazem, azathioprine, cyclosporine, and aspirin. Recent lipid analysis found an LDL of 103 mg/dL and an HDL of 41 mg/dL.

CARDIAC CATHETERIZATION

The right heart pressures were normal. Selective coronary angiography revealed nonobstructive, mild atheromatous disease in the right coronary artery, unchanged from the previous year (Figure 15-2). The left coronary artery showed progression of the lesion in the left anterior descending artery. This lesion now appeared to significantly narrow the lumen (Figure 15-3 and Video 15-1). The circumflex appeared angiographically normal.

Based on the observed progression of his disease and the known natural history of transplant-associated vasculopathy, his transplant cardiologist recommended percutaneous intervention of the left anterior descending artery. Using an intravenous bolus and infusion of bivalirudin followed by an oral load of 600 mg of clopidogrel, the operator inserted a 3.5 mm diameter by 16 mm long paclitaxel-eluting stent, and postdilated the stent with a 4.0 mm diameter by 9 mm long noncompliant balloon, achieving an excellent angiographic result (Figure 15-4 and Video 15-2). He had no complications and was observed overnight.

POSTPROCEDURAL COURSE

He was discharged the next morning with the addition of long term clopidogrel to his medical regimen. He remained symptom- and event-free during follow-up. A routine coronary angiogram performed 1 year later found no progression of the disease in the right coronary artery and a widely patent stent in the left anterior descending artery without evidence of restenosis (Figure 15-5).

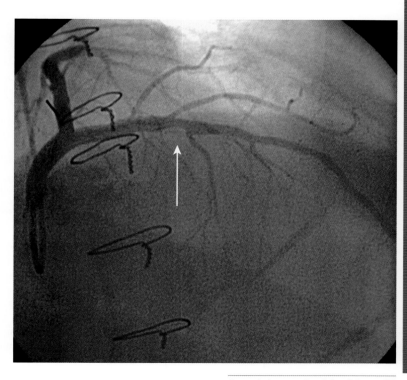

FIGURE 15-1. This is a representative image of the left coronary artery in the right anterior oblique projection with cranial angulation obtained 1 year earlier. There is mild luminal narrowing noted in the proximal segment (arrow).

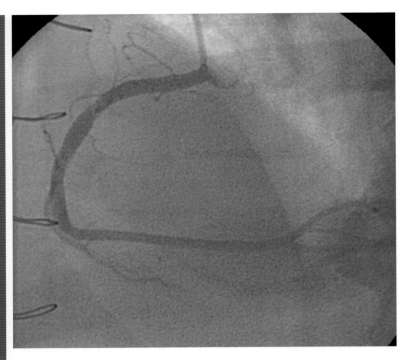

FIGURE 15-2. A right coronary angiogram revealed only mild luminal irregularities.

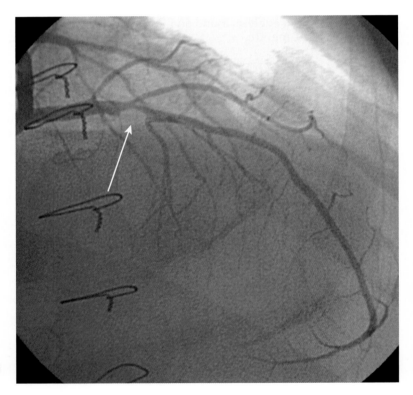

FIGURE 15-3. The left anterior descending artery showed marked progression of disease (*arrow*).

DISCUSSION

Cardiac allograft vasculopathy is a progressive atherosclerotic condition that limits long-term survival after cardiac transplantation. Angiographic evidence of allograft vasculopathy is observed in nearly half of patients within 8 to 10 years of transplant. The prevalence is even higher when intravascular ultrasound, a more sensitive method for detecting atherosclerosis, is used.[1,2] The pathophysiology is complex and related to both immune and nonspecific insults and has been extensively reviewed elsewhere.[1,3] Often described as a diffuse obliterative process affecting the distal vasculature, it may also manifest as focal lesions in proximal vessels, such as the one presented in this case.[4]

The patient presented in this case is fairly typical for cardiac allograft vasculopathy. Patients are usually asymptomatic and the disease is identified by performing

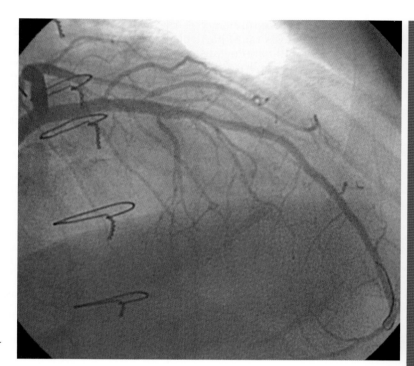

FIGURE 15-4. This angiogram demonstrates the result after stent insertion in the proximal left anterior descending artery.

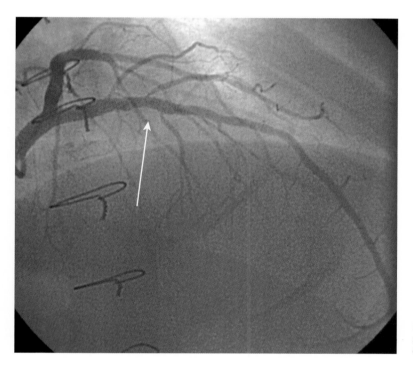

FIGURE 15-5. A routine angiogram performed 1 year later showed no evidence of restenosis or progression of disease elsewhere (*arrow*).

routine coronary angiograms, usually at 12-month intervals following cardiac transplantation at most transplant centers. Due to cardiac denervation, chest pain and classic angina are unusual; the most common symptom is dyspnea from heart failure caused by ischemic left ventricular dysfunction. Arrhythmias and sudden death are other possible manifestations.

Great effort has been invested in prevention, but only statin therapy reliably lowers the rate of development of transplant-associated vasculopathy.[5] Once the disease is angiographically evident, it progresses rapidly.

Retransplantation is the only definitive treatment, but is not practical due to the limited donor pool and is associated with poor long-term survival.

Revascularization is a palliative technique that has not been convincingly shown to change the natural history of the disease or extend the life of the allograft. Coronary bypass surgery can be performed, but is often not feasible because of poor distal targets from the diffuse obliterative disease; it is also associated with a high procedural mortality. Based on limited case series, percutaneous revascularization techniques appear safe and feasible. The high procedural success rates are tempered by excessive restenosis rates, particularly following balloon angioplasty and bare-metal stents.[6] Although there is no randomized comparison between bare-metal and drug-eluting stents, small series suggest lower restenosis rates with drug-eluting stents.[6,7]

KEY CONCEPTS

1. Cardiac allograft vasculopathy is an atherosclerotic disease affecting the coronary arteries of the transplanted heart and is evident by angiography in 50% of patients after 10 years.
2. Retransplantation is the only definitive treatment.
3. Percutaneous revascularization is safe and feasible but is associated with high restenosis rates; also, it is not known if revascularization extends the life of the allograft.
4. Nonrandomized trials suggest that drug-eluting stents offer a lower risk of restenosis than bare-metal stents.

Selected References

1. Schmauss D, Weis M: Cardiac allograft vasculopathy. Recent developments, Circulation 117:2131–2141, 2008.
2. Tuzcu EM, DeFranco AC, Goormastic M, et al: Dichotomous pattern of coronary atherosclerosis 1 to 9 years after transplantation: insights from systematic intravascular ultrasound imaging, J Am Coll Cardiol 27:839–846, 1996.
3. Mehra MR: Contemporary concepts in prevention and treatment of cardiac allograft vasculopathy, Am J Transplant 6:1248–1256, 2006.
4. Gao SZ, Alderman EL, Schroeder JS, Silverman JF, Hunt SA: Accelerated coronary vascular disease in the heart transplant patient: coronary arteriographic findings, J Am Coll Cardiol 12:334–340, 1988.
5. Wenke K, Meiser B, Thiery J, et al: Simvastatin initiated early after heart transplantation: 8-year prospective experience, Circulation 107:93–97, 2003.
6. Tanaka K, Li H, Curran PJ, Takano Y, Arbit B, Currier JW, Yeatman LA, Kobashigawa JA, Tobis JM: Usefulness and safety of percutaneous coronary interventions for cardiac transplant vasculopathy, Am J Cardiol 97:1192–1197, 2006.
7. Lee MS, Kobashigawa J, Tobis J: Comparison of percutaneous coronary intervention with bare-metal and drug-eluting stents for cardiac allograft vasculopathy, J Am Coll Cardiol Intv 1:710–715, 2008.

SECTION TWO

Complications

Complications of percutaneous coronary intervention are a lot like motor vehicle accidents. While both can strike without warning or arise from an avoidable cause, most are, in fact, predictable. Just as most motor vehicle accidents are caused by speed, inattention, and conditions of the car, road, weather, and driver, most complications of percutaneous coronary intervention are due to procedural haste, inattention to detail, and conditions of the patient, artery, and operator. However, even if the most highly skilled operator meticulously selects and prepares patients for an intervention, complications will inevitably arise. Thus, it is imperative for all interventional cardiologists to obtain knowledge of the incidence, risk factors, recognition, and management of the commonly observed complications associated with percutaneous cardiovascular procedures.

Coronary interventional procedures are subject to all of the complications associated with diagnostic catheterization and angiography (Table II-1). In addition, there are multiple complications unique to coronary intervention (Table II-2). The incidence of these complications depends on the definition used to characterize the complication. For example, periprocedural acute myocardial infarction (MI) may be defined as the development of a new Q wave postprocedure, as a rise in CK-MB three times baseline, or as any rise in troponin I. Thus,

TABLE II-1 Selected Complications Associated with Diagnostic Catheterization and Angiography

Common Complications (1-5%)

Renal failure

Heart failure

Oversedation

Hypotension

Transient arrhythmia

Contrast reaction (hives)

Vascular complications

  Access site bleeding/hematoma

  Femoral pseudoaneurysm

  Arteriovenous fistula

  Retroperitoneal bleed

  Arterial dissection/thrombosis/occlusion

Rare Complications (<1%)

Catheter-induced vessel injury or perforation

Cerebrovascular accident

Contrast reaction (anaphylaxis)

Cholesterol embolization

Myocardial infarction

Death

Catheter entrapment

TABLE II-2 Selected Complications Unique to Percutaneous Coronary Interventions

Coronary dissection

Abrupt vessel closure

Emergency CABG

Periprocedural MI

  No-reflow phenomenon

  Side-branch occlusion

  Coronary thrombus

  Distal embolization

Perforation and tamponade

Coronary vasospasm

Complications related to adjunctive pharmacology

  Increased bleeding from antiplatelet and antithrombin use

  Thrombocytopenia from glycoprotein IIb/IIIa inhibitors

Miscellaneous

  Stent or other equipment embolization

depending on the definition, the rate of periprocedural MI will vary from less than 1% to more than 20%. The National Cardiovascular Data Registry established by the American College of Cardiology (ACC-NCDR) created standard definitions of common complications, allowing individual laboratories and operators to compare their own complication rates to other institutions and national benchmarks. Although this registry data is limited by self-reporting and there is no auditing of data quality, at the least it allows an individual institution to track its own complication rates in a consistent manner and foster practice improvement.

Bleeding and vascular problems continue to represent one of the most commonly observed complications associated with percutaneous coronary intervention. Bleeding is increased mainly from adjunctive use of potent antiplatelet and antithrombin agents, necessary to reduce ischemic complications from coronary intervention. Recently, periprocedural bleeding has been identified as an important independent predictor of increased mortality following intervention, and thus, efforts to reduce bleeding may improve patient outcomes.[1,2]

Coronary dissection is perhaps the most commonly observed complication unique to percutaneous coronary intervention. Importantly, it is often the underlying cause for other serious complications such as abrupt vessel closure, perforation and tamponade, need for emergency bypass surgery, and periprocedural MI. Coronary dissections are created during intervention by several mechanisms. The guide catheter may result in arterial injury if the catheter is engaged improperly or is not coaxial to the origin. Large-bore guides, aggressive curves, or deep engagement within the artery to achieve better backup for device delivery may also cause dissection. Guidewire dissections are caused when the wire is inadvertently positioned in a subintimal position or when stiff-tipped or hydrophilic-tipped guidewires are used to cross highly stenosed or totally occluded arteries. Finally, dissections may be balloon, stent, or device-related and caused by excessive barotrauma or oversized balloons. During the balloon era, coronary dissections were classified based on their likelihood of progressing to abrupt closure and need for emergency bypass (Table II-3).[3] While stents have greatly reduced the adverse sequelae of a coronary dissection, there remain situations where a stent cannot be deployed or a dissection goes unrecognized, and thus these unfavorable consequences remain tangible risks of a coronary intervention.

In the balloon era, dissection and abrupt vessel closure led to an emergent bypass operation in 2% to 3% of cases.[4,5] Coronary stents and optimization of adjunctive pharmacology reduced this to much less than 0.5% in the current era.[6] Presently, the most common indications for emergency CABG include extensive dissection (54%), perforation or tamponade (20%), recurrent acute closure (20%), hemodynamic instability (3%), aortic dissection (2%), and guidewire fracture (1%).[6]

The very low rate of emergency bypass surgery today has led many to question the recommendation that percutaneous coronary intervention only be performed at institutions with the capacity to perform open heart surgery. Although the rate of this complication is very low, it is often entirely unpredictable[4] and, when emergency surgery is needed, the delay required to transfer a patient to an institution with this capacity may lead to disastrous consequences. In fact, centers without on-site surgical backup may be unable to stabilize a severely hemodynamically compromised patient, thereby not allowing transfer and offering the patient no chance at survival. It has been estimated that 1 in 4 patients referred for emergency CABG would be placed at increased risk by a change in this practice.[7]

RISK FACTORS FOR DEVELOPING COMPLICATIONS FROM PERCUTANEOUS CORONARY INTERVENTION

There are important clinical, procedural, and anatomic variables associated with PCI-related complications. The clinical variables include patient instability at the time of the procedure (for example, acute infarction, cardiogenic shock, Class IV heart failure), reduced left ventricular function, advanced age, presence of renal failure, and female gender. Patients undergoing emergency procedures are at a higher risk than stable patients undergoing elective procedures. Certain procedural variables are associated with a higher risk. For example, the atheroablative techniques such as rotational and directional atherectomy have a higher risk of perforation, periprocedural MI, and dissection than balloon or stenting procedures. Finally, several important anatomic variables are associated with increased risk of PCI. These include degenerated saphenous vein graft lesions, bifurcation stenoses, presence of visible thrombus, chronic total occlusions, presence of diffuse disease, heavy coronary calcification, lesion eccentricity, vessel tortuosity, and small caliber arteries.

The cases presented in this section were chosen to provide the reader an overview of the full spectrum of complications seen in the modern era of coronary intervention, including several uncommon complications. It is important to recognize that the author has made no attempt at providing the "best" method of managing each case. The clinical decisions presented for each case reflects one operator's approach; other methods may have been equally or even more efficacious at managing these complications.

Selected References

1. Ndrepepa G, Berger PB, Mehilli J, Seyfarth M, Neumann FJ, Schomig A, Kastrati A: Periprocedural bleeding and 1-year outcome after percutaneous coronary interventions. Appropriateness of including bleeding as a component of a quadruple endpoint, J Am Coll Cardiol 51:690–697, 2008.
2. Doyle BJ, Rihal CS, Gastineau DA, Holmes DR: Bleeding, blood transfusion, and increased mortality after percutaneous coronary intervention. Implications for contemporary practice, J Am Coll Cardiol 53:2019–2027, 2009.
3. Huber MS, Mooney FJ, Madison J, Mooney MR: Use of a morphologic classification to predict clinical outcome after dissection from coronary angioplasty, Am J Cardiol 68:467–471, 1991.
4. Shubrooks SJ, Nesto RW, Leeman D, Waxman S, Lewis SM, Fitzpatrick P, Dib N: Urgent coronary bypass surgery for failed percutaneous coronary intervention in the stent era: Is backup still necessary? Am Heart J 142:190–196, 2001.
5. Detre K, Holubkov RS, Kelsey , Cowley M, Kent K, Williams D, Myler R, Faxon D, Holmes D, Bourassa M, et al: Percutaneous transluminal coronary angioplasty in 1985-1986 and 1977-1981. The National Heart, Lung, and Blood Institute Registry, N Engl J Med 318:265–270, 1988.
6. Seshadri N, Whitlow PL, Acharya N, Houghtaling P, Blackstone EH, Ellis SG: Emergency coronary artery bypass surgery in the contemporary percutaneous coronary intervention era, Circulation 106:2346–2350, 2002.
7. Lotfi M, Mackie K, Dzavik V, Seidelin PH: Impact of delays to cardiac surgery after failed angioplasty and stenting, J Am Coll Cardiol 43:337–342, 2004.

TABLE II-3 NHLBI Classification of Coronary Dissection

Type	Angiographic Description
A	Radiolucency within lumen during contrast injection with no or minimal persistent contrast staining
B	Parallel tracts or double lumen separated by radiolucency during injection with minimal or no persistent contrast staining
C	Contrast outside the lumen with persistent staining after clearance of dye injection
D	Spiral luminal filling defects with extensive contrast staining
E	Intraluminal filling defects with >50% luminal obstruction
F	Dissection with closure

Risk of Developing Serious Adverse Outcome[3]

Type	Emergency CABG	Abrupt Closure
B	0.7%	3.1%
C	9.7%	9.7%
D	66.7%	30.3%
E	27.8%	38.9%
F	62.9%	68.6%

Coronary Perforation

Michael Ragosta, MD, FACC, FSCAI

CASE PRESENTATION

An otherwise healthy and active 65-year-old man, with a past history notable for coronary artery bypass surgery 14 years earlier consisting of a right internal mammary artery graft to the right coronary artery, presents for cardiac catheterization. Five years earlier, he presented with an acute inferolateral wall myocardial infarction and underwent bare-metal stent placement to the first obtuse marginal artery and to his first diagonal artery; a long occluded segment of the distal circumflex artery was noted and deemed not treatable percutaneously. He remained free of cardiac symptoms until 3 months prior to his presentation, when he developed effort angina. Anginal symptoms progressed and began limiting his ability to work in his yard or to engage in hunting and fishing. Medical therapy, consisting of metoprolol, long-acting nitrates, aspirin, clopidogrel, and simvastatin, failed to improve his symptoms and he was referred for cardiac catheterization. Physical examination and routine laboratory evaluations were unremarkable. His baseline electrocardiogram revealed a prior inferolateral infarction and an incomplete right bundle branch block.

CARDIAC CATHETERIZATION

Left ventricular systolic function was preserved, with an estimated ejection fraction of 60% and only mild inferior wall hypokinesis. A widely patent right internal mammary artery graft provided an excellent distal blood supply to a severely diseased right coronary artery (Figure 16-1). Stents placed in the diagonal and obtuse marginal arteries were widely patent and the previously-noted long occluded segment of the distal circumflex remained unchanged (Figure 16-2). A long, tubular stenosis of moderate severity was apparent in the midportion of the left anterior descending artery (Figure 16-3 and Videos 16-1, 16-2). Given the uncertainty of the stenosis severity, the operator measured fractional flow reserve using a pressure wire and intracoronary adenosine to achieve maximal hyperemia. With classic anginal symptoms despite maximal medical therapy and a fractional flow reserve measuring 0.78, the physician decided to revascularize the left anterior descending artery percutaneously. Following administration of intravenous heparin and eptifibatide, the operator directly stented the diseased segment using a 6 French left coronary

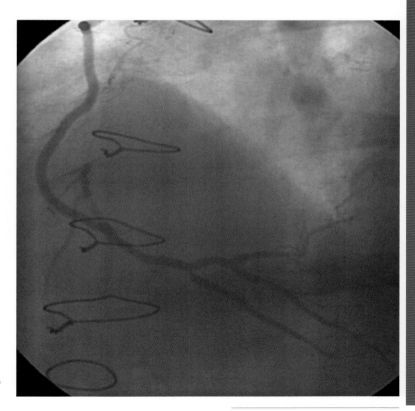

FIGURE 16-1. Patent right internal mammary artery graft to the severely diseased right coronary artery.

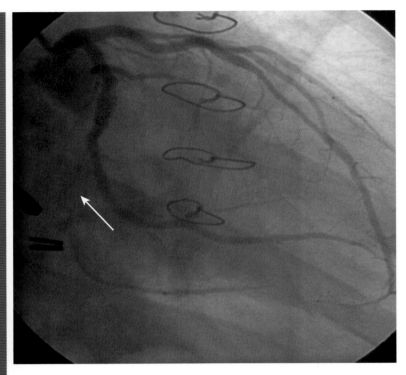

FIGURE 16-2. A large first obtuse marginal artery is free of disease; there is occlusion of a long segment of the distal circumflex artery (*arrow*).

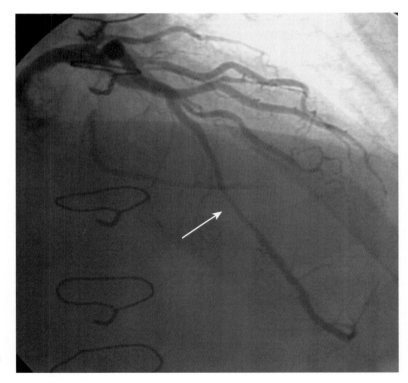

FIGURE 16-3. Long, tubular stenosis in the midportion of the left anterior descending artery (*arrow*).

guide catheter with a 3.0 mm diameter by 32 mm long sirolimus-eluting stent inflated to 12 atmospheres (Figure 16-4).

Immediately following stent deployment, the angiogram demonstrated free extravasation of contrast emanating from the midportion of the stented segment consistent with a coronary artery perforation (Figure 16-5 and Video 16-3). The patient reported substernal chest

and left shoulder pain; ST-segment elevation was apparent on the monitored leads. Central aortic pressure fell to a systolic pressure of 70 mmHg and the heart rate increased to 110 beats per minute. A 3.0 mm diameter by 20 mm long compliant balloon was immediately advanced over the 0.014 inch guidewire and inflated at the site of contrast extravasation (Figure 16-6). This maneuver, along with simultaneous infusion of saline

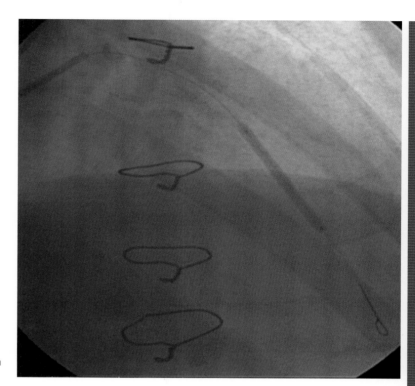

FIGURE 16-4. Position of the stent at the site of the lesion in the left anterior descending artery.

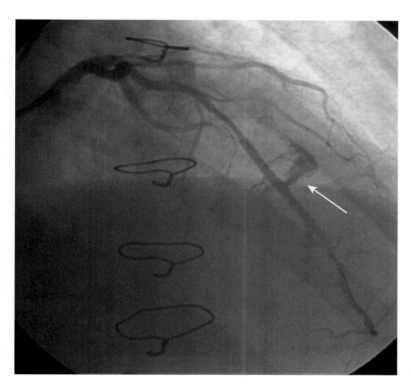

FIGURE 16-5. Free extravasation of contrast (*arrow*) is noted from the midportion of the stent, consistent with perforation of the coronary artery.

and initiation of intravenous dopamine, led to immediate stabilization of blood pressure.

At this point, the operator stopped the eptifibatide infusion and performed an emergent echocardiogram. This revealed a small, loculated effusion over the anterior wall. The patient remained hemodynamically stable with the balloon inflated for 10 minutes. Repeat

angiography following this prolonged balloon inflation showed continued, free-flowing contrast extravasation (Video 16-4), and the balloon was reinflated at the site.

Working quickly, the operator deflated the balloon, removed the guidewire, and replaced the 6 French sheath and guide catheter with an 8 French system. After repositioning an exchange-length, 0.014 inch

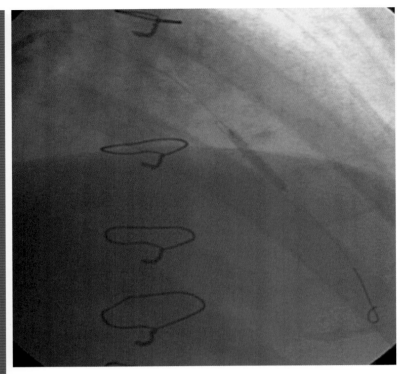

FIGURE 16-6. Balloon inflated at the site of the perforation temporarily halted further hemorrhage into the pericardial space.

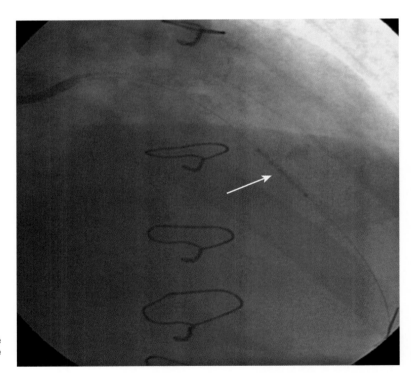

FIGURE 16-7. Position of the PFTE-covered stent at the site of the perforation. Note the contrast staining at the site of the perforation (arrow).

guidewire in the left anterior descending artery, the physician centered a 3.0 mm diameter by 19 mm long polytetrafluoroethylene-covered (PTFE) stent (Jostent Graftmaster) centered on the site of contrast extravasation (Figure 16-7), successfully sealing the perforation (Video 16-5). The dopamine infusion was stopped with no further hypotension and he was observed in the cardiac catheterization laboratory for an additional 15 minutes; a final angiogram revealed no further evidence of contrast extravasation.

POSTPROCEDURAL COURSE

Following the procedure, the patient was admitted to the coronary care unit for observation. He remained hemodynamically stable, but noted pleuritic chest and shoulder pain for 24 hours following the procedure that responded to nonsteroidal antiinflammatory agents. Echocardiography performed the day after the procedure showed a small effusion. The postprocedure troponin level peaked at 34 ng/mL. He was discharged the second day postprocedure and returned for follow-up 2 months later feeling well and without angina.

DISCUSSION

Coronary artery perforation complicates less than 0.5% of coronary interventions[1] but is potentially lethal, particularly in the event of free extravasation into the pericardial space as exemplified in this case. More commonly seen with ablative techniques such as rotational or directional atherectomy, coronary perforation may be caused by vessel disruption from barotrauma (the likely cause in this case) or from deep dissection extending through the adventitia. Guidewire perforations may occur at the site of the lesion during attempts at crossing a stenosis or may occur distally from migration of the wire tip into a small vessel, with subsequent perforation.

Freely extravasating contrast, as seen in this case, is a true emergency. Once identified, the operator must work rapidly to control the hemorrhage into the pericardial space. Immediate balloon expansion proximal to or directly at the perforation site effectively halts the hemorrhage, allowing time to plan subsequent management. At this point, anticoagulation should be stopped or reversed. Platelet transfusion is necessary if abciximab was used and protamine administration may be considered if unfractionated heparin was given and the activated clotting time is excessive. Pericardiocentesis should be performed if there is ongoing hemodynamic instability despite fluid and pressor support. While all this activity is taking place, it is a good idea to notify a cardiothoracic surgeon; this will limit delays if attempts to seal the perforation fail and the patient requires emergency surgery. In the case presented here, the history of prior bypass surgery may have helped maintain stability by limiting the extent of tamponade due to the presence of pericardial adhesions.

Small perforations may seal with reversal of anticoagulation and prolonged balloon inflation at the perforation site. Large, free-flowing rents in the artery, like the one shown in this case, usually require sealing with a PTFE-covered stent.[2,3] These devices consist of a thin layer of PTFE sandwiched between two stents. They are fairly bulky and may be difficult to position and are not available in sizes smaller than 2.5 mm diameter. Importantly, they require large-bore guides, usually necessitating a change in the sheath and guide during an emergency. If the patient cannot tolerate release of the inflated balloon used to temporarily staunch the bleeding, then access should be obtained in the contralateral femoral artery and the appropriately sized sheath and guide catheter placed while the balloon remains inflated.

Major perforations are fairly morbid events with a high rate of periprocedural infarction of about 10% to 15% of patients. Infarction is often caused by the prolonged balloon inflation needed to stabilize a patient, but may also be due to the presence of external compression by a subepicardial hematoma. Death occurs in about 10% to 15% of major perforations, and about 10% require surgery to repair them. Pericarditis, arrhythmia, and need for blood transfusion are additional consequences. The PFTE-covered stents have a high restenosis rate, particularly at the edges.

KEY CONCEPTS

In the event of an obvious coronary perforation:
1. Initial efforts should concentrate on maintaining patient stability. This includes fluid resuscitation and initiation of pressor agents, insertion of a balloon either proximal to the perforation or at the perforation site to stop bleeding, and pericardiocentesis if there is continued instability.
2. Reverse anticoagulation.
3. Promptly notify a cardiothoracic surgeon early in the course of events, so as to be ready in the event that attempts to seal the perforation are unsuccessful and there is continued hemodynamic instability requiring emergency surgery.
4. If there is free extravasation of contrast, a PTFE-covered stent should be placed at the perforation site.
5. Ongoing bleeding despite reversal of anticoagulation and attempts to seal the perforation require emergency surgery.

Selected References

1. Fasseas P, Orford JL, Panetta CJ, et al: Incidence, correlates, management and clinical outcome of coronary perforation: analysis of 16,298 procedures, *Am Heart J* 147:140–145, 2004.
2. Briguori C, Nishida T, Anzuini A, DiMario C, Grube E, Colombo A: Emergency polytetrafluoroethylene-covered stent implantation to treat coronary ruptures, *Circulation* 102:3028–3031, 2000.
3. Lansky AJ, Yank Y, Khan Y, Costa RA, Pietras C, Tsuchiya Y, Cristea E, Collins M, Mehran R, Dangas GD, Moses JW, Leon MB, Stone GW: Treatment of coronary artery perforations complicating percutaneous coronary intervention with a polytetrafluoroethylene-covered stent graft, *Am J Cardiol* 98:370–374, 2006.

Extensive Coronary Dissection

Michael Ragosta, MD, FACC, FSCAI

CASE PRESENTATION

A 61-year-old woman with hypertension, diabetes mellitus, hyperlipidemia, and a strong family history of premature coronary disease presents with a 2-month history of exertional angina. The presence of an abnormal noninvasive test with an inferolateral stress-induced perfusion defect, along with continued symptoms despite medical therapy, prompted referral for cardiac catheterization. Medications included 325 mg of aspirin, high-dose niacin, omega-3 fatty acid, metoprolol, and sublingual nitrates as needed for angina. Her physical examination, 12-lead electrocardiogram, and routine preprocedural laboratory evaluations were unrevealing.

CARDIAC CATHETERIZATION

Cardiac catheterization revealed preserved left ventricular systolic function and multivessel coronary disease, with severe discrete stenoses of the proximal right coronary artery and left anterior descending artery and an angiographically normal circumflex artery (Figures 17-1, 17-2 and Videos 17-1, 17-2). The attending physician discussed revascularization options, and the patient chose percutaneous coronary intervention of both the right coronary and left anterior descending coronary arteries with drug-eluting stents instead of bypass surgery. She returned to the cardiac catheterization laboratory the next morning following a dose of 300 mg of clopidogrel taken the night before. The operator began with the left anterior descending artery. This was successfully treated with a 2.5 mm diameter by 18 mm long, drug-eluting stent (zotarolimus), with an excellent angiographic result (Figure 17-3). The operator engaged a 6 French right Judkins 4.0 guide catheter in the right coronary artery and easily crossed the stenosis with a floppy-tipped guidewire and predilated the lesion to 10 atmospheres with a 2.5 mm diameter by 15 mm long compliant balloon. The operator then attempted, but failed to pass, a 2.5 mm diameter by 24 mm long drug-eluting stent (zotarolimus) across the lesion. The stent met significant resistance at the site of a bend in the proximal right coronary artery (see Figure 17-1, arrow), and the attempt caused the guide to inadvertently disengage, resulting in loss of guidewire access to the distal right coronary artery. Angiography following reengagement of the guide catheter showed no obvious dissection but a persistent residual stenosis at the site of the balloon-dilated lesion (Video 17-3).

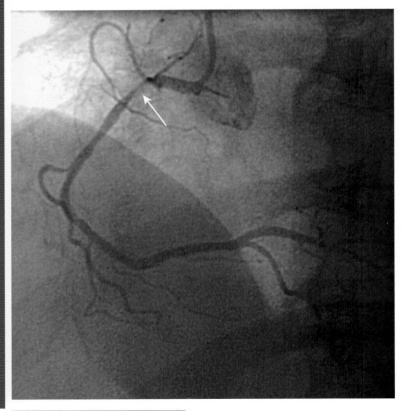

FIGURE 17-1. This is a left anterior oblique projection of the right coronary artery demonstrating a severe stenosis in the proximal segment (*arrow*).

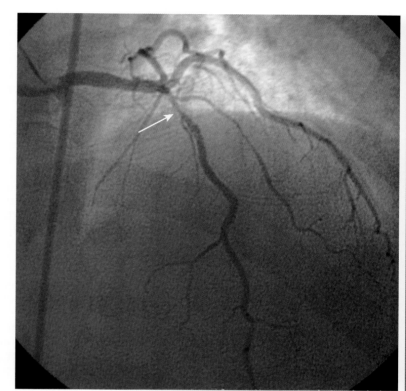

FIGURE 17-2. This angiogram of the left coronary artery in a right anterior oblique projection with cranial angulation reveals a severe stenosis of the proximal segment of the left anterior descending coronary artery (*arrow*) at the bifurcation of a small caliber diagonal artery.

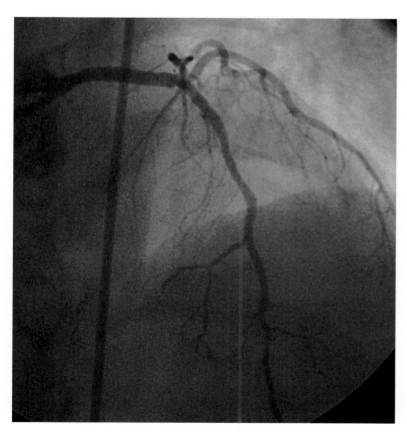

FIGURE 17-3. Following stenting of the left anterior descending artery, an excellent angiographic result was noted; the small diagonal branch occluded after stenting.

At this point, the operator chose an extra-support guidewire to facilitate stent placement (Mailman, Boston Scientific). Although the wire advanced with ease to a distal location in the posterolateral branch of the artery, the patient soon complained of severe chest pain associated with ST-segment elevation on the monitored leads. Fearing abrupt vessel closure, the operator repeated right coronary angiography, and noted an extensive spiral dissection along the entire course of the right coronary artery with closure of the posterolateral branch (Figure 17-4 and Video 17-4). The operator removed the extra-support wire, replacing it with a floppy wire, and successfully positioned this wire in the posterior descending artery (Video 17-5). Unable to pass short bare-metal stents beyond the proximal lesion, the operator consulted surgery for consideration of emergency bypass surgery.

POSTPROCEDURAL COURSE

An intraaortic balloon pump was placed and, although the patient remained hemodynamically stable, chest pain and ST-segment elevation continued and she was emergently transferred from the cardiac catheterization laboratory to the operating room, where she underwent a single-vessel bypass consisting of an off-pump, saphenous vein graft to the posterior descending artery. Her postoperative course was uneventful and she was discharged 7 days later. She remained free of angina at 6-month follow-up.

DISCUSSION

Well known to experienced interventional cardiologists, this case exemplifies the fact that a case cannot be declared "easy" until it is successfully completed. The operator's difficulty in passing the stent and the subsequent development of an extensive dissection could not be anticipated by the deceptively straightforward angiographic appearance of the right coronary artery.

Coronary dissection represents a unique complication of percutaneous coronary intervention and, if untreated, can lead to serious sequelae including abrupt vessel closure, periprocedural myocardial infarction, closure of major side branches, vessel perforation, and tamponade. Coronary stents successfully treat most dissections so that, in the current era, the risk of sustained vessel closure or the need for emergency bypass surgery due to a dissection is very rare.

Arterial injury and dissection can be induced by any of the components of the procedure; including insertion of the guide catheter, use of the device to treat the lesion, and placement of the guidewire. Guide-related dissections are often related to the use of large-bore (i.e., 8 French) or aggressive guides (such as an Amplatz curve) in order to provide extra backup. Similarly, dissection may arise when the operator requires additional support and deeply inserts the guide into the artery. Attempts to deeply engage the artery when the guide is not coaxial to the vessel is particularly likely to cause this complication. Coronary dissection may be due to the balloon, stent, or device used to treat a coronary stenosis. Oversizing the balloon or stent, application of high inflation pressure (particularly when a compliant balloon is used), and the use of atherectomy devices are commonly associated with dissection. This is particularly true when certain lesion characteristics are present, including heavy calcification, lesion eccentricity, and severe angulation.

Coronary dissection may be caused by the 0.014 inch guidewire used to direct the balloon and stent catheters;

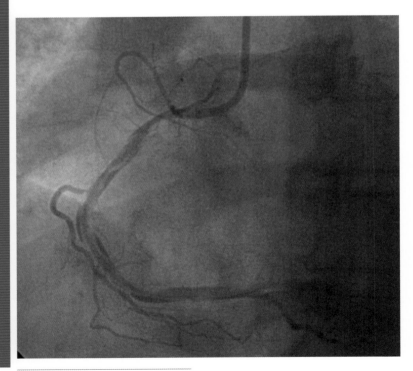

FIGURE 17-4. The extensive spiral dissection of the right coronary artery is shown on this left anterior oblique projection.

this was the likely mechanism involved in the present case. Any guidewire, but particularly the polymer-tipped and stiff-tipped guidewires employed to cross highly stenosed or occluded arteries, may burrow beneath the plaque and intima, dissecting the artery. In the present case, the initially placed guidewire fell out of the artery when the guide catheter became disengaged and the operator recrossed the freshly ballooned segment with another (and stiffer) guidewire. It is likely that balloon angioplasty created a small, undetected dissection and the wire tip entered the subintimal space via a false lumen within the ballooned segment. Unaware of the malposition of the wire tip, the operator advanced the wire, thus extending the false lumen and propagating the dissection along the entire length of the artery. The stiff shaft of the extra-support wire likely exacerbated this process.

Focal dissections respond well to stenting. It is important to identify the extent of the dissection and to cover both ends of the dissection with a stent. In this case, dissection affected nearly the entire artery; in addition, the initially-encountered difficulty in advancing a stent across the lesion would not allow a stenting option.

In the present era, the need to perform emergency coronary bypass surgery to treat a complication from percutaneous coronary intervention has become very rare.[1] Currently, most emergency bypass operations occur when a dissection in a major artery cannot be stented or when a coronary perforation cannot be controlled by percutaneous means. Unfortunately, emergency bypass surgery in the setting of a failed percutaneous coronary intervention is associated with a high rate of in-hospital death, myocardial infarction, and stroke. Thus, in the event of a large, untreatable dissection, the risk-benefit ratio of surgery must be carefully weighed against the risk of leaving the artery closed

and treating the resulting infarction medically. In the present case, the involved physicians and surgeons struggled with the decision to salvage the artery with emergency coronary bypass surgery. Although her continued chest pain and ST-segment elevation suggested the need for surgical treatment, the procedure likely offered only a modest benefit given the size of the right coronary artery. The decision to operate is easier when the affected artery supplies a larger vascular territory. In addition, the involved physicians feared stent thrombosis in the freshly placed stent in the left anterior descending artery induced by the stress of surgery.

KEY CONCEPTS

1. Coronary dissections may complicate percutaneous coronary interventions and can be caused by guide catheters, guidewires, and the devices used to treat coronary stenoses.
2. Extensive coronary dissection may not be treatable with stents. If left untreated, they are associated with increased risk of myocardial infarction, side-branch closure, perforation and tamponade, and periprocedural mortality.
3. Inability to stent an extensive dissection in a major artery remains one of the ongoing indications for emergency bypass surgery.

Selected References

1. Seshadri N, Whitlow PL, Acharya N, Houghtaling P, Blackstone EH, Ellis SG: Emergency coronary artery bypass surgery in the contemporary percutaneous coronary intervention era, *Circulation* 106:2346–2350, 2002.

Unsuccessful Coronary Intervention

Michael Ragosta, MD, FACC, FSCAI

CASE PRESENTATION

A 77-year-old woman presented to the hospital emergency department with chest pain at rest. Fourteen years earlier, she underwent coronary bypass surgery consisting of a left internal mammary graft to the left anterior descending artery and saphenous vein grafts to both the right coronary artery and the first obtuse marginal artery. She did well until 1 year earlier when she developed substernal chest pain occurring with exertion and relieved by rest. This symptom progressed and led to diminished exercise tolerance. Her physician evaluated her progressive anginal symptoms by pharmacologic stress perfusion scintigraphy, which confirmed ischemia in the inferior and lateral walls. Based on these results, her physician scheduled her for an outpatient elective cardiac catheterization. However, several prolonged episodes of rest chest pain resolving only after nitroglycerin prompted this hospital visit.

Upon arrival, her chest pain had already resolved and she did not report any other symptoms. In addition to the prior coronary bypass surgery, review of her past medical history was notable for the presence of a left bundle branch block on electrocardiogram, Factor V Leiden with several occurrences of deep vein thrombosis, hypercholesterolemia, and prior tobacco abuse. Home medications included warfarin, atenolol, aspirin, and fluvastatin. Physical examination found no abnormalities. Routine laboratory evaluation confirmed normal renal function, a hematocrit of 43%, and an International Normalized Ratio (INR) of 2.4. Initial troponin I was 0.02 ng/mL, subsequently increasing to 0.21 ng/mL. She was admitted to a telemetry unit and treated with unfractionated heparin in addition to aspirin, beta blockers, and nitrates; warfarin was held to allow the INR to return to baseline, at which point she underwent cardiac catheterization.

CARDIAC CATHETERIZATION

The diagnostic angiograms demonstrated occlusion of the native right coronary and left anterior descending coronary artery with occlusion of both saphenous vein grafts. A widely patent left internal mammary graft supplied a large left anterior descending artery. Severe disease of the proximal segment of a large first obtuse marginal artery as well as severe disease of a smaller-caliber second obtuse marginal artery likely accounted for her clinical presentation (Figures 18-1, 18-2 and Video 18-1). Based on these angiograms, stress test results, and her symptoms of progressive angina, her physician decided to revascularize the first obtuse marginal artery percutaneously.

After selective engagement of the left coronary ostium with a 6 French JCL 4.5 guide catheter, and following administration of an intravenous bolus followed by an infusion of bivalirudin, a floppy-tipped 0.014 inch guidewire was advanced to the lesion. The wire tip successfully crossed the two lesions but was unable to advance around the sharply angulated segment, due to tethering of the vessel from the previously placed saphenous vein graft (Figure 18-3). Despite prolonged attempts and the incorporation of various curves applied to the wire tip, followed by the use of a hydrophilic-tipped guidewire (Boston Scientific, PT2), the operator failed to successfully gain access to the distal part of the artery. Additional manipulations ultimately closed the artery (Figure 18-3 and Videos 18-2, 18-3) and the patient experienced chest discomfort but remained hemodynamically stable. Fortunately, removal of the guidewire and administration of intracoronary nitroglycerin led to restoration of vessel patency (Video 18-4); there also appeared to be small dissection flaps within the diseased segment caused by the attempts. The operator abandoned further attempts at percutaneous revascularization and the patient left the cardiac catheterization laboratory with no electrocardiographic changes and noting only minimal chest discomfort.

POSTPROCEDURAL COURSE

The patient was admitted to the coronary care unit for further observation. She remained free of chest pain. Serial troponin I assays demonstrated a further rise in troponin, peaking at 11.30 ng/mL the following morning. Since percutaneous attempts failed and the risk-benefit ratio of repeat coronary bypass surgery appeared prohibitive, she was treated medically with the addition of long-acting nitroglycerin and clopidogrel along with an increase in her beta-blocker dose. She remained symptom-free and was discharged 48 hours later. She remained free of limiting symptoms at a follow-up visit 6 months postprocedure.

DISCUSSION

In the current era, the success rate of percutaneous coronary interventions exceeds 90%, a testimony to the remarkable advances in pharmacology, equipment, and techniques over the past several decades. Several terms are used to define success: 1) angiographic success, 2) procedural success, and 3) clinical success. Angiographic

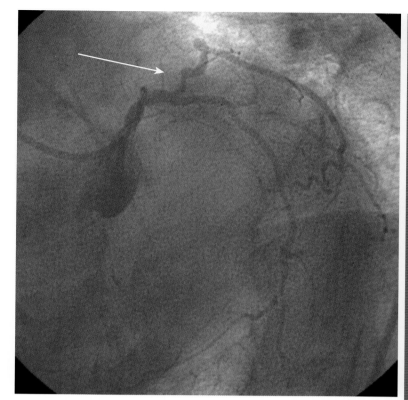

FIGURE 18-1. This is a left anterior oblique projection with caudal angulation of the left coronary artery demonstrating a severe stenosis in the proximal segment of the first obtuse marginal artery (*arrow*). There is also occlusion of the left anterior descending artery.

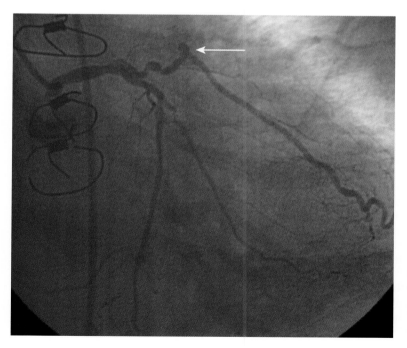

FIGURE 18-2. This angiogram of the left coronary artery in a right anterior oblique projection with caudal angulation reveals two severe stenoses of the proximal segment of the first obtuse marginal artery. There is tethering of the vessel due to the previously placed saphenous vein graft (*arrow*). The left anterior descending coronary artery is occluded and there is also severe stenosis of a small-caliber second obtuse marginal artery.

success indicates the presence of less than 20% residual stenosis at the treated lesion. Procedural success is defined as the presence of angiographic success along with the absence of a major complication (death, myocardial infarction, or need for emergency bypass surgery), and clinical success is present when there is procedural success plus improvement in symptoms. Current rates of angiographic and procedural success rates are very high, approaching 95% and 92% respectively.[1]

Failure to cross a lesion with a guidewire is one of the most frequent causes of an unsuccessful intervention; it is usually due to the presence of a chronic occlusion, where success rates, even in the best hands, rarely exceed 70%. The present case illustrates the point that failure to cross may also occur in the setting of a patent vessel when there is great complexity to the lesion. In the case described here, difficulty crossing was due to severe angulation from tethering of the vessel from a

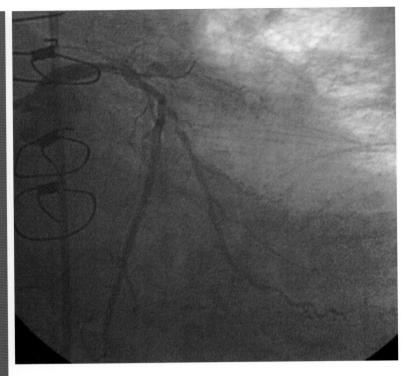

FIGURE 18-3. Attempts at crossing the lesion with a guidewire were unsuccessful, because of the presence of severe angulation due to the tethering of the vessel from the previously placed saphenous vein graft.

previously placed saphenous vein graft. Although the operator was able to cross the severe stenosis, the guidewire would not advance around the sharply angulated segment. In such cases, guidewire passage may be difficult or impossible because the wire becomes bound by the stenosis and the operator loses the ability to change the direction of the tip. Additional reasons contributing to an operator's failure to cross include the presence of marked lesion eccentricity, the presence of a side branch at the site of a severe stenosis, creation of a false lumen or achieving a subintimal position with the wire tip, and the presence of an unrecognized chronic occlusion.

In this case, the attempt to cross with a guidewire led to abrupt vessel closure and a periprocedural myocardial infarction; fortunately the artery reopened spontaneously, limiting the extent of myocardial damage. Guidewire-induced trauma is one cause of abrupt closure after a coronary intervention; additional mechanisms include elastic recoil, dissection, spasm, and thrombus. In the pre-stent era, abrupt vessel closure complicated 2% to 8% of coronary balloon angioplasties. The morbidity of these events was substantial; nearly one third of these required emergency bypass surgery, and there was a high rate of Q-wave myocardial infarction and death.[2] The advances in pharmacology preventing procedural thrombus and the routine use of coronary stents targeting recoil and dissection reduced the incidence of sustained abrupt vessel closure to less than 1% and the need for emergency bypass surgery to the current, nearly negligible levels.

Fortunately, this patient responded to medical therapy. Since failure to cross with a guidewire excludes percutaneous options, the only revascularization alternative is bypass surgery. In the event of a failed intervention, indications for emergent bypass surgery would include the presence of ongoing ischemic chest pain, hemodynamic instability, or the presence of a large vascular territory at risk from the closed or severely stenotic artery. In this case, based on the relatively small size of the vascular territory, and in the absence of chest pain or hemodynamic instability, her physicians did not feel that the potential benefits warranted the risk of a reoperation.

KEY CONCEPTS

1. Failure to cross a lesion with a guidewire remains one of the most common reasons for a failed percutaneous coronary intervention. In most cases, this is due to the presence of a chronic total occlusion, but complex lesion morphology or excessive angulation may also lead to unsuccessful wire crossing.
2. Unsuccessful attempts at crossing a lesion with a guidewire may lead to abrupt vessel closure and the potential for serious adverse events, including periprocedural myocardial infarction, need for emergency bypass surgery, and death.

Selected References

1. Anderson HV, Shaw RE, Brindis RG, Hewitt K, Krone RJ, Block PC, McKay CR, Weintraub WS: A contemporary overview of percutaneous coronary interventions. The American College of Cardiology-National Cardiovascular Data Registry (ACC-NCDR), *J Am Coll Cardiol* 39:1096–1103, 2002.
2. Klein LW: Coronary complications of percutaneous coronary intervention: A practical approach to the management of abrupt vessel closure, *Catheter Cardiovasc Interv* 64:395–401, 2005.

Coronary Dissection Involving the Aortic Root

Michael Ragosta, MD, FACC, FSCAI

CASE PRESENTATION

A 63-year-old woman with hypertension, tobacco abuse, and dyslipidemia, but no prior coronary events, developed stable angina pectoris. Her physician evaluated these symptoms with an exercise stress test. During the stress test, chest discomfort began at a low workload and the scintigraphic images revealed reversible perfusion defects in multiple zones, including the inferior and anterior walls and the apex. She was referred for an elective cardiac catheterization.

CARDIAC CATHETERIZATION

Diagnostic catheterization found normal left ventricular function and significant stenoses in the proximal segment of the right coronary artery (Figure 19-1 and Video 19-1) and in the left anterior descending artery (Figures 19-2, 19-3 and Video 19-2). The left circumflex artery appeared angiographically normal. Coronary calcification was noted in both the right coronary and left anterior descending arteries. After discussing the options of medical therapy, coronary bypass surgery, and percutaneous coronary intervention, the patient chose a percutaneous revascularization strategy.

After administration of a bolus of 70 U/kg of unfractionated heparin followed by a double bolus and infusion of eptifibatide, the operator first approached the left anterior descending artery. The lesion was first dilated with a balloon and then treated with a sirolimus-eluting stent (Figure 19-4). The operator then turned attention to the right coronary artery. Anticipating the need for extra backup to support the intervention, due to the presence of coronary calcification noted on the diagnostic study, the operator chose a left Amplatz guide catheter (AL-2), as shown in Video 19-1. Although this guide catheter appeared to provide excellent support, pressure damping and retention of contrast in the arterial wall was observed in the proximal segment consistent with a guide-related dissection, leading to the exchange of the Amplatz guide for a right Judkins guide catheter. Upon engagement, the physician noted distal extension of the dissection, with retention of contrast nearly to the

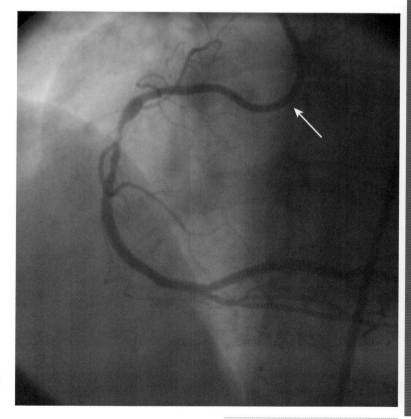

FIGURE 19-1. This is a left anterior oblique projection of the right coronary artery demonstrating the severe stenosis in the proximal segment. An Amplatz guide catheter was used to acquire this image (*arrow*).

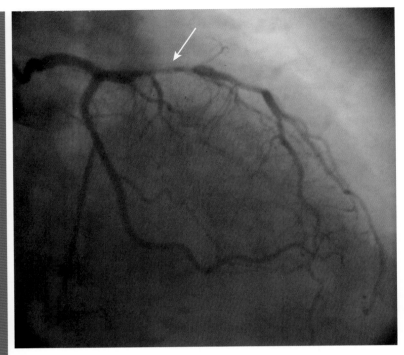

FIGURE 19-2. This angiogram of the left coronary artery in a right anterior oblique projection with caudal angulation depicts the severe stenosis of the left anterior descending coronary artery after a first septal perforator (*arrow*). The circumflex is free of angiographic disease.

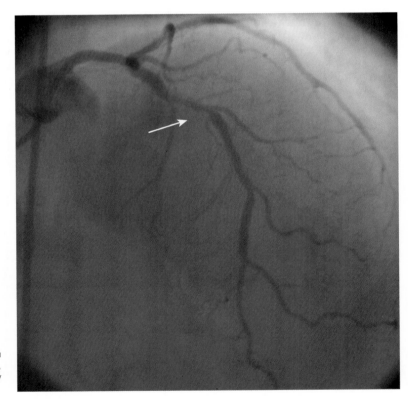

FIGURE 19-3. Angiography of the left coronary artery in the right anterior oblique projection with cranial angulation, demonstrating the lesion in the left anterior descending artery (arrow).

bifurcation of the posterior descending and posterolateral branches (Figure 19-5 and Video 19-3). The right coronary artery appeared to have reduced distal flow; ST-segment elevation was apparent on the monitored leads, and the patient reported severe substernal chest pain.

Fortunately, the 0.014 inch guidewire entered the true lumen distally and the physician was able to position a bare-metal stent, successfully sealing the distal extent of the dissection. Additional stents were placed in the midsection, successfully restoring flow to the distal right coronary artery and eliminating the patient's chest

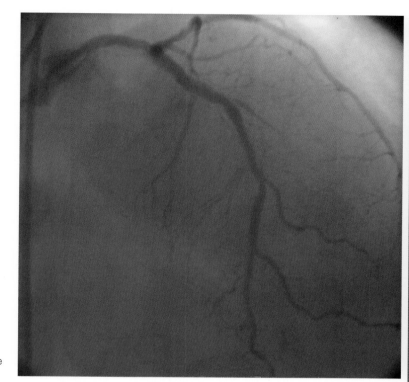

FIGURE 19-4. Angiogram obtained following stenting of the left anterior descending artery.

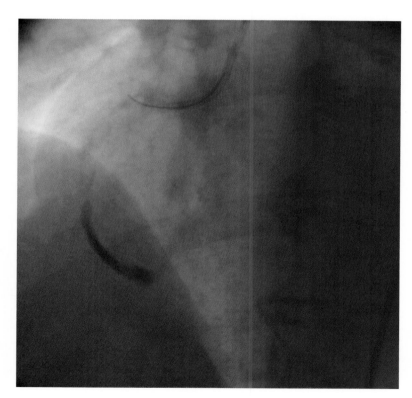

FIGURE 19-5. Retention of contrast is observed in the midportion of the right coronary artery. The previously placed Amplatz guide catheter created an extensive dissection of the proximal and midportion of this artery, leading to abrupt vessel closure. The extent of coronary calcification can be appreciated on this image.

discomfort and ST-segment changes. A substantial dissection remained in the proximal segment (Video 19-4). While deploying a stent in the proximal segment, the operator noted staining of the aortic cusp, suggesting that the dissection had propagated to the aorta (Figure 19-6). A final stent was placed to cover the ostium. The final angiographic result was excellent, but a large arc of contrast retention was noted in the aortic cusp (Figure 19-7 and Videos 19-5, 19-6). The patient remained asymptomatic except for mild residual chest discomfort, and suffered no hemodynamic consequences. Repeat angiography 15 minutes later showed patency of the artery but persistent contrast staining in the aorta (Figure 19-8).

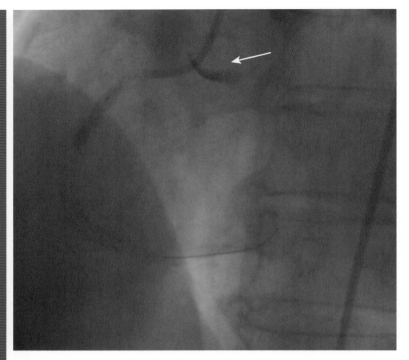

FIGURE 19-6. A guidewire was successfully positioned in the true lumen, and stenting of the dissection successfully restored patency of the vessel. However, contrast retention now appeared in the aortic cusp, suggesting extension of the dissection into the aorta (*arrow*).

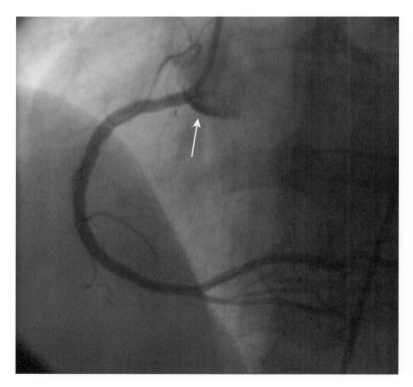

FIGURE 19-7. Final angiographic result obtained after stenting to the ostium of the right coronary artery. Retention of contrast within the aortic cusp remained present (*arrow*).

POSTPROCEDURAL COURSE

The patient was observed overnight in an intensive care unit. She remained free of symptoms and was discharged on the second day postprocedure. One week later, she was admitted with atypical chest pain occurring at rest that was judged by her physicians to be noncardiac in nature. This event was not associated with electrocardiographic changes or biomarker release; however, the uncertainty related to the natural history of her complex intervention the week before led to a repeat coronary angiogram. This showed wide patency of the stents in the left anterior descending and right coronary arteries. Upon injection of the right coronary artery, the previously observed retention of contrast in the aortic cusp was no longer apparent (Videos 19-7, 19-8).

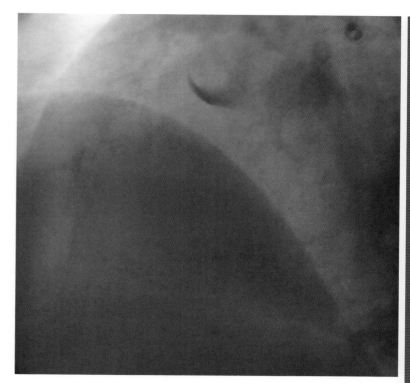

FIGURE 19-8. Persistent retention of contrast within the aorta.

DISCUSSION

Coronary artery dissection is one of the most commonly occurring complications of percutaneous coronary intervention. Most commonly caused by direct barotrauma from the balloon or stent, arterial dissection may also be created by the guidewire or from an injury created by a guide catheter. Most dissections are focal and limited to the site of the injury; rarely, they extend and propagate from the original site of injury, affecting much more of the artery. The term "spiral dissection" is often used to describe a dissection that spreads from the site of the original intimal tear and extends the length of the artery. Usually, dissections propagate in the direction of arterial blood flow. Thus, they typically extend distal to the site of the initial injury; it is very unusual for a dissection to propagate proximally.

In this case, the operator anticipated the need for greater backup and chose an aggressive guide catheter. While these guides help accomplish a difficult intervention, they may engage traumatically and disrupt the intimal lining. Amplatz guides, in particular, have a tendency to engage suddenly with a lunging motion and thus have a greater risk of a dissection. This is particularly true if there is proximal disease, as evidenced by the present case.

The development of an aortic dissection complicating a coronary dissection is very rare. A review of iatrogenic aortic dissection due to catheterization or coronary intervention found 9 cases out of 43,143 catheterizations (which included 20,475 coronary interventions) for an incidence of 0.02%.[1] In this largest series to date, the authors described three types of dissection. Type I involved only the aortic cusp, similar to the example shown in this case. Type II involved the aortic cusp and extended up the aorta less than 40 mm, and Type III extended up the aorta greater than 40 mm. Similar to the case described here, all 9 events reported in this series involved the right coronary artery; the authors also comment that, of the 17 previously reported cases in the literature, 15 involved arose from a dissection in the right coronary artery. Also of note, the authors found that 44% of cases involved the use of an Amplatz catheter. Outcomes were excellent for Type I and II dissections but were poor for Type III dissections. Thus, if the aorta is involved in a limited manner, then optimal management consists of stenting of the dissection at its entry. Extensive involvement of the aorta (greater than 40 mm up the aorta), may require surgical intervention.

KEY CONCEPTS

1. Guide dissections may arise from the use of an aggressive guide catheter, particularly if there is proximal disease.
2. Dissections most commonly extend distally. Rarely, a dissection involving the right coronary artery may propagate proximally and affect the aorta.
3. If an aortic dissection from a guide dissection occurs and is limited to the aortic cusp and less than 40 mm of the ascending aorta, outcomes are generally good with therapy directed at stenting the aorto-ostium. Surgery may be needed if more extensive involvement of the aorta is present.

Selected References

1. Dunning DW, Kahn JK, Hawkins ET, O'Neill WW: Iatrogenic coronary artery dissections extending into and involving the aortic root, *Catheter Cardiovasc Interv* 51:387–393, 2000.

No-Reflow After Coronary Intervention

Michael Ragosta, MD, FACC, FSCAI

CASE PRESENTATION

An active and healthy 66-year-old man with no prior cardiac history developed acute onset of midsternal chest pain radiating to his back and left shoulder, associated with nausea. He presented to the emergency department after experiencing symptoms for 45 minutes and rapidly became pain-free following administration of nitroglycerin. His medical history is notable for hypertension, dyslipidemia, a family history of premature coronary disease, and remote tobacco use. His medications on presentation included metoprolol, amlodipine, hydrochlorothiazide, and atorvastatin. Physical exam found no important abnormalities, and the initial electrocardiogram obtained without pain showed nonspecific ST-T wave changes. Serial troponins peaked at 1.7 ng/dL; the remaining routine laboratory studies were normal.

CARDIAC CATHETERIZATION

Diagnosed with a non-ST segment elevation acute myocardial infarction, he was admitted to a telemetry unit and treated with aspirin, enoxaparin, nitroglycerin, atorvastatin and metoprolol. He remained pain-free and underwent cardiac catheterization the following day. Left ventriculography was normal. Coronary angiography noted nonobstructive luminal irregularities in the right coronary and left circumflex arteries and severe narrowing in the proximal segment of the left anterior descending artery (Figure 20-1). Compared to the circumflex artery, angiographic flow appeared reduced at baseline (Video 20-1). After the intravenous administration of unfractionated heparin and eptifibatide, balloon angioplasty was performed using a 2.5 mm diameter by 20 mm long compliant balloon. Angiography performed after balloon dilatation showed complete occlusion of the left anterior descending artery at the site of the intervention (Video 20-2). The patient developed chest pressure but remained hemodynamically stable. An intracoronary bolus dose of 100 mcg of adenosine delivered through the guide catheter improved flow slightly; however, the entire artery did not fill with contrast (Video 20-3). There did not appear to be a dissection or other luminal problem responsible for the reduced flow, and the activated clotting time (ACT) was

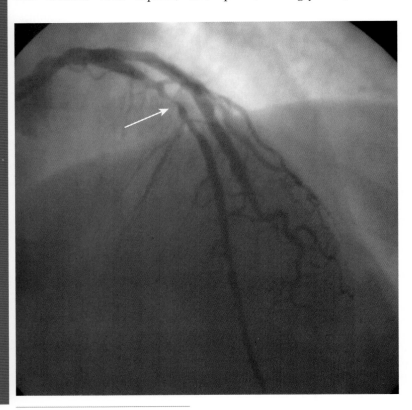

FIGURE 20-1. Coronary angiography performed in a right anterior oblique projection with cranial angulation, showing a severe stenosis in the proximal left anterior descending artery (*arrow*).

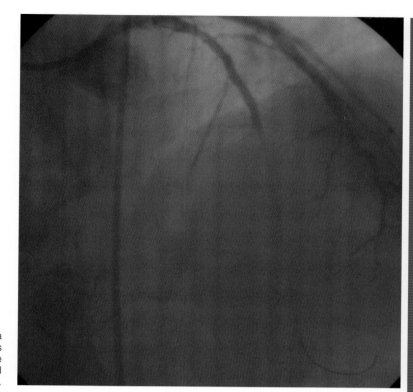

FIGURE 20-2. This angiogram of the left coronary artery in a right anterior oblique projection with cranial angulation was obtained after stent placement and shows no flow past the stent. The site of the previous stenosis shows no residual luminal narrowing and there does not appear to be a dissection.

280 seconds. The operator then deployed a tacrolimus-eluting stent (3.0 mm diameter by 28 mm long). Flow remained reduced, and the patient continued to experience chest pain after stenting despite repeated bolus injections of 100 mcg of adenosine (total of 500 mcg) injected through the guide catheter (Figure 20-2 and Video 20-4). At this point, the operator positioned an infusion catheter (Rapid Transit Catheter, Cordis Corporation) in the distal left anterior descending artery and injected an additional 100 µg adenosine. Subsequent angiography demonstrated nearly normal flow (Video 20-5) and the patient's chest discomfort resolved.

POSTPROCEDURAL COURSE

Following the procedure, the patient had no further symptoms and was discharged the next morning on aspirin, clopidogrel, atorvastatin, metoprolol, lisinopril, and hydrochlorothiazide. He continued to remain active and reported no symptoms 6 months later.

DISCUSSION

The angiographic appearance of markedly reduced coronary flow in the absence of luminal obstruction is termed the "no-reflow" phenomenon. No reflow implies patency of the epicardial artery but inadequate tissue perfusion. Two distinct clinical entities are associated with the no-reflow phenomenon: 1) following reperfusion therapy for acute myocardial infarction, and 2) as a complication of a coronary intervention.

Although related, the dominant mechanism responsible for no reflow in these two settings differ.[1,2] The no-reflow observed after reperfusion for an acute myocardial infarction is likely a consequence of ischemic

microvascular dysfunction, myocardial edema, inflammation, and reperfusion injury; there also may be a component of distal embolization due to thrombus or necrotic plaque. No-reflow observed as a complication of percutaneous coronary intervention is usually due to microvascular obstruction from embolization of plaque components, platelets, and thrombi.

Coronary dissection, vasospasm, and air embolism may masquerade as no–reflow, and these conditions should be carefully excluded. Although the no-reflow phenomenon complicates less than 5% of all coronary interventions, there is a higher frequency of no-reflow following interventions associated with distal embolization, including saphenous vein graft lesions, atheroablative procedures such as rotational atherectomy, and coronary intervention performed in the setting of acute coronary syndromes. In addition, several plaque characteristics are associated with an increased risk of no-reflow (Table 20-1).[1,2]

TABLE 20-1 Characteristics Associated with No-Reflow After Coronary Intervention

Angiographic Characteristics
Plaque ulceration
Thrombus
Long lesion length
Total coronary occlusion
Plaque Characteristics (by intravascular ultrasound)
Ruptured plaque
Large lipid pool
Thrombus
Large plaque burden

The case presented here is typical for no-reflow complicating a coronary intervention. The angiographic appearance is classic and is characterized by slow penetration of a widely patent artery with failure to rapidly and completely fill the artery. The patient presented with an acute coronary syndrome and the culprit lesion appeared irregular and long with diminished flow at baseline. Another important feature exemplified by this case is the fact that flow appeared to worsen with each additional coronary manipulation. This behavior is typical and the operator should always be wary of performing ancillary inflations during an intervention complicated by no-reflow. This is true even if flow is restored, since additional manipulations may cause further deteriorations in flow that may not reverse. In the case presented here, the no-reflow was, fortunately, well-tolerated and reversed by the completion of the case, resulting only in prolonged chest pain. Prolonged and sustained no-reflow may lead to serious sequelae such as hemodynamic collapse, arrhythmia, periprocedural myocardial infarction, and death.

Among pharmacologic agents successful at restoring or improving flow, intracoronary administration of nitroprusside (200 mcg), adenosine (24 to 1000 mcg), and verapamil (50 to 900 mcg) are most popular.[3-5] Intracoronary nitroglycerin is not effective, primarily because of its lack of effect on the resistance arterioles. The platelet glycoprotein IIb/IIIa receptor antagonists have a role in preventing this complication in the setting of acute coronary syndrome, and distal protection devices reduce the no-reflow phenomenon in the case of saphenous vein graft interventions.

In the case presented here, intracoronary administration of high doses of adenosine failed to improve flow. This was likely due to the profound flow reduction present and the inability of the drug to reach the target site (the microcirculation vessels) by intracoronary injection. Adenosine became effective only when the drug was delivered directly into the distal arterial bed by injection through the transit catheter.

KEY CONCEPTS

1. No-reflow may complicate coronary intervention in the setting of acute coronary syndrome and may lead to serious ischemic complications, including prolonged ischemic pain, periprocedural myocardial infarction, hemodynamic compromise, arrhythmia, and death.
2. Intracoronary delivery of vasodilators such as nitroprusside, verapamil, and adenosine may improve flow.
3. In the setting of profound no-reflow, if intracoronary injection of a vasodilator fails to improve flow, administration of a vasodilator agent directly into the distal arterial bed by use of a transit catheter or balloon catheter may reverse the condition and improve flow.

Selected References

1. Jaffe R, Charron T, Puley G, Dick A, Strauss BH: Microvascular obstruction and the no-reflow phenomenon after percutaneous coronary intervention, *Circulation* 117:3152–3156, 2008.
2. Rezkalla SH, Kloner RA: No-reflow phenomenon, *Circulation* 105:656–662, 2002.
3. Iijima R, Shinji H, Ikeda N, Itaya H, Makino K, Funatsu A, Yokouchi T, Komatsu H, Ito N, Nuruki H, Nakajima R, Nakamura M: Comparison of coronary arterial finding by intravascular ultrasound in patients with "transient no-reflow" versus "reflow" during percutaneous coronary intervention in acute coronary syndrome, *Am J Cardiol* 97:29–33, 2006.
4. Hillegass WB, Dean NA, Liao L, Rhinehart RG, Myers PR: Treatment of no-reflow and impaired flow with the nitric oxide donor nitroprusside following percutaneous coronary interventions: Initial human clinical experience, *J Am Coll Cardiol* 37:1335–1343, 2001.
5. Kelly RV, Cohen MG, Stouffer GA: Incidence and management of "no-reflow" following percutaneous coronary interventions, *Am J Med Sci* 329:78–85, 2005.

Tamponade Following a Coronary Intervention

Michael Ragosta, MD, FACC, FSCAI

CASE PRESENTATION

An active 76-year-old man underwent elective coronary angiography for evaluation of a several-month history of exertional chest pain. This identified a severe stenosis in the midportion of a large caliber right coronary artery and a normal appearing left coronary artery. He was referred for percutaneous coronary intervention of the right coronary artery. Past medical history was notable only for hypertension, gout, and paroxysmal atrial fibrillation, and his medications included aspirin, atenolol, atorvastatin, and amlodipine. Physical examination was unremarkable, and his baseline electrocardiogram was notable for sinus rhythm and bifascicular block (right bundle branch and left anterior fascicular block).

CARDIAC CATHETERIZATION

He was administered 300 mg of clopidogrel as a loading dose prior to the intervention, and procedural anticoagulation was accomplished with a bolus of 6000 units of heparin, followed by eptifibatide bolus and infusion. An activated clotting time measured 230 seconds prior to intervention. An 8 French, Judkins 4.0 guide catheter was positioned in the right coronary ostium and a 0.014 inch floppy-tipped guidewire placed distally in the posterior descending artery. After predilating the stenosis with a 4.0 mm diameter by 15 mm long balloon, a 5.0 mm diameter by 24 mm bare-metal stent was positioned and successfully deployed and postdilated with a 5.0 mm diameter by 22 mm long semicompliant balloon. The operator achieved an excellent angiographic result with no residual stenosis and no apparent angiographic complications. The patient felt well and was hemodynamically stable and transferred to a recovery room adjacent to the catheterization laboratory with the arterial sheath in place to await his hospital bed.

Shortly after arrival in the recovery room, the patient developed diaphoresis and nausea. His blood pressure fell to 52/30 mmHg with a heart rate of 60 beats per minute. Physical exam demonstrated marked elevation of his jugular veins. The monitor leads (lead II) showed no ST-segment abnormalities. An infusion of normal saline was initiated and additional venous access obtained in order to infuse dopamine. An emergent echocardiogram confirmed a large circumferential pericardial effusion and the patient was immediately transported back to the cardiac catheterization laboratory. The patient was given 30 mg of protamine intravenously and the eptifibatide infusion was discontinued. The operator performed an emergent pericardiocentesis and aspirated a large volume of blood from the pericardial space. This stabilized the patient's hemodynamic status, with a rise in systolic blood pressure to 100 mmHg. The pigtail catheter remained in the pericardial space and blood was continually aspirated. Meanwhile, a blood sample was collected and sent to the blood bank for transfusion crossmatching.

The operator performed right coronary angiography to determine the source of the bleeding. This showed wide patency of the stent in the right coronary artery with no evidence of a perforation at the site of the stent (Figure 21-1); however, contrast was observed in the pericardial space (Video 21-1) and the pigtail catheter continued to drain blood. Additional views were performed; free-flowing contrast was apparent from the distal tip of the posterior descending artery in an anteroposterior view with cranial angulation (Video 21-2). A 2.5 mm balloon was inflated in the posterior descending artery proximal to the perforation and effectively stopped the bleeding (Figure 21-2). While the balloon remained inflated, the patient remained hemodynamically stable with no additional blood accumulation from the pericardial drain. A cardiothoracic surgeon was informed of the patient's condition and alerted to the possible need for emergency surgery to correct the problem. Meanwhile, 12 units of platelets were rapidly infused and an infusion of packed red blood cells begun. After 10 minutes, the balloon in the posterior descending artery was deflated. Repeat angiography showed ongoing contrast extravasation from the distal posterior descending artery. The balloon was then reinflated for 20 minutes. Angiography after balloon deflation confirmed no further evidence of contrast extravasation (Video 21-3). The patient was observed in the cardiac catheterization laboratory and another angiogram performed 10 minutes later showed no further contrast extravasation. No additional blood was aspirated from the pericardial catheter. In total, 2.6 L of blood drained from the pericardial catheter and he received a total of 4 units of packed red blood cells in the cath lab.

POSTPROCEDURAL COURSE

The patient left the cath lab off pressors with the pericardial drain secured in place. Except for pleuritic chest pain, he remained clinically stable. He was maintained on clopidogrel and aspirin. There was no rise in serial biomarkers and no electrocardiographic changes. After 24 hours, no additional fluid could be aspirated from the drain and no effusion was observed on echocardiography, prompting

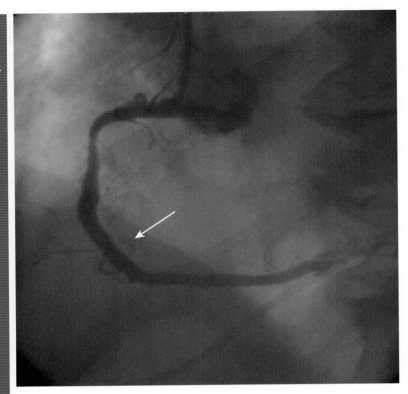

FIGURE 21-1. Right coronary angiogram performed after pericardiocentesis showing wide patency of the coronary stent (*arrow*) placed earlier with no apparent perforation at the site of the stent. A pigtail catheter is present in the pericardial space.

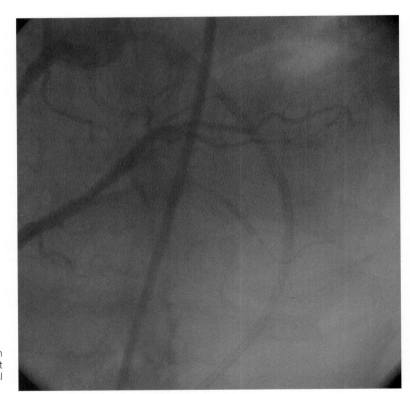

FIGURE 21-2. This figure depicts the site of balloon inflation in the posterior descending artery proximal to the site of contrast extravasation, resulting in successful control of additional bleeding.

removal of the drain. The remainder of his hospital stay was uncomplicated and he was discharged on the second day postprocedure. He was seen at follow-up at 1 and 7 months later feeling well with no further angina.

DISCUSSION

When a patient develops hypotension after a successful coronary intervention, the physician must work quickly to determine if it is caused by benign etiologies such as dehydration or procedural sedation, or from life-threatening etiologies such as retroperitoneal bleed, contrast-related anaphylaxis, abrupt vessel closure, and tamponade. In the present case, elevated neck veins and the absence of ischemic chest pain or ST-segment changes prompted the physician to immediately consider tamponade. An emergency echocardiogram confirmed this suspicion and led to rapid treatment of tamponade, identification and treatment of the bleeding source, and an excellent ultimate outcome.

Tamponade is a very rare complication of coronary intervention, with an incidence in one recent study of 0.12%.[1] Coronary perforation caused by the guidewire, balloon, stent, or other interventional device is responsible for nearly all cases of tamponade. Rarely, tamponade may occur from perforation from a temporary pacemaker lead used to support the intervention or from free-wall rupture complicating an acute myocardial infarction.

Overall, tamponade occurs in 12% to 25% of coronary perforations, but is dependent upon the type of perforation present.[2,3] Ellis and colleagues[3] classified perforations by angiographic criteria as follows: Type I are limited to a crater extending outside of the lumen; Type II are characterized by the presence of a contrast blush in the pericardium or myocardium without an exit hole greater than 1 mm in diameter; and Type III perforations are present when there is free-flowing contrast through an exit hole greater than 1 mm. A variation of Type III is known as "Type III cavity-spilling," defined as perforation into an anatomic chamber such as a ventricle or the coronary sinus. Tamponade complicates about 10% of Type I and II perforations, but occurs in about 60% of Type III perforations.[3] The patient shown in this case had a Type II perforation, with contrast seen in the pericardium but with a very small exit hole caused by the guidewire. Guidewire perforations are more commonly seen when hydrophilic or stiff-tipped wires are used to cross complex lesions or chronic total occlusions. In this case, the tip of a conventional, floppy-tipped guidewire perforated a very distal vessel. This case emphasizes the importance of carefully monitoring the location of the wire tip during the course of an intervention to be sure the tip does not stray into a small branch where it may perforate if advanced inadvertently.

When a perforation is immediately recognized at the time of the intervention, steps may be promptly taken to prevent the development of tamponade. In this case, the wire perforation was not appreciated and hypotension from tamponade developed after he left the catheterization laboratory, resulting in a medical emergency. This is not unusual. Tamponade may result from a slow, steady, unrecognized bleeding caused by an occult wire perforation or from a deep dissection at the site of the intervention. This process may be fueled by powerful platelet antagonists such as the platelet glycoprotein IIb/IIIa receptor antagonists. Only about half of cases of tamponade develop in the cath lab. In the remaining cases, tamponade may not be manifest until many hours after the intervention.[1] Thus, tamponade from an occult perforation should be strongly suspected in a patient with progressive hypotension after a coronary intervention.

Once identified, the first priority is to correct the hemodynamic derangement of tamponade. Rapid infusion of saline along with pressor support can temporarily stabilize a critically ill patient while preparing for pericardiocentesis. In the event of a coronary perforation, rapid accumulation of only a small volume of blood in the pericardium may cause tamponade; this may be difficult to remove, particularly in an obese patient. In addition, rarely, some patients with coronary perforation develop an epicardial hematoma causing local tamponade. In such cases, pericardiocentesis will not relieve compression. However, in most patients, pericardiocentesis rapidly stabilizes the patient, allowing the physician to concentrate on correcting the underlying problem.

In the presence of tamponade due to coronary perforation (or any other life-threatening bleed, for that matter), it is crucial to promptly reverse the procedural anticoagulation. Unfractionated heparin may be reversed with protamine. Low-molecular-weight heparin will only be partially corrected by protamine. Bivalirudin, a direct thrombin inhibitor, cannot be easily reversed, requiring cryoprecipitate, fresh frozen plasma, or factor VIIa infusion for correction; fortunately, it has a short half-life when discontinued. Pharmacologic differences in the platelet glycoprotein IIb/IIIa inhibitors create problems when bleeding requires reversal. The high affinity and irreversible binding property of abciximab means that there is little free drug circulating; this agent can be reversed by replacing all of the patient's circulating, inhibited platelets with transfused platelets (10 to 12 units). The smaller molecules (eptifibatide and tirofiban) are low affinity and bind reversibly to platelets and thus there is a great amount of circulating drug present; transfused platelets will also be affected thus limiting the benefit of platelet transfusion. Fortunately, these drugs are short-acting and their antiplatelet effect drops off rapidly once discontinued.

Repair of the perforation site requires precise identification of the location. In the event of a distal wire perforation as shown in this case, a covered stent is not an option. Proximal occlusion of the vessel with a balloon catheter successfully stops the hemorrhage. Prolonged stasis results in clotting of the exit hole; this may require 10 to 20 minutes of balloon occlusion to accomplish. If prolonged balloon inflation coupled with reversal of anticoagulation does not successfully seal the perforation, surgical repair should be considered. This is necessary in only about 10% of cases.

KEY CONCEPTS

1. Distal guidewire perforations may be inapparent during the procedure and may cause tamponade in the early postprocedural period. Tamponade may present several hours later in the event of a slow bleed, particularly when a platelet glycoprotein IIb/IIIa inhibitor is used.
2. The initial management of tamponade complicating a coronary intervention is focused on patient resuscitation. This includes performance of emergency pericardiocentesis, fluid and pressor support, and reversal of anticoagulation.

Subsequent management includes identifying and treating the source of bleeding.

3. In the event of a distal wire perforation, occlusion of the artery proximal to the site of perforation with a balloon usually stops the bleeding, allowing time to restore clinical stability, transfuse blood products, and reverse anticoagulation.

4. Once anticoagulants are reversed, prolonged balloon inflations are often necessary to seal the perforation site. Surgical repair may be needed if these efforts fail.

Selected References

1. Fejka M, Dixon SR, Safian RD, O'Neill WW, Grines CL, Finta B, Marcovitz PA, Kahn JK: Diagnosis, management, and clinical outcome of cardiac tamponade complicating percutaneous coronary intervention, *Am J Cardiol* 90:1183–1186, 2002.

2. Fasseas P, Orford JL, Panetta CJ, Bell MR, Kenktas AE, Lennon RJ, Holmes DR, Berger PB: Incidence, correlates, management, and clinical outcome of coronary perforation: Analysis of 16,298 procedures, *Am Heart J* 147:140–145, 2004.

3. Ellis SG, Ajluni S, Arnold AZ, Popma JJ, Bittl JA, Eigler NL, Cowley MJ, Raymond RE, Safian RD, Whitlow PL: Increased coronary perforation in the new device era: Incidence, classification, management and outcome, *Circulation* 90:2725–2730, 1994.

Saphenous Vein Graft Rupture

Michael Ragosta, MD, FACC, FSCAI

CASE PRESENTATION

While preparing for bed, an active and healthy 66-year-old man developed sudden-onset substernal chest pain radiating to his jaw. This pain reminded him of the angina he had experienced 14 years earlier, prior to coronary bypass surgery consisting of a left internal mammary artery graft to the left anterior descending artery, a right internal mammary artery graft to the right coronary artery, and a saphenous vein graft to a large second obtuse marginal artery. The pain lasted for 15 minutes and resolved with nitroglycerin. Evaluation in the hospital emergency department found no electrocardiographic abnormalities or rise in cardiac biomarkers. Following hospital admission and treatment with aspirin, unfractionated heparin, atenolol, and long-acting nitrates, his cardiologist performed a stress echocardiogram. During this test, he developed recurrent chest pain along with marked ST depression at a low workload with stress-induced lateral wall hypokinesis on echocardiography. Physical examination and routine laboratory studies were normal and he was referred for cardiac catheterization.

CARDIAC CATHETERIZATION

Angiography found wide patency of both internal mammary artery grafts and a severe proximal stenosis and moderately severe, more distal stenosis in the body of the 14-year-old vein graft to the obtuse marginal artery (Figures 22-1, 22-2 and Videos 22-1, 22-2). The operator planned to stent both the proximal and midgraft lesions with distal embolic protection afforded by the Percu-Surge Guardwire (Medtronic) temporary balloon occlusion and aspiration system.[1] An 8 French, right Judkins guide catheter was inserted in the vein graft. The operator chose unfractionated heparin and eptifibatide for procedural anticoagulation, and the Guardwire was positioned distally in the vein graft. The occlusion balloon was inflated to allow distal embolic protection. After first dilating with a 3.5 mm diameter balloon, a 4.5 mm diameter by 18 mm long bare-metal stent was deployed in the proximal lesion (Figure 22-3). The operator then positioned and deployed a 4.0 mm diameter by 28 mm long bare-metal stent in the midgraft lesion. Aspiration was performed, the distal occlusion balloon deflated, and angiography performed. To the operator's

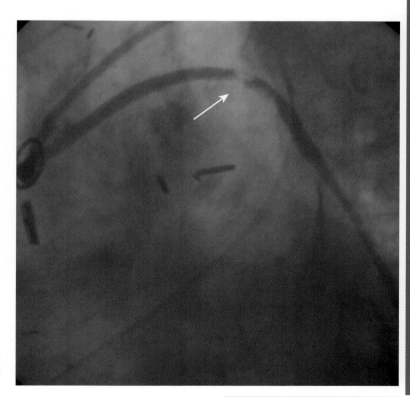

FIGURE 22-1. Left anterior oblique projection of the saphenous vein graft to the obtuse marginal artery. A severe stenosis is apparent in the body of the vein graft (arrow).

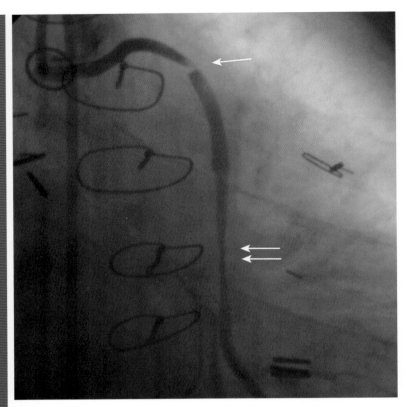

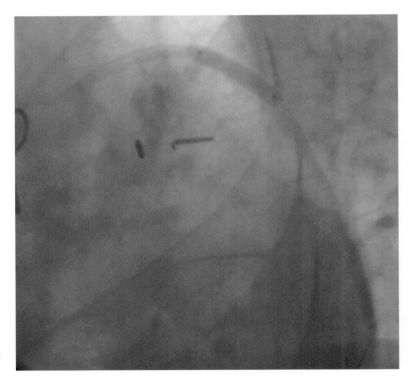

FIGURE 22-2. Right anterior oblique view of the saphenous vein graft to the obtuse marginal artery. There is a severe stenosis in the body of the vein graft (*arrow*) followed by a long tubular narrowing more distally (*double arrow*).

FIGURE 22-3. Inflation of the stent balloon in the more proximal lesion in the saphenous vein graft.

horror, free-flowing contrast was observed extravasating from a large defect in the midportion of the vein graft within the stented segment (Video 22-3). The patient developed marked hypotension with arterial pressure falling to 50/30 mmHg. To staunch the hemorrhage, a

3.5 mm perfusion balloon was positioned and inflated in the vein graft at the site of the defect, eptifibatide was discontinued, and 30 mg of protamine was administered intravenously. This greatly decreased the amount of contrast extravasation, and the perfusion balloon allowed distal perfusion; however, there remained evidence of ongoing hemorrhage by angiography (Video 22-4). Fluid resuscitation and dopamine infusion restored blood pressure, but each time the balloon was deflated for even a few seconds, the patient developed marked hypotension. Since the operator did not feel there was sufficient time to safely exchange the perfusion balloon for a PTFE-covered stent nor felt confident that the large defect could be successfully sealed with this device, cardiothoracic surgery agreed to operate on the patient emergently.

POSTPROCEDURAL COURSE

To maintain hemodynamic stability and prevent further hemorrhage, the perfusion balloon remained inflated during transport to the operating room. Through a left thoracotomy, the surgeon first evacuated a large amount of blood in the pleural space, then repaired the perforation and placed a saphenous vein graft from the descending thoracic aorta to the circumflex marginal artery, just distal to the previous placed graft, which was subsequently ligated. The patient's postoperative course was remarkably benign and he was ultimately discharged on postoperative day five. He had no additional angina during follow-up.

DISCUSSION

Distal embolization, no-reflow, and periprocedural myocardial infarction are the operator's major concerns when performing an intervention on a lesion in an old saphenous vein graft. Although the occurrence of rupture of a saphenous vein graft, as presented in this case, is very rare, the operator may encounter a rigid lesion in a saphenous vein graft. In such cases, full stent expansion may require high-pressure inflations and may result in perforation.

A saphenous vein graft perforation may behave differently than one involving a native coronary artery. A saphenous vein graft may be more prone to perforation since, in a native coronary artery, the presence of a thicker muscular layer, as well as a more robust adventitia and an overlying layer of subepicardial fat, may help contain a deep dissection or smaller perforation that might lead to free bleeding if a similar injury involved a vein graft, which lacks these protective layers. Alternatively, in the event of a definite breach of the vessel during intervention, a perforation of a saphenous vein graft may be less likely to cause tamponade. If the lesion involves the proximal segment of the vein graft, a rupture may cause bleeding into the pleural instead of the pericardial space. Furthermore, the existence of pericardial adhesions or the persistence of a pericardiotomy created at the time of bypass surgery might protect the patient from developing tamponade, should the bleeding enter the pericardial space. Although the case presented here bled into the pleural space and the patient did not develop tamponade, the rupture still led to dramatic hemodynamic collapse from free bleeding into the pleural space. In addition, tamponade may still occur in these cases because the pericardium may reflect high onto the ascending aorta, there

may be minimal adhesions, and the pericardial opening made during surgery may close.[2]

Treatment strategies for native coronary artery perforation have been discussed in other cases in this section involving perforation. These basic principles are also applicable to a saphenous vein graft perforation. Similar to native coronary arteries, the outcome of the perforation will depend on the size of the defect.[3] The case presented here is an example of a Type III perforation with freely flowing contrast from an exit hole greater than 1 mm in diameter. Simple measures, such as reversal of anticoagulation and prolonged balloon inflation at the site of the perforation, could not be expected to effectively seal such a large defect. A covered stent might have succeeded; however, the operator chose surgery, primarily based on the large size of the defect and the concern that a covered stent might not necessarily seal the rupture. Furthermore, release of the occluding balloon for even a few seconds led to prompt hemodynamic instability. An attempt at a covered stent would have been technically challenging under these circumstances.

As exemplified in this case, emergency surgery is necessary when there is ongoing bleeding from a coronary perforation despite reversal of anticoagulation and institution of measures to treat the perforation, such as prolonged balloon inflation or use of a covered stent graft. Overall, between 10% and 40% of patients with coronary perforation are treated surgically black[4-6]; surgery is less likely to be necessary when the perforation is small and not associated with tamponade or hemodynamic instability. In this case, a perfusion balloon was used to occlude the bleeding site while allowing distal perfusion of the artery, thereby limiting ischemia during the time required for transport to the operating room. Unfortunately, perfusion balloons are no longer commercially available, thereby removing this strategy as an option in the current era.

KEY CONCEPTS

1. Perforation of a saphenous vein graft is a rare complication and may lead to dramatic hemodynamic collapse from the resulting hemorrhage.
2. Although a saphenous vein graft perforation may cause pleural space rather than pericardial hemorrhage, tamponade may still be possible.
3. Emergency surgery is necessary in 10% to 40% of coronary perforations, and is more commonly needed when there is associated tamponade or a large perforation.

Selected References

1. Baim DS, Wahr D, George B, Leon MB, Greenberg J, Cutlip DE, Kaya U, Popma JJ, Ho KKL, Kuntz RE: Randomized trial of a distal embolic protection device during percutaneous intervention of saphenous vein aorto-coronary bypass grafts, *Circulation* 105: 1285–1290, 2002.
2. Lowe R, Hammond C, Perry RA: Prior CABG does not prevent pericardial tamponade following saphenous vein graft perforation associated with angioplasty, *Heart* 91:1052, 2005.

3. Ellis SG, Ajluni S, Arnold AZ, Popma JJ, Bittl JA, Eigler NL, Cowley MJ, Raymond RE, Safian RD, Whitlow PL: Increased coronary perforation in the new device era: Incidence, classification, management and outcome, *Circulation* 90:2725–2730, 1994.

4. Fasseas P, Orford JL, Panetta CJ, Bell MR, Kenktas AE, Lennon RJ, Holmes DR, Berger PB: Incidence, correlates, management, and clinical outcome of coronary perforation: Analysis of 16,298 procedures, *Am Heart J* 147:140–145, 2004.

5. Fejka M, Dixon SR, Safian RD, O'Neill WW, Grines CL, Finta B, Marcovitz PA, Kahn JK: Diagnosis, management, and clinical outcome of cardiac tamponade complicating percutaneous coronary intervention, *Am J Cardiol* 90:1183–1186, 2002.

6. Stankovic G, Orlic D, Corvaja N, Airoldi F, Chieffo A, Spanos V, Montorfano M, Carlino M, Finci L, Sangiorgi G, Colombo A: Incidence, predictors, in-hospital, and late outcomes of coronary artery perforations, *Am J Cardiol* 93:213–216.

Coronary Perforation

Michael Ragosta, MD, FACC, FSCAI

CASE PRESENTATION

A remarkably healthy and independent 89-year-old woman, with a prior history of hypertension and carotid atherosclerosis treated with lisinopril, hydrochlorothiazide, and aspirin, reported a 6-month history of progressive fatigue and dyspnea. Previously able to regularly walk several miles at a time, her symptoms caused a marked restriction in her exercise capacity and, at the time of presentation, she was no longer able to walk more than a block without having to stop to rest. Additionally, over the preceding 3 weeks, she developed chest tightness with minimal exertion. This symptom prompted her to seek medical attention. Her physician scheduled a stress test but she developed rest chest pain along with severe dyspnea and diaphoresis before this test could be performed and was admitted to the hospital.

Upon presentation in the emergency department, she was symptom-free and a 12-lead electrocardiogram showed Q waves inferiorly without acute ischemic changes. Serum cardiac biomarkers were not elevated. Her physical examination was notable for systolic hypertension with a blood pressure of 214/77 mmHg in both arms, a heart rate of 73 beats per minute, bilateral carotid bruits, and a systolic murmur of aortic sclerosis. The routine admission laboratory studies were normal, including renal function.

Given her advanced age, negative cardiac isoenzymes, and marked systolic hypertension on presentation without a trial of adequate medical therapy, a beta-blocker, statin, and long-acting nitrates were added to her medical regimen. A pharmacologic stress perfusion scan was performed the next day. During the test she developed severe chest pain associated with diffuse ST-segment depression and reversible ischemia in the anterior wall. The patient agreed to undergo catheterization.

CARDIAC CATHETERIZATION

Coronary angiography revealed multivessel coronary disease with severe disease in the proximal segment of the right coronary artery and severe disease of the midportion of the left anterior descending coronary artery (Figures 23-1, 23-2 and Video 23-1). The operator judged the right coronary artery suitable for percutaneous

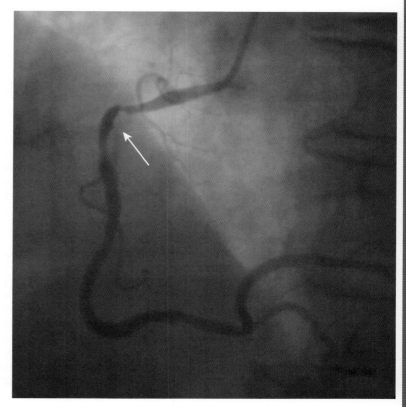

FIGURE 23-1. This is a left anterior oblique coronary angiogram of the right coronary artery, showing a severe stenosis in the proximal segment (*arrow*).

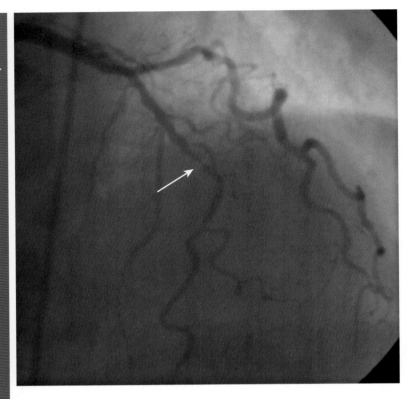

FIGURE 23-2. This angiogram of the left coronary artery in a right anterior oblique projection with cranial angulation depicts the severe stenosis in the midportion of the artery (*arrow*). Notice the diffuse nature of the disease, the small caliber vessel, and the presence of vessel angulation and tortuosity.

coronary intervention; however, the left anterior descending artery provided several challenges. Not only did the vessel appear small in caliber, there was also marked tortuosity with diffuse disease surrounding the severely stenosed segment. Prior to the catheterization, the patient dismissed the option of bypass surgery and agreed only to percutaneous revascularization. The patient confirmed this after she was presented with the catheterization results, and the operator proceeded with a multivessel intervention on the right coronary artery and left anterior descending artery.

Following administration of a bolus and infusion of the direct thrombin inhibitor bivalirudin, the operator began with the right coronary artery. This lesion was first dilated with a 3.0 mm diameter by 15 mm long compliant balloon and a 3.5 mm diameter by 28 mm long sirolimus-eluting stent was deployed successfully with an acceptable angiographic result (Figure 23-3). The operator then turned to the left anterior descending artery. A 6 French, 45 C-curve guide catheter was engaged and a 0.014 inch floppy-tipped guidewire advanced to the distal portion of the vessel. The 3.0 mm by 15 mm compliant balloon used to predilate the right coronary lesion was advanced to the lesion and inflated to 8 atmospheres for 30 seconds (Figure 23-4). The operator deflated the balloon and observed contrast extravasation at the balloon angioplasty site (Figure 23-5 and Video 23-2). The vessel was immediately tamponaded using the same balloon inflated to 6 atmospheres and the infusion of bivalirudin was discontinued. The patient developed transient hypotension and bradycardia. This corrected quickly with 1 mg of atropine and a 500 cc bolus of fluid. An urgent echocardiogram revealed a small pericardial effusion. The balloon remained inflated for 15 minutes and repeat angiography confirmed successful sealing

of the perforation. The operator noted some difficulty advancing the previously-inflated balloon to the lesion because of vessel angulation. Subsequently, two short bare-metal stents (2.5 mm diameter by 13 mm long distally and a 2.5 mm diameter by 12 mm long proximally) were deployed to 12 atmospheres and covered the diseased segment of the mid-LAD. Postdeployment, the stents appeared well-deployed with no further evidence of contrast extravasation (Figure 23-6 and Video 23-3). The patient left the catheterization laboratory hemodynamically stable with minimal chest discomfort.

POSTPROCEDURAL COURSE

She returned to a monitored bed and was watched carefully overnight. She remained stable with normal vital signs and eventual resolution of her chest pain. A repeat echocardiogram performed the following morning showed no change in the size of the small pericardial effusion. The patient was observed an additional day and discharged 48 hours after the coronary intervention feeling well. She remains active with no angina 5 years later at the age of 94 years.

DISCUSSION

The perforation in this case was likely caused by employing an oversized balloon in an angulated artery in an elderly woman. In an effort to economize resources in a patient undergoing a multivessel intervention, the operator chose to predilate the left anterior descending artery with the balloon used earlier to predilate the right coronary artery. In addition, vessel rigidity required higher inflation pressures causing further growth in diameter of the compliant balloon. The end result was

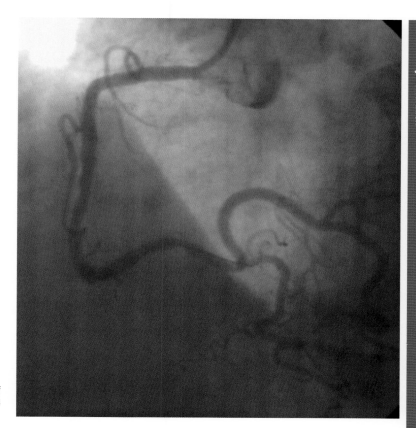

FIGURE 23-3. Following stenting of the proximal segment of the right coronary artery, an excellent angiographic result was obtained.

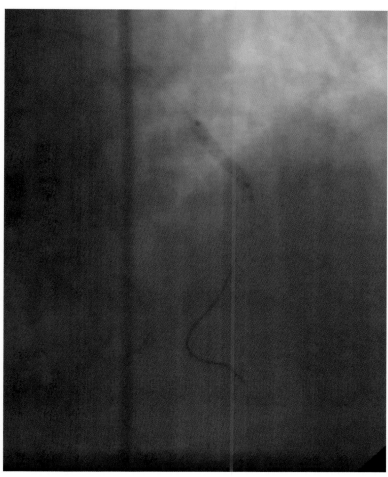

FIGURE 23-4. Balloon angioplasty was performed to predilate the lesion in the left anterior descending artery.

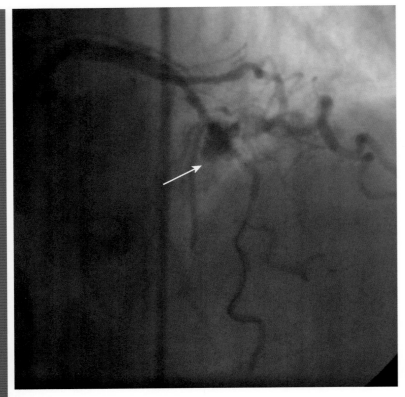

FIGURE 23-5. Following balloon angioplasty, there is extravasation of contrast noted emanating from the site of balloon dilatation, consistent with a perforation (*arrow*).

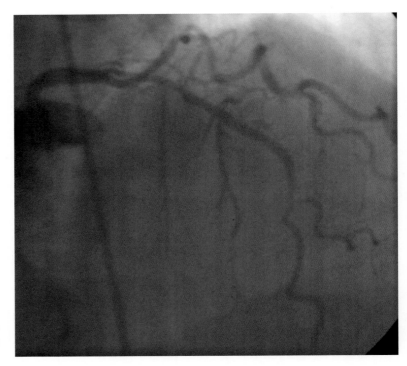

FIGURE 23-6. This is the final angiogram obtained after prolonged balloon inflation sealed the perforation and two stents were deployed.

an oversized balloon creating an extensive and deep dissection, resulting in the observed perforation.

The ultimately favorable outcome in this case emphasizes several important concepts in the management of a patient with a coronary perforation. Based on the classification system described by Ellis and colleague the Type II perforation present in this case would be expected to result in tamponade in 10% to 15% of cases.[1,2] Rapid recognition and management by the operator prevented this. The operator acted quickly, rapidly repositioning and inflating the balloon at the site of the perforation while simultaneously discontinuing the infusion of bivalirudin. This quick response allowed only a small amount of blood to enter the pericardium, thus preventing tamponade. Even a small delay might have caused enough blood to accumulate in the pericardial space to cause dramatic hemodynamic deterioration requiring patient resuscitation and a potentially less favorable outcome. Note that the brief period of hypotension and bradycardia occurring immediately after the perforation likely represented a vagal reaction, a common sequelae of an acute perforation. In this case, the brief period of hypotension and bradycardia responded immediately to atropine and fluid bolus.

Reversal of anticoagulation and prolonged balloon inflation successfully sealed the perforation in this case. In the event of ongoing bleeding despite these measures, a polytetrafluoroethylene (PTFE)-covered stent is indicated; however, this might have been very difficult or impossible to deliver based on the small caliber and marked tortuosity of the artery. Surgical correction, necessary in 10% to 30% of perforations, is another option should these measures fail to control bleeding, but would not have been desirable given the patient's advanced age.

KEY CONCEPTS

1. A common cause of a perforation is use of an oversized balloon or stent inflated to high pressures causing deep dissection and vessel disruption.
2. Prompt recognition and treatment of a coronary perforation may prevent tamponade. Prolonged balloon inflation with cessation of anticoagulation is often successful in the event of a small perforation.
3. Vagal reactions are common and, in the absence of tamponade, respond well to atropine and fluid infusion.

Selected References

1. Ellis SG, Ajluni S, Arnold AZ, Popma JJ, Bittl JA, Eigler NL, Cowley MJ, Raymond RE, Safian RD, Whitlow PL: Increased coronary perforation in the new device era: Incidence, classification, management and outcome, *Circulation* 90:2725–2730, 1994.
2. Fasseas P, Orford JL, Panetta CJ, Bell MR, Kenktas AE, Lennon RJ, Holmes DR, Berger PB: Incidence, correlates, management, and clinical outcome of coronary perforation: Analysis of 16,298 procedures, *Am Heart J* 147:140–145, 2004.

Early Stent Thrombosis

Michael Ragosta, MD, FACC, FSCAI

CASE PRESENTATION

The onset of chest pain occurring during heavy exertion prompted a healthy 44-year-old man to seek medical attention. For 6 weeks, he had noted symptoms occurring only when running or performing strenuous labor. The chest pain always promptly resolved with rest. For many years he had maintained a high level of fitness for his job as a physical trainer, and he had no significant medical history except for a family history of premature coronary disease (both father and paternal grandfather suffered fatal acute myocardial infarctions at age 52 and 55, respectively). A 12-lead electrocardiogram was notable for T-wave inversions inferiorly (Figure 24-1). To further evaluate his symptoms, his family physician ordered an exercise stress test. He exercised to 12.9 METS but experienced chest pain in the third stage and developed 2 mm of downsloping ST-segment depression. His physician prescribed aspirin and metoprolol and referred him for cardiac catheterization.

CARDIAC CATHETERIZATION

A severe stenosis present in the proximal right coronary artery explained his symptoms (Figure 24-2 and Videos 24-1, 24-2). Atherosclerotic disease evident in the left coronary artery did not appear to cause significant luminal obstruction (Figures 24-3, 24-4). The operator proceeded with percutaneous intervention of the right coronary artery using a bolus and infusion of bivalirudin as the procedural anticoagulant. The patient received 325 mg of aspirin prior to catheterization and was dosed with 600 mg of clopidogrel at the start of the percutaneous coronary intervention. Using first a

2.5 mm diameter by 20 mm long compliant balloon to predilate the lesion, the operator then deployed a 3.0 mm diameter by 23 mm long sirolimus-eluting stent (Figure 24-5). Not satisfied with the angiographic result, the operator postdilated the stent with a 3.0 mm diameter noncompliant balloon to 18 atmospheres (Figure 24-6). This resulted in a satisfactory angiographic result (Figure 24-7 and Videos 24-3, 24-4) and the patient left the cardiac catheterization laboratory without chest pain. An electrocardiogram obtained approximately 1 hour after the procedure showed no changes compared to baseline (Figure 24-8).

Over the course of the afternoon, the patient reported continual low-grade chest discomfort, but repeat electrocardiograms showed no changes. Although the pain was attributed to noncardiac causes, it continued throughout the afternoon and failed to respond to nitrates, antacids, or positional changes. Approximately 6 hours after the intervention, the chest pain suddenly became acutely worse and was associated with diaphoresis, nausea, and bradycardia. An electrocardiogram obtained at this point revealed normalization of the previously present inferior T-wave changes and new ST-segment elevation in leads III and aVF (Figure 24-9). Emergency coronary angiography confirmed occlusion of the right coronary stent (Figure 24-10 and Video 24-5).

Balloon angioplasty using a 3.0 mm diameter by 15 mm long noncompliant balloon rapidly restored normal flow to the right coronary artery, relieving the patient's chest pain and resolving the ST-segment elevation. Vasospasm observed distal to the stent (Video 24-6) resolved after administration of intracoronary nitroglycerin (Video 24-7). Because the operator thought there might be a small dissection at the proximal end of the earlier-placed stent, an

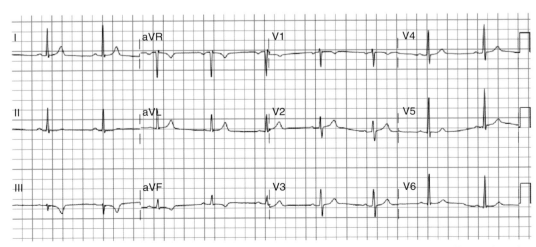

FIGURE 24-1. Baseline 12-lead electrocardiogram obtained prior to catheterization. There are inferior T-wave inversions noted.

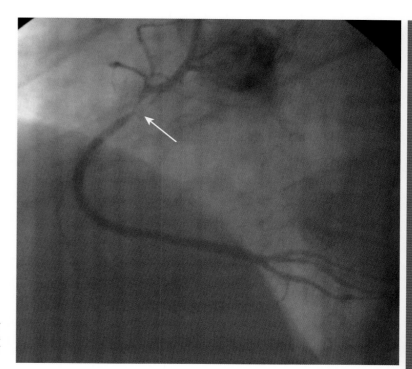

FIGURE 24-2. A representative image of the right coronary artery obtained in the left anterior oblique projection. There is a severe stenosis of the proximal segment of the right coronary artery (*arrow*).

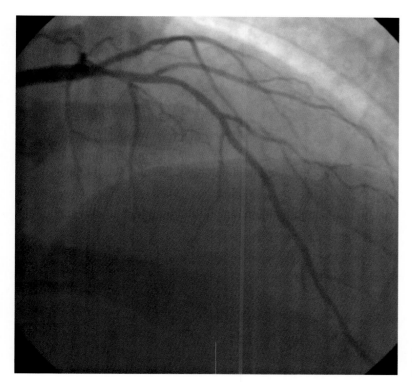

FIGURE 24-3. A representative image of the left coronary artery obtained in the right anterior oblique projection with cranial angulation. There is nonobstructive coronary disease present.

additional stent (3.0 mm diameter by 8 mm long) was deployed. The final angiographic result is shown in Figure 24-11 and Videos 24-8 and 24-9.

POSTPROCEDURAL COURSE

Following the second procedure, he left the cardiac catheterization laboratory without chest pain and was observed in the coronary care unit. Serial troponin I assays confirmed a periprocedural infarction, peaking 12 hours after the second intervention at 33.23 ng/mL (normal <0.10 ng/mL); a 12-lead electrocardiogram obtained the next day demonstrated inferior Q waves (Figure 24-12). The remainder of his hospital stay was uneventful, and he was discharged free of symptoms on the third day postprocedure.

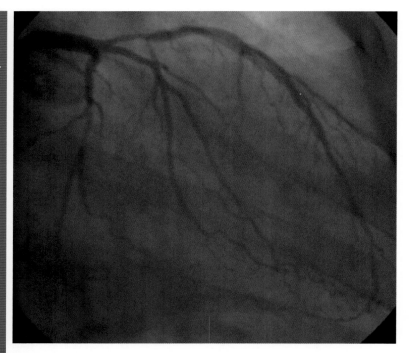

FIGURE 24-4. A representative image of the left coronary artery obtained in the right anterior oblique projection with caudal angulation. The distal circumflex is diseased and there is nonobstructive disease present in the proximal left anterior descending artery.

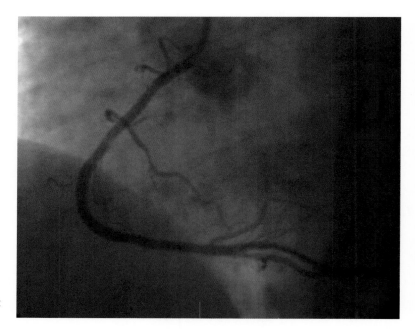

FIGURE 24-5. This angiogram was obtained following stent placement in the proximal portion of the right coronary artery.

DISCUSSION

This case provides an example of early stent thrombosis. In the current era, stent thrombosis is a rare but potentially catastrophic complication of stent implantation. Stent thrombosis is called "acute" when it occurs within 24 hours of stent placement and "subacute" when it happens 24 hours to 30 days after intervention.[1] These two groups are often combined and described as "early" stent thrombosis. The term "late" stent thrombosis describes events happening 30 days to 1 year after intervention; stent thrombosis occurring after 1 year is called "very late".[1]

Initial clinical experiences with coronary stents witnessed early stent thrombosis rates of around 10%. The incorporation of routine high-pressure balloon inflations during stent deployment along with the adjunctive use of dual antiplatelet therapy reduced the rate of early stent thrombosis to the current level of less than 1% and similar rates for bare-metal and drug-eluting stents.[1-4]

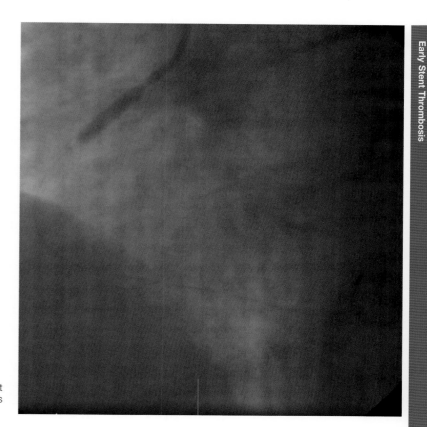

FIGURE 24-6. Following stent deployment, the proximal right coronary artery underwent balloon inflation to high pressures using a noncompliant balloon.

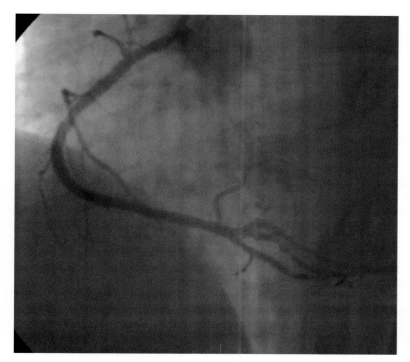

FIGURE 24-7. This is a representative image of the final angiographic result following stent placement in the proximal right coronary artery.

Patient factors relating to early stent thrombosis include the presence of an acute coronary syndrome, diabetes mellitus, chronic renal failure, and premature discontinuation of antiplatelet drugs.[1] Procedural factors include bifurcation stenting, presence of residual dissection or thrombus, stent underexpansion, tissue protrusion, long lesion and stent length, small vessel or stent diameter, and smaller postprocedural luminal diameter.[2,3,5] Intravascular ultrasound studies have shown that an underlying cause is present in 78% of

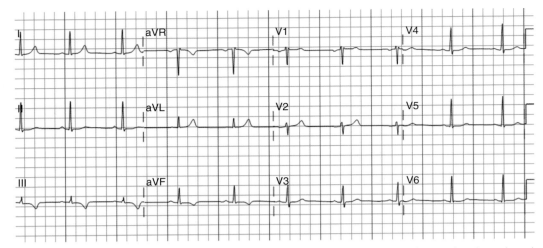

FIGURE 24-8. The 12-lead electrocardiogram recorded after the successful right coronary intervention showed no changes compared to baseline.

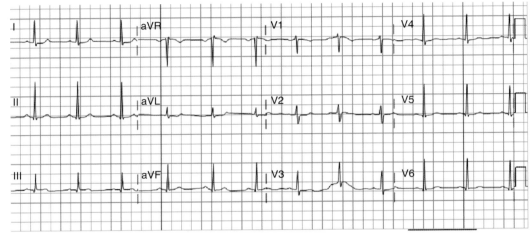

FIGURE 24-9. An electrocardiogram obtained 6 hours after intervention during chest pain shows changes in the inferior leads with normalization of the T waves and ST-segment elevation in leads III and aVF suggesting closure of the right coronary artery.

events and no cause apparent in 22% of cases.[5] The most common abnormality observed on intravascular ultrasound is underexpansion of the stent, resulting in a smaller minimal luminal area compared to patients without stent thrombosis. Additionally, residual dissection, thrombus, or tissue protrusion may be evident. Interestingly, incomplete stent apposition found on intravascular ultrasound is not related to stent thrombosis.[6]

The underlying cause of the stent thrombosis observed in this case cannot be readily discerned. Angiographically, the stent appeared well-deployed with no evidence of dissection, tissue prolapse, or thrombus. The operator performed high-pressure balloon inflation post-stenting. Intravascular ultrasound was not performed during the initial intervention or when the patient returned with stent thrombosis, which might have provided a clue to the cause. Inadequate adjunctive pharmacology may have played a role. Based on the REPLACE-2 trial, elective coronary intervention in low-risk lesions using bivalirudin and aspirin with a 300 mg clopidogrel load 2 to 12 hours prior to intervention is associated with similar ischemic endpoints as with unfractionated heparin plus glycoprotein IIb/IIIa inhibitors, but with a lower rate of

bleeding.[7] The optimal dose and time of clopidogrel load relative to the coronary intervention is not clearly defined. Maximum inhibition of platelet aggregation is achieved 2 hours after a load of 600 mg of clopidogrel, and the ISAR-REACT trial enrolling low-risk and intermediate-risk patients undergoing elective intervention who received 600 mg of clopidogrel at least 2 hours prior to stenting found no benefit from the platelet glycoprotein IIb/IIIa inhibitor abciximab suggesting that this dose and timing provides adequate levels of platelet inhibition to safely allow elective stenting in the absence of high-risk features.[8] In the present case, clopidogrel was loaded just prior to the intervention, and it is interesting to note that stent thrombosis occurred 6 hours after intervention when the dose of clopidogrel should have already achieved optimal platelet inhibition. Thrombosis in this case may have been caused by aspirin or clopidogrel resistance, estimated to be present in as high as 10% to 15% of patients undergoing coronary intervention.

Stent thrombosis typically manifests as an ST-segment elevation acute myocardial infarction. These are very serious events associated with death in 10% to 15% of cases at 30 days and myocardial infarction in about

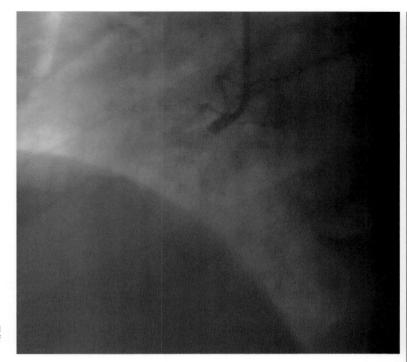

FIGURE 24-10. Right coronary angiogram obtained during chest pain 6 hours after stent placement revealed occlusion of the stent consistent with acute stent thrombosis.

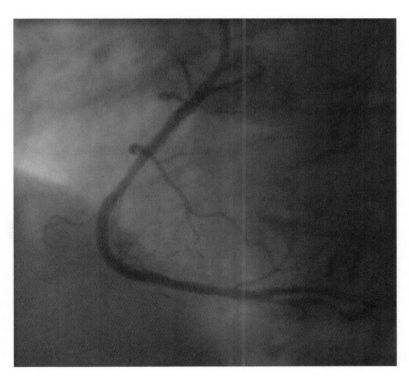

FIGURE 24-11. This is the final result after repeat intervention on the right coronary artery.

60%.[2,3] In the present case, although the problem was identified and treated promptly, the patient suffered a sizeable event and developed new Q waves on his electrocardiogram. Obviously, thrombosis of a stent placed in a large proximal artery and stent thrombosis occurring after hospital discharge, resulting in delays in recognition and management, may have devastating and fatal consequences.

Restoration of vessel patency is the major goal of management; most operators begin with balloon angioplasty to achieve this. Adjunctive use of glycoprotein IIb/IIIa inhibitors is strongly recommended unless contraindicated, particularly because the thrombus causing stent occlusion is rich in platelets. Large, visible thrombi may be effectively removed with one of the commercially available aspiration catheters. Once reperfusion

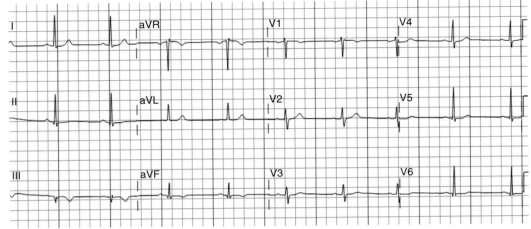

FIGURE 24-12. This electrocardiogram obtained prior to discharge confirmed the presence of new inferior Q waves.

has been accomplished, evaluation of the stent and adjacent arterial segments with intravascular ultrasound may provide valuable insight into the mechanism of stent thrombosis and may directly impact management. For example, intravascular ultrasound may demonstrate an edge dissection unrecognized on angiography requiring additional stenting, or may reveal an inadequate luminal area necessitating dilatation with a larger diameter balloon. If ultrasound is not used, it is advisable to perform additional balloon inflations within the stent using either a larger diameter, noncompliant balloon or a noncompliant balloon inflated to higher pressure than originally used.

KEY CONCEPTS

1. In the current era, early stent thrombosis, defined as occurring within 30 days of an intervention, complicates less than 1% of coronary stent procedures and the rate is similar for bare-metal and drug-eluting stents.
2. Predictors of early stent thrombosis include stenting in the presence of an acute coronary syndrome, bifurcation lesions, long stent length, stent underexpansion, tissue protrusion, small vessel or stent diameter, and smaller postprocedural luminal diameter. Incomplete stent apposition alone is not associated with stent thrombosis.
3. Stent thrombosis often manifests as an acute ST-segment elevation myocardial infarction and carries substantial morbidity and mortality.
4. Management of stent thrombosis centers on prompt reperfusion of the occluded vessel. Balloon angioplasty alone is often successful and glycoprotein IIb/IIIa inhibitors are advisable. Intravascular ultrasound is an important tool to help define the responsible mechanism leading to stent thrombosis.

Selected References

1. Lemesle G, Delhaye C, Bonello L, de Labriolle A, Waksman R, Pichard A: Stent thrombosis in 2008: Definition, predictors, prognosis and treatment, *Arch Cardiovasc Dis* 101:769–777, 2008.
2. Cutlip DE, Baim DS, Ho KKL, Popma JJ, Lansky AJ, Cohen DJ, Carozza JP, Chauhan MS, Rodriguez O, Kuntz RE: Stent thrombosis in the modern era: A pooled analysis of multicenter coronary stent clinical trials, *Circulation* 103:1967–1971, 2001.
3. Ong ATL, Hoye A, Aoki J, van Mieghem CAG, Granillo GAR, Sonnenschein K, Regar E, McFadden EP, Sianos G, van der Giessen WJ, de Jaegere PPT, de Feyter P, van Domburg RT, Serruys PW: Thirty-day incidence and six-month clinical outcome of thrombotic stent occlusion after bare-metal, sirolimus, or paclitaxel stent implantation, *J Am Coll Cardiol* 45:947–953, 2005.
4. Daemen J, Wenaweser P, Tsuchida K, Abrecht L, Vaina S, Morger C, Kukreja N, Juni P, Sianos G, Hellige G, van Domburg RT, Hess OM, Boersma E, Meier B, Windecker S, Serruys PW: Early and late coronary stent thrombosis of sirolimus-eluting and paclitaxel-eluting stents in routine clinical practice: Data from a large two-institutional cohort study, *Lancet* 369:667–678, 2007.
5. Cheneau E, Leborge L, Mintz GS, Kotani J, Pichard AD, Satler LF, Canos D, Castagna M, Weissman NJ, Waksman R: Predictors of subacute stent thrombosis: Results of a systematic intravascular ultrasound study, *Circulation* 108:43–47, 2003.
6. Tanabe K, Serruys PW, Degertekin M, et al, for the TAXUS II Study Group: Incomplete stent apposition after implantation of paclitaxel-eluting stents or bare-metal stents: Insights from the randomized TAXUS II trial, *Circulation* 111:900–905, 2005.
7. Lincoff AM, Bittl JA, Harrington RA, et al, for the REPLACE-2 Investigators: Bivalirudin and provisional glycoprotein IIb/IIIa blockade compared with heparin and planned glycoprotein IIb/IIIa blockade during percutaneous coronary intervention. REPLACE-2 randomized trial, *JAMA* 289:853–863, 2003.
8. Kastrati A, Mehilli J, Schuhlen H, et al, for the Intracoronary Stenting and Antithrombotic Regimen-Rapid Early Action for Coronary Treatment (ISAR-REACT) Study Investigators: A clinical trial of abciximab in elective percutaneous coronary intervention after pretreatment with clopidogrel, *N Engl J Med* 350:232–238, 2004.

Retroperitoneal Bleed

Michael Ragosta, MD, FACC, FSCAI

CASE PRESENTATION

A healthy, active, nonsmoking 40-year-old man with a history of hypertension and dyslipidemia noted midsternal chest pain while dragging a heavy deer he had just hunted out of the woods and to his car. He stopped to rest, but the pain increased in severity and was associated with diaphoresis. He drove himself to a local hospital's emergency department, where an electrocardiogram showed sinus tachycardia and ST elevation in the anterior precordial leads. Shortly after the electrocardiogram was obtained, he became unresponsive from ventricular fibrillation and required cardioversion. After administration of 325 mg of aspirin, 5 mg of intravenous metoprolol, an intravenous bolus of unfractionated heparin, and 4 mg of morphine sulfate, he was flown by helicopter to a tertiary care hospital 40 miles away for emergency coronary angiography.

CARDIAC CATHETERIZATION

Angiography confirmed proximal occlusion of the left anterior descending artery (Figure 25-1). The operator successfully restored normal flow in this vessel with balloon angioplasty (2.5 mm diameter by 20 mm long balloon) followed by insertion of a 3.5 mm diameter by 15 mm long bare-metal stent (Figure 25-2). Adjunctive

pharmacology included an additional bolus of unfractionated heparin and a bolus and infusion of eptifibatide. The left circumflex and right coronary arteries were angiographically normal. At the end of the procedure, 600 mg of clopidogrel was administered orally. The activated clotting time measured 260 seconds. An angiogram of the right femoral artery performed through the arterial sheath is shown in Figure 25-3 and Video 25-1. The operator successfully achieved access site hemostasis using a closure device (Starclose, Abbott Medical). The patient left the cardiac catheterization laboratory feeling well, with a blood pressure of 110/70 mmHg.

POSTPROCEDURAL COURSE

Upon arrival to the coronary care unit, he remained free of chest pain but became nauseated and reported right lower abdominal and scrotal pain. His heart rate fell to 51 beats per minute and his blood pressure dropped to 81/56 mmHg. He appeared pale and diaphoretic but denied chest pain. An electrocardiogram confirmed resolution of ST-segment elevation. Examination of the access site did not reveal any abnormalities; however, there was significant tenderness noted in the right lower quadrant, and scrotal swelling was observed. The operator again reviewed the femoral artery angiogram shown in Figure 25-3 and became concerned about

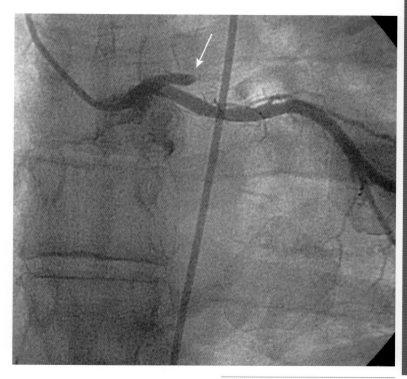

FIGURE 25-1. This is the initial left coronary angiogram demonstrating total occlusion of the proximal left anterior descending coronary artery (*arrow*).

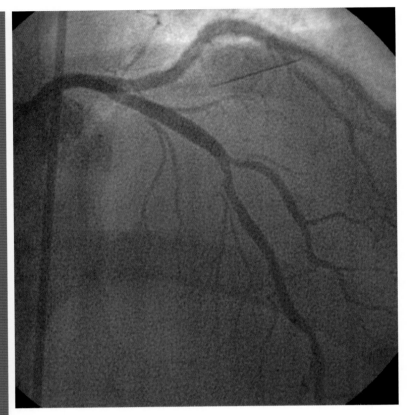

FIGURE 25-2. Representative left coronary angiogram showing the final angiographic result after balloon angioplasty and stenting.

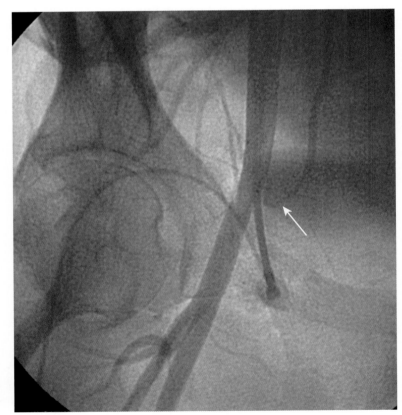

FIGURE 25-3. This is a right femoral artery angiogram obtained in a right anterior oblique projection. The insertion site of the sheath appears to enter the artery just above the lower border of the inferior epigastric artery (*arrow*) consistent with a high puncture above the inguinal ligament.

the possibility of a retroperitoneal bleed. The infusion of eptifibatide was stopped and manual pressure was applied to the access site for 30 minutes. A bolus of 500 cc of normal saline and 1 mg of atropine restored the blood pressure and heart rate to normal. The hematocrit slowly fell from an immediate postcatheterization value of 36.0% to 27.1%, and increased to 34% after a two unit transfusion of packed red cells. Blood pressure, heart rate, and hematocrit remained stable and right lower abdominal discomfort improved. The right lower abdominal discomfort and scrotal swelling gradually resolved over the subsequent 3 days. He remained symptom-free and was discharged 4 days after admission.

DISCUSSION

Few complications of percutaneous coronary intervention are as insidious as a retroperitoneal bleed. Retroperitoneal bleeds complicate about 0.5% to 0.7% of coronary interventions performed via the femoral artery.[1-3] Although they are relatively rare, they are associated with a high incidence of serious adverse outcomes, including death in 10% to 12% of cases.[2,3] Clearly, the most common cause of a retroperitoneal bleed is from inadvertent puncture of the artery above the inguinal ligament when obtaining femoral artery access. Rarely, a retroperitoneal bleed may be caused by spontaneous hemorrhage from anticoagulation, puncture of a vein, or from perforation of the iliac artery or aorta when advancing guide catheters or sheaths through tortuous vessels. Risk factors for development of retroperitoneal bleed have been well-studied and include female gender, high arterial puncture, chronic renal insufficiency, low body weight, and the use of glycoprotein IIb/IIIa inhibitors.[1-3]

The diagnosis of a retroperitoneal bleed may prove challenging, as the initial symptoms are often subtle and mimic other conditions. Often, the only clue to a retroperitoneal bleed is sustained or fluctuating hypotension, present in nearly all cases. The retroperitoneal space is intensely innervated with vagal afferents and thus, symptoms of increased vagal tone such as bradycardia, nausea, diaphoresis, and pallor are very frequently observed. Lower abdominal pain is more common than back pain. Subtle symptoms attributable to other causes may predominate including urinary difficulties, suprapubic discomfort, and symptoms from compression of the femoral nerve. A drop in hematocrit is universally seen but may not be immediately observed, mandating the need for serial assessments when suspecting this complication. Because the bleeding is directed internally, the access site usually appears normal without an associated hematoma.

In most cases, the diagnosis is based on clinical assessment. This complication should be considered in any patient with unexplained hypotension, vagal symptoms, and anemia following the removal of a femoral artery sheath. Computed tomography imaging is diagnostic and confirms the extent of the bleed as well as the precise site of hemorrhage, but this test should be used cautiously as these patients may be too unstable to allow transfer to a radiographic suite.

The patient presented here demonstrated many of the classic manifestations of a postprocedural retroperitoneal bleed. Femoral artery angiography demonstrated a high puncture; additionally, the patient was treated with a glycoprotein IIb/IIIa inhibitor. Symptoms were classic and began soon after sheath removal. Fortunately, this complication was recognized rapidly and aggressive management prevented serious sequelae.

In addition to the high mortality rate, retroperitoneal bleeding is associated with significant morbidity. Many adverse events are related to prolonged hypotension including renal failure, hepatic or acute lung injury, and multisystem failure. Blood transfusion is needed in 60% to 90% of patients.[1,2] Stent thrombosis may arise from hypotension, as well as from abrupt reversal of anticoagulation and transfusion of blood products. Vascular surgical repair may be necessary in 5% to 15% of cases, usually for ongoing bleeding despite conservative measures or for the development of compressive neuropathy or uropathy.[1-4]

Although not entirely preventable, this dreaded complication can be minimized by using fluoroscopy to guide femoral artery access. Puncture should be directed no higher than the middle of the femoral head. Femoral artery angiography performed by injecting contrast through the side arm of the femoral sheath confirms the puncture site in most cases. The lower border of the loop created by the inferior epigastric artery defines the lower border of the retroperitoneal space (Figure 25-3); arterial access above this site may lead to a retroperitoneal bleed following sheath removal. Without a firm base formed by the bony mass of the femoral head, application of manual pressure cannot effectively compress the artery. Bleeding is directed internally and, reassured by the absence of bleeding from the incision site or development of a hematoma, the operator falsely assumes hemostasis has been achieved. The role of vascular closure devices in the development of this complication is controversial. Operators are urged to avoid them in the event of high puncture.

Prompt and aggressive management of a retroperitoneal bleed may prevent the serious consequences described above. Initial attention is directed at hemodynamic resuscitation. Infusion of saline followed by transfusion of blood products and pressor support as needed to maintain blood pressure, urine output, and hematocrit represents the mainstay of initial therapy. In most cases, anticoagulants such as heparin and the glycoprotein IIb/IIIa inhibitors should be stopped and their action reversed. The decision to stop clopidogrel and aspirin in a patient with a recently placed stent should be made with great caution; in general, these agents should be continued. Additional manual compression at the site may help staunch the ongoing hemorrhage. While it is prudent to involve vascular surgery early in the management of these patients, surgery is indicated in only 5% to 15% of cases, usually because of ongoing hemodynamic instability or transfusion requirement. Endovascular management includes obtaining access from the contralateral side and placing a covered stent across the puncture site in the vessel to stop the bleeding and eliminate the need for complex surgery.

KEY CONCEPTS

1. A retroperitoneal bleed should be suspected in a patient with unexplained hypotension, vagal reaction, and lower abdominal discomfort following removal of a femoral artery sheath.

2. Although rare, this complication is associated with significant morbidity and mortality. Prompt recognition and management are crucial to avoid adverse outcomes. Diagnosis is usually made on clinical grounds; imaging with CT scan may be useful in patients stable for transfer.

3. Risk factors for retroperitoneal bleeding include high arterial puncture, low body weight, chronic renal insufficiency, female gender, and use of glycoprotein IIb/IIIa inhibitors. Performance of fluoroscopy to guide arterial puncture to the middle of the femoral head may reduce the occurrence of this dreaded complication.

4. Management options include cessation of anti-coagulants, volume resuscitation, blood transfusions, and endovascular repair. Vascular surgery is needed in 5% to 15% of patients because of ongoing bleeding and hemodynamic instability.

Selected References

1. Farouque HMO, Tremmel JA, Shabari FR, Aggarwal M, Fearon WF, Ng MKC, Rezaee M, Yeung AC, Lee DP: Risk factors for the development of retroperitoneal hematoma after percutaneous coronary intervention in the era of glycoprotein IIb/IIIa inhibitors and vascular closure devices, *J Am Coll Cardiol* 45:363–368, 2005.

2. Ellis SG, Bhatt D, Kapadia S, Lee D, Yen M, Whitlow PL: Correlates and outcomes of retroperitoneal hemorrhage complicating percutaneous coronary intervention, *Catheter Cardiovasc Interv* 67:541–545, 2006.

3. Tiroch KA, Arora N, Matheny ME, Liu C, Lee TC, Resnic FS: Risk predictors of retroperitoneal hemorrhage following percutaneous coronary intervention, *Am J Cardiol* 102:1473–1476, 2008.

4. Kent KC, Moscucci M, Mansour KA, DiMattia S, Gallagher S, Kuntz R, Skillman JJ: Retroperitoneal hematoma after cardiac catheterization: prevalence, risk factors and optimal management, *J Vasc Surg* 20:905–913, 1994.

Severe Thrombocytopenia After Coronary Intervention

Michael Ragosta, MD, FACC, FSCAI

CASE PRESENTATION

An active 94-year-old retired psychiatrist with prior acute myocardial infarction 3 years earlier presented to the emergency department after awakening from sleep with severe chest pain. He was transported by ambulance where an electrocardiogram confirmed an acute anterior ST-segment elevation myocardial infarction. History obtained from his wife along with a quick review of the records revealed that, 3 years earlier, he presented with an acute anterior infarction complicated by cardiogenic shock and underwent emergent catheterization. That examination uncovered moderate disease in the right coronary artery, chronic occlusion of the proximal circumflex artery, and an acutely occluded, proximal left anterior descending artery. Reperfusion of the left anterior descending artery was successfully established by balloon angioplasty followed by placement of a 2.5 mm diameter by 16 mm long paclitaxel-eluting stent and he remained symptom-free until presentation.

Soon after arrival, his rhythm deteriorated to polymorphic ventricular tachycardia and he was successfully cardioverted to normal sinus rhythm. Two additional episodes of sustained ventricular tachycardia requiring cardioversion followed by progressive hypotension and diminished mental status led to endotracheal intubation and mechanical ventilation. He was administered intravenous infusions of amiodarone and dopamine and transported emergently to the cardiac catheterization laboratory.

CARDIAC CATHETERIZATION

Coronary angiography confirmed complete occlusion of the previously placed stent in the proximal left anterior descending artery and total occlusion of the left circumflex, as previously noted (Figure 26-1 and Video 26-1). There was moderate disease in the right coronary artery (Figure 26-2). After administration of a heparin bolus of 50 units/kg and an eptifibatide bolus (12.6 mg) followed

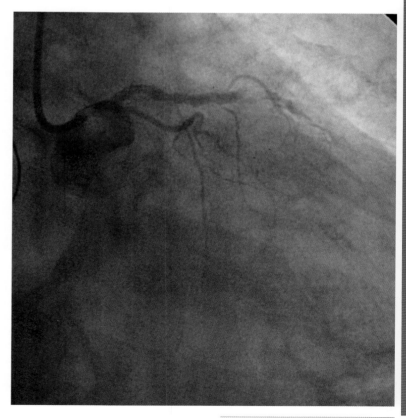

FIGURE 26-1. This angiogram of the left coronary artery shows the acute occlusion of the proximal left anterior descending artery stent and chronic occlusion of the left circumflex artery.

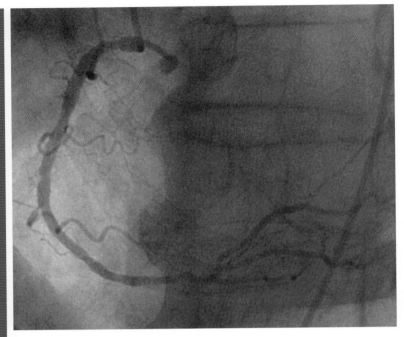

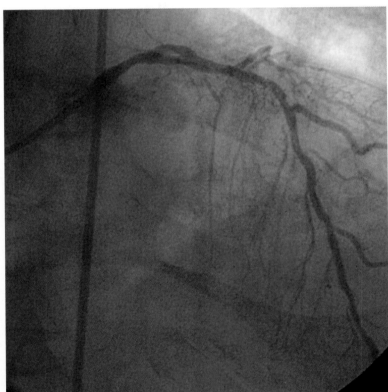

FIGURE 26-2. This is an angiogram of the right coronary artery. There is moderate nonobstructive disease noted in the proximal segment of the artery.

FIGURE 26-3. Angiogram obtained following balloon angioplasty of the occluded stent showing restoration of flow.

by an infusion (2 mcg/kg/min), balloon angioplasty using a 2.5 mm diameter by 20 mm long balloon inflated to high pressures was performed. This restored TIMI-3 flow (Figure 26-3 and Video 26-2).

POSTPROCEDURAL COURSE

The patient was transported to the coronary care unit, requiring dopamine and dobutamine for blood pressure support. He remained intubated but was awake and

responsive and denied chest pain. Routine admission blood analysis found normal renal function and a platelet count of 144×10^9/L. However, the platelet count 2 hours later dropped to 65×10^9/L and the eptifibatide infusion was discontinued. Five hours after receiving eptifibatide, the platelet count decreased to $<10 \times 10^9$/L. Hematology consultation recommended platelet transfusion. This raised the level to 35×10^9/L. Fortunately, the patient had no mucosal, access site, or other evidence of bleeding and platelets recovered to 83×10^9/L by the fourth day, and to $155 \times 10^9/L$ by the sixth day. Meanwhile, his hemodynamic status rapidly improved and the patient was removed from mechanical ventilation and inotropic support within 24 hours. Low dose beta-blocker, angiotensin-converting-enzyme inhibitor, statin, aspirin, and clopidogrel therapy were prescribed and the patient was ultimately discharged home.

DISCUSSION

Although this case dramatically displays the potentially deadly consequences of late stent thrombosis after drug-eluting stent placement, more importantly, this case provides a classic example of the rare complication of acute, profound thrombocytopenia after glycoprotein IIb/IIIa inhibition.

Originally described with abciximab, thrombocytopenia has been associated with all three of the available glycoprotein IIb/IIIa receptor antagonists (abciximab, eptifibatide, and tirofiban). The mechanism is poorly understood but is believed to be an immune-mediated phenomenon.[1] For patients receiving abciximab, thrombocytopenia, defined as a platelet count of less than $100 \times 10^9/L$, occurs in 2.7% of patients. Severe thrombocytopenia (platelet count less than $50 \times 10^9/L$) occurs in 0.8% of patients receiving abciximab and profound thrombocytopenia (platelet count less than $20 \times 10^9/L$) is observed in 0.3% of patients.[2] Severe thrombocytopenia may be less frequent with infusions of eptifibatide and tirofiban than with abciximab, with platelet counts under $50 \times 10^9/L$ occurring in 0.2% to 0.5% of patients after receiving these agents.[1]

It is important to distinguish true thrombocytopenia from "pseudothrombocytopenia"; the latter is due to artifactual clumping of platelets due to the anticoagulants used in the blood collection tubes and for the assay to measure platelets. Identification of platelet clumping on a blood smear and demonstration of a normal platelet count using a different anticoagulant confirms the diagnosis of pseudothrombocytopenia. It is also important to consider heparin-associated thrombocytopenia if this agent has been administered, although the clinical course and level of thrombocytopenia usually differ from that seen with glycoprotein IIb/IIIa receptor antagonists.

As observed in this case, most occurrences of severe and profound thrombocytopenia develop within the first few hours after administration of the drug bolus; for this reason, it is recommended that clinicians measure platelet counts 2 to 4 hours after the bolus is administered and again at 24 hours.[1] Risk factors for the development of thrombocytopenia have been studied and include advanced age, lower body weight, and lower baseline platelet count.[2,3]

Patients developing severe thrombocytopenia are at increased risk of bleeding and have increased mortality compared to those without thrombocytopenia.[2,3] The management of severe thrombocytopenia includes maintaining platelet counts with platelet transfusions and close monitoring for bleeding complications. Immediate discontinuation of the glycoprotein IIb/IIIa receptor antagonist is obviously necessary. Adjunctive use of heparin or other anticoagulants should be avoided until platelet counts recover. The clinician is often faced with a dilemma regarding continued use of clopidogrel and aspirin. Although the cessation of these agents may result in stent thrombosis, continuation in the case of profound thrombocytopenia may lead to life-threatening bleeding and thus the risks and benefits of discontinuation of antiplatelet therapy should be carefully considered. Transfusion of platelets is recommended for platelet counts less than $20 \times 10^9/L$. Platelet counts recover fairly rapidly with cessation of the agent. The case presented here is typical, with full recovery of the platelet count by 5 to 7 days after eptifibatide and 3 to 14 days for abciximab.[1]

KEY CONCEPTS

1. Severe, profound thrombocytopenia occurs in less than 1% of patients treated with any of the currently available glycoprotein IIb/IIIa inhibitors, although it may be more commonly observed with abciximab.
2. Most cases of severe, profound thrombocytopenia are apparent 2 to 4 hours after administration of the agent. Some cases may occur 12 to 24 hours after administration.
3. Patients with severe thrombocytopenia after glycoprotein IIb/IIIa inhibition are at increased risk of bleeding and mortality. Platelet counts recover with cessation of the agent. Normal counts are present by 7 days, in most cases.
4. Management is conservative and includes prompt cessation of the agent, careful monitoring for bleeding complications, and platelet transfusions if counts fall below $20 \times 10^9/L$.

Selected References

1. Huxtable LM, Tafreshi MJ, Rakkar ANS: Frequency and management of thrombocytopenia with the glycoprotein IIb/IIIa receptor antagonists, *Am J Cardiol* 97:426–429, 2006.
2. Berkowitz SD, Sane DC, Sigmon KN, Shavender JH, Harrington RA, Tcheng JE, Topol EJ, Califf RM: Occurrence and clinical significance of thrombocytopenia in a population undergoing high risk percutaneous coronary revascularization, *J Am Coll Cardiol* 32:311–319, 1998.
3. Kereiakes DJ, Berkowitz SD, Lincoff AM, Tcheng JE, Wolski K, Achenbach R, Melsheimer R, Anderson K, Califf RM, Topol EJ: Clinical correlates and course of thrombocytopenia during percutaneous coronary intervention in the era of abciximab platelet glycoprotein IIb/IIIa blockade, *Am Heart J* 140:74–80, 2000.

Loss of Side Branch During Right Coronary Intervention

Michael Ragosta, MD, FACC, FSCAI

CASE PRESENTATION

A 43-year-old woman with untreated hypertension and ongoing tobacco use presented with 2 hours of chest pain occurring at rest and associated with diaphoresis and nausea. An electrocardiogram revealed inferior Q waves and nonspecific inferolateral ST-segment changes. Initially normal, her serum troponin I rose to 0.11 ng/mL. After treatment with aspirin, metoprolol, topical nitrates, atorvastatin, and 1 mg/kg of enoxaparin subcutaneously twice a day, she remained pain-free and was referred for cardiac catheterization.

CARDIAC CATHETERIZATION

Catheterization was performed during the hospital admission. Left ventricular function appeared normal and there was no significant disease noted in the left coronary artery (Figure 27-1); however, collateral filling of the distal right coronary artery was noted. The right coronary artery arose aberrantly high and anterior in the right coronary sinus. Heavy calcification along with severe atherosclerotic narrowing affected the midportion of the right coronary artery, and atherosclerotic disease

also narrowed the ostium of the posterolateral side branch (Figures 27-2, 27-3 and Videos 27-1, 27-2).

Her physician decided to proceed with percutaneous coronary intervention of the right coronary artery. Adequate backup for intervention required a left Amplatz 2.0 guide catheter. Procedural anticoagulation included intravenous bolus of heparin (50 U/kg) and double bolus plus infusion of eptifibatide using standard doses. The operator predilated the stenotic segment with a 2.5 mm diameter by 30 mm long compliant balloon, and chose bare-metal stents because of concern about the patient's compliance with long-term clopidogrel. Two stents successfully treated the diseased segment with a 2.5 mm diameter by 18 mm long stent placed distally and a 3.0 mm diameter by 28 mm long stent deployed proximally (Figure 27-4 and Video 27-3). At this point, the ostium of the posterolateral branch appeared narrowed but remained patent. Noncompliant balloons (2.5 mm diameter by 20 mm long distally and 3.5 mm diameter by 15 mm long proximally) inflated to high pressure were used to postdilate the stented segment. Angiography after high-pressure balloon inflations demonstrated improved appearance of the stented

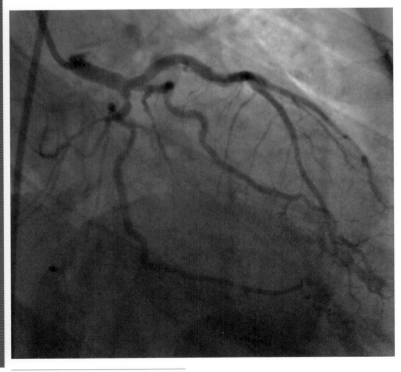

FIGURE 27-1. This is a representative left coronary angiogram. There is no significant obstructive disease noted.

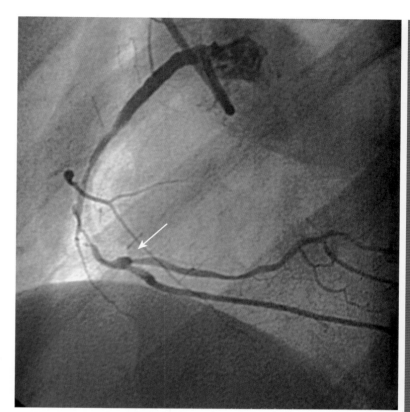

FIGURE 27-2. This is a left anterior oblique (LAO) image of the right coronary artery. There is severe disease of the mid portion of the right coronary artery with heavy calcification noted as well as narrowing of the ostium of the posterolateral branch (*arrow*).

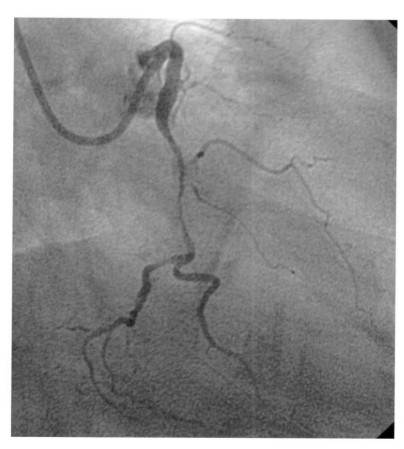

FIGURE 27-3. This right anterior oblique (RAO) projection with caudal angulation shows the severely diseased segment of the right coronary artery.

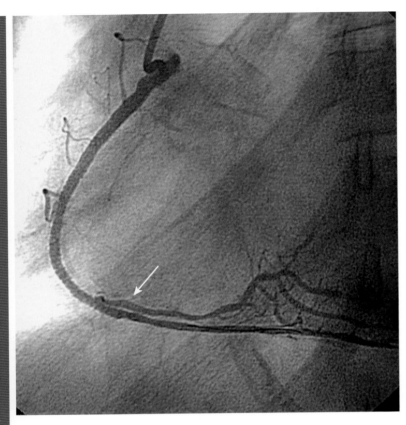

FIGURE 27-4. Right coronary angiogram (LAO projection) after placement of stents. Note continued patency of the posterolateral branch (*arrow*).

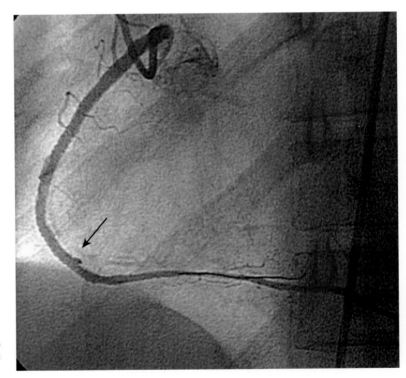

FIGURE 27-5. After postdilatation with a high-pressure balloon, loss of the posterolateral branch was noted on this LAO angiogram (*arrow*).

segment but occlusion of the posterolateral side branch (Figures 27-5, 27-6 and Videos 27-4, 27-5). Although the operator was able to pass a hydrophilic guidewire into the side branch, it was not possible to pass a 2.0 mm diameter by 15 mm long compliant balloon and the

side branch remained closed. The patient left the cardiac catheterization laboratory with ongoing mild chest pain, but her rhythm and blood pressure remained stable and she was transferred to a telemetry unit for monitoring.

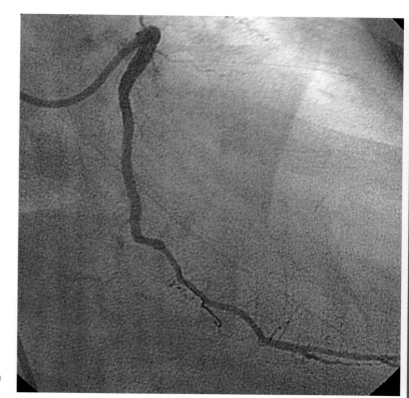

FIGURE 27-6. RAO angiogram post high-pressure balloon showing loss of posterolateral side branch.

POSTPROCEDURAL COURSE

Postprocedure electrocardiogram remained unchanged and chest pain resolved 1 hour after the procedure. She ambulated without any further symptoms. Serial creatine phosphokinase assays rose from a normal baseline (86 U/L with MB fraction of 2.5 ng/mL) to a peak of 253 U/L with MB fraction 21.8 ng/mL 18 hours after the procedure. She was discharged the second day postprocedure on 325 mg aspirin, 75 mg of clopidogrel, metoprolol, and atorvastatin. She remained well with no further chest pain at follow-up 6 months later.

DISCUSSION

Percutaneous management of lesions involving the bifurcation of a side branch can prove challenging. The chief concern relates to the potential loss of the side branch; this event may cause a periprocedural myocardial infarction and result in significant morbidity if the side branch is large. The risk of side branch closure depends on the location of the atheroma. The highest risk of closure occurs when atheroma surrounds and also involves the ostium of the side branch; in such cases, almost 70% of side branches will close following stenting of the main vessel.[1] The risk is lowest when the side branch ostium is free of involvement; closure complicates only about 6% of such cases.[1] As shown in the case presented here, most side branches occlude after post-stent dilatation with a high-pressure balloon. However, closure may also occur after pre-stent balloon inflation or after initial stent deployment.

The wide variety of methods proposed over the years to preserve the side branch is a testimony to the ineffectiveness of most of them. Placing a guidewire into the side branch before stenting the main branch might help maintain patency in some cases but, in the event of closure after stenting, this wire cannot be used for balloon angioplasty or stenting of the side branch because it lies trapped behind the stent in the main artery. At a minimum, this wire will help guide the operator to the location of the side branch ostium and may facilitate recrossing with a new guidewire. In the author's experience, pretreatment of the side branch with either balloon angioplasty or rotational atherectomy before deploying the stent in the main artery is not a guaranteed method of preserving the side branch. Again, closure of the side branch most commonly occurs after the stent is placed or after high-pressure balloon inflation of the stent has been performed, due to the plaque shifts occurring with these events; pre-stent treatment of the side branch (particularly with a balloon) is unlikely to influence this.

Different treatment strategies to treat bifurcation lesions have been proposed, but it appears that optimal outcomes are obtained using a simple strategy of stenting only the main vessel with provisional stenting of the side branch performed only if an unacceptable result is obtained in the side branch.[2] In the author's experience, the "crush" stent technique is the most reliable method of preserving large side branches, but is associated with a high rate of restenosis and stent thrombosis particularly if a final "kissing" balloon cannot be performed.[3]

In the event of side branch closure, a guidewire can often be successfully negotiated through the stent struts and passed distally into the side branch, particularly if there is some residual patency of the side branch. Hydrophilic wires may be successful if a floppy-tipped guidewire fails. Once a guidewire is positioned, low-pressure balloon angioplasty of the ostium can improve the lumen and restore patency. A satisfactory result is defined by restoration of patency without dissection or significant luminal narrowing. It is usually not necessary to strive for a "perfect" angiographic result. Aggressive attempts to enlarge the lumen may dissect the artery and lead to a more complex repair than otherwise necessary. In the case shown here, complete occlusion of the side branch was present and, although a guidewire successfully crossed into the side branch, a low-profile, compliant balloon failed to pass the stent struts and the side branch remained closed. When this occurs, the operator may try removing and repositioning the side branch guidewire in the hope that it passes by a different set of struts, thus allowing passage of the balloon.

KEY CONCEPTS

1. Side branch closure may complicate anywhere from 5% to 70% of bifurcation interventions, depending on the nature of the bifurcation. The greatest risk is present when there is atheroma involving the ostium of the side branch.

2. Closure of a side branch is a major cause of periprocedural myocardial infarction. Not all side branch closures can be successfully reopened.

3. Successful methods of preserving the side branch include positioning a second guide wire into the side branch and the "crush" stent technique.

Selected References

1. Aliabadi D, Tillis FV, Bowers TR, Benjuly KH, Safian RD, Goldstein JA, Grines CL, O'Neill WW: Incidence and angiographic predictors of side branch occlusion following high-pressure intracoronary stenting, *Am J Cardiol* 80:994–997, 1997.

2. Steigen TK, Maeng M, Wiseth R, et al: Nordic PCI Study Group Randomized study on simple versus complex stenting of coronary artery bifurcation lesions: the Nordic Bifurcation Study, *Circulation* 114:1955–1961, 2006.

3. Hoye A, Iakovou I, Ge L, van Mieghem CAG, Ong ATL, Cosgrave J, Sangiorgi GM Airoldi F, Montorfano M, Michev I, Chieffo A, Carlino M, Corvaja N, Aoki J, Granillo GAR, Valgimigli M, Sianos G, van der Giessen WJ, de Feyter PJ, van Domburg RT, et al: Long-term outcomes after stenting of bifurcation lesions with the "crush" technique: Predictors of an adverse outcome, *J Am Coll Cardiol* 47:1949–1958, 2006.

Coronary Perforation Caused by a Guidewire

Michael Ragosta, MD, FACC, FSCAI

CASE PRESENTATION

A 43-year-old man with multiple risk factors for coronary artery disease, including severe dyslipidemia, family history of premature coronary disease, and ongoing tobacco abuse, was referred for cardiac catheterization after presenting with a prolonged episode of rest ischemic chest pain and an elevated troponin I (1.3 ng/mL). Coronary angiography demonstrated three-vessel coronary disease consisting of complex and severe narrowing of the proximal to midsegment of the left anterior descending artery involving a diagonal branch (Figure 28-1 and Video 28-1), severe obstructive disease of the first obtuse marginal artery, total occlusion of the second obtuse marginal and distal left circumflex, and moderate obstructive disease of the posterior descending branch of the right coronary artery, with preserved left ventricular function. After a lengthy discussion regarding therapeutic options, the patient chose to undergo percutaneous revascularization of the lesions in the left anterior descending artery and first obtuse marginal artery.

CARDIAC CATHETERIZATION

In an effort to avoid closure of the diagonal side branch, the operator chose a "crush stent" technique to treat the left anterior descending artery and diagonal branch. Using an 8 French, left Judkins 4.0 guide catheter and procedural anticoagulation consisting of unfractionated heparin (5300 units) and eptifibatide (two boluses of 15.8 mg followed by an infusion of 2 mcg/kg/min), the operator positioned a floppy-tipped 0.014 inch guidewire into both the left anterior descending artery and diagonal branch and predilated the stenosis in the left anterior descending artery with a 2.5 mm diameter by 15 mm long compliant balloon, resulting in further compromise of the lumen of the diagonal artery (Figures 28-2, 28-3 and Video 28-2). Balloon dilation of the diagonal was performed, and during the catheter manipulations, the operator noted that the tip of the diagonal wire appeared to have migrated either into a small branch or outside of the lumen of the diagonal artery (Figure 28-4). The wire was repositioned and angiography demonstrated contrast staining emanating from the diagonal branch

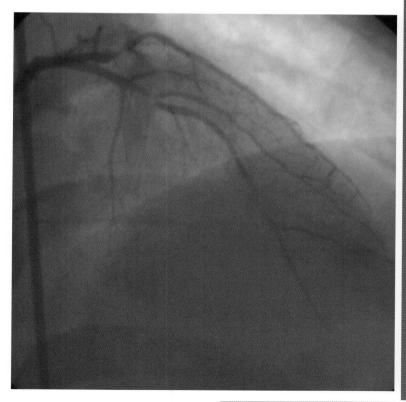

FIGURE 28-1. This coronary angiogram obtained in the right anterior oblique projection with cranial angulation depicts the complex stenosis involving the proximal left anterior descending artery and diagonal branch.

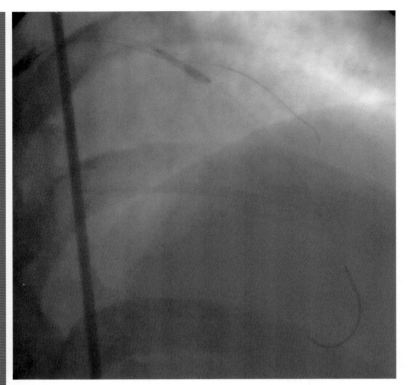

FIGURE 28-2. A floppy-tipped guidewire was placed in both the diagonal branch and the left anterior descending artery and balloon angioplasty of the left anterior descending artery was performed.

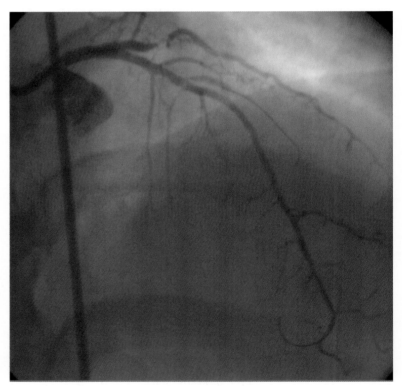

FIGURE 28-3. This angiogram shows the result of balloon angioplasty. While the left anterior descending stenosis responded well to balloon angioplasty, there is compromise of the ostium of the first diagonal branch.

consistent with a wire perforation (Figure 28-5 and Video 28-3). The patient remained asymptomatic and hemodynamically stable with no evidence of tamponade. The operator continued the eptifibatide infusion after repeat angiography 5 minutes later showed persistent contrast staining but no evidence of active bleeding from the site. The "crush stent" procedure was performed with a 3.0 mm diameter by 18 mm long sirolimus-eluting stent placed in the left anterior descending artery and a 2.25 mm diameter by 12 mm long bare-metal stent placed in the diagonal branch (Figure 28-6). The final angiographic appearance was excellent with no evidence of additional contrast extravasation from the wire perforation site (Figure 28-7 and Video 28-4). The obtuse marginal lesion was then treated with another drug-eluting stent without complication.

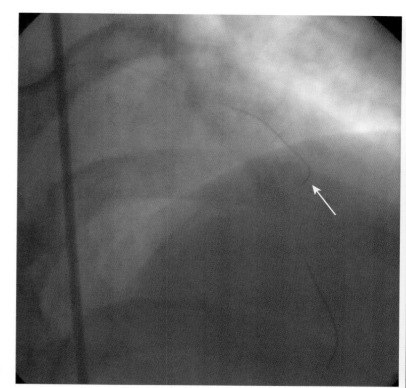

FIGURE 28-4. The tip of the diagonal wire appears to have deviated from the main lumen (*arrow*).

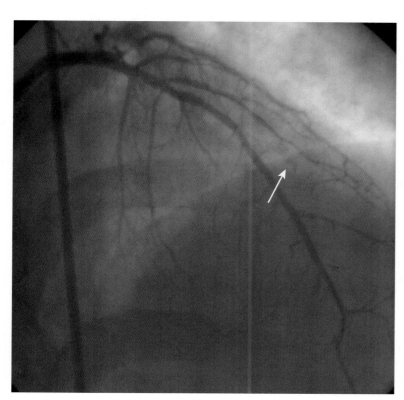

FIGURE 28-5. Extravasation of contrast was noted after the wire tip was repositioned (*arrow*).

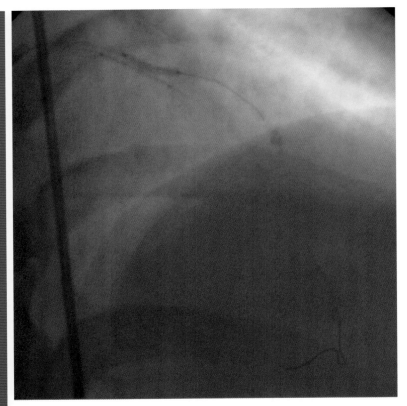

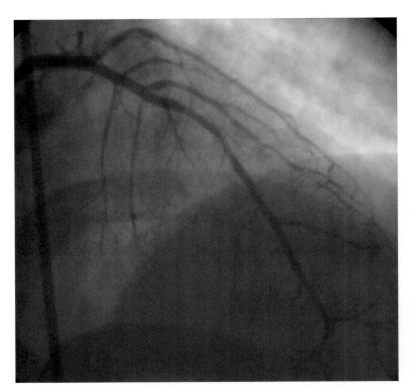

FIGURE 28-6. This figure depicts the configuration of the stents positioned to perform the "crush stent" procedure.

FIGURE 28-7. Angiogram obtained after stent deployment. There was no change in the appearance of contrast staining throughout the procedure.

POSTPROCEDURAL COURSE

His postprocedural course was uncomplicated. After overnight observation, he was discharged on metoprolol, atorvastatin, aspirin, and clopidogrel. He remained free of angina 1 year later. Interestingly, he developed recurrent angina nearly 3 years later and was found to have progressive disease in the right coronary artery; however, the stents placed in the left anterior descending and diagonal arteries remained widely patent (Figure 28-8).

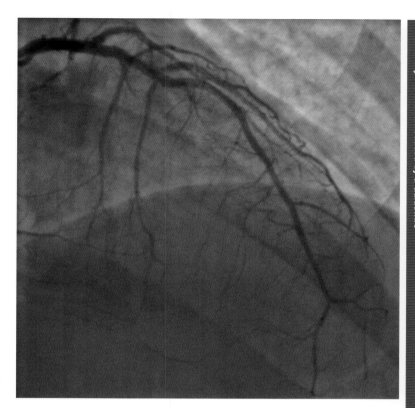

FIGURE 28-8. This angiogram was obtained 3 years later and showed wide patency of the bifurcation stents.

DISCUSSION

Perforation of the coronary artery is a potentially deadly complication of coronary intervention.[1] The clinical consequences range from a benign angiographic finding to dramatic cardiovascular collapse from tamponade caused by frank bleeding into the pericardial space from a large tear in the artery. The perforation shown in the case presented here was caused by the 0.014 inch guidewire and is an example of the benign side of the spectrum of coronary perforation.

Most guidewire perforations are caused by attempts at crossing a severe stenosis or from aggressive attempts at crossing a chronic occlusion with stiff-tipped guide wires. Another common cause, as demonstrated by this case, is from the inadvertent distal migration of the wire tip into a small side branch and subsequent perforation. Meticulous attention to the distal location of the wire tip and ensuring that the tip remains in the main artery during advancement of balloon and stent catheters helps prevent this type of guidewire perforation.

Guidewire perforations are generally well-tolerated because the hole is very small (0.014 inch). However, tamponade may result if the perforation communicates with the pericardial space and if there is continued bleeding, particularly if glycoprotein IIb/IIIa inhibitors are used. In this case, there was no evidence that the perforation extended beyond the perivascular tissues and the patient did not develop a pericardial effusion or evidence of tamponade. This case only required close observation and wire repositioning for effective management.

In the event of free contrast extravasation and tamponade, management of a guidewire perforation is similar to that caused by other mechanisms. Depending on the patient's clinical status, management may include pericardiocentesis, cessation and reversal of procedural anticoagulants, and immediate balloon inflation in the vessel proximal to the perforation site. Prolonged balloon inflation (10 to 20 minutes) may be required to staunch bleeding while efforts are taken to correct the procedural coagulopathy. The PTFE-covered stents do not have a role since the site of perforation is distal and not amenable to this strategy.[2,3] Rarely, surgery is necessary for guidewire perforations; this is more likely in the presence of a chronic occlusion with perforation from unsuccessful attempts at crossing the occlusion with a guidewire. In this situation, there may be back-bleeding from collaterals or the operator may find it difficult or impossible to inflate a balloon proximal to the perforation without distal wire access.

KEY CONCEPTS

1. Guidewire perforations are usually caused by attempts to cross a severe stenosis or chronic occlusion with stiff-tipped guide wires or from the inadvertent distal migration of a wire tip in a small branch during catheter advancement.

2. Many cases of guidewire perforations are well-tolerated; particularly if they result only in perivascular staining without communication to the pericardial space. However, if there is

communication with the pericardial space, guidewire perforations may result in tamponade, particularly in the presence of potent procedural anticoagulants.

3. The principles of management of guidewire perforation are similar to the management of any coronary perforation and include concentration on the patient's hemodynamic status, cessation and reversal of procedural anticoagulants, and prolonged balloon inflations to seal the perforation site. Surgery may be necessary if these steps do not stop bleeding.

Selected References

1. Fasseas P, Orford JL, Panetta CJ, et al: Incidence, correlates, management and clinical outcome of coronary perforation: Analysis of 16,298 procedures, *Am Heart J* 147:140–145, 2004.
2. Briguori C, Nishida T, Anzuini A, DiMario C, Grube E, Colombo A: Emergency polytetrafluoroethylene-covered stent implantation to treat coronary ruptures, *Circulation* 102:3028–3031, 2000.
3. Lansky AJ, Yank Y, Khan Y, Costa RA, Pietras C, Tsuchiya Y, Cristea E, Collins M, Mehran R, Dangas GD, Moses JW, Leon MB, Stone GW: Treatment of coronary artery perforations complicating percutaneous coronary intervention with a polytetrafluoroethylene-covered stent graft, *Am J Cardiol* 98:370–374, 2006.

Acute Vessel Closure During Coronary Intervention

Michael Ragosta, MD, FACC, FSCAI

CASE PRESENTATION

A 57-year-old woman with prior bypass surgery consisting of a left internal mammary graft to the left anterior descending artery and a saphenous vein graft to the right coronary artery presented with the acute onset of prolonged rest chest pain and an elevated troponin I (7.0 ng/mL). In addition to the prior bypass surgery, other important medical history included diabetes, end-stage renal disease treated with hemodialysis, and a prior episode of ventricular tachycardia resulting in implantation of a defibrillator.

Coronary angiography performed at another hospital demonstrated patent bypass grafts but severe disease in the ungrafted ramus intermedius and left circumflex arteries. Initially treated medically, she reported ongoing severe angina and was referred for coronary intervention of the ramus and circumflex arteries.

CARDIAC CATHETERIZATION

Representative angiograms of her left coronary artery are shown in Figures 29-1, 29-2 and Videos 29-1, 29-2. A complex lesion was present in the proximal portion of the ramus intermedius at a bifurcation. The proximal to midsegment of the circumflex was also severely diseased. Importantly, this artery branched from the left main with marked angulation, clearly seen in the left anterior oblique view with caudal angulation (see Figure 29-1).

Procedural anticoagulation was accomplished with an intravenous heparin bolus to achieve an activated clotting time greater than 300 seconds and a supportive guide catheter was chosen (6 French JCL 4.5). The operator began with the ramus intermedius (Figure 29-3). This lesion was successfully treated with balloon angioplasty (2.5 mm diameter by 15 mm long compliant balloon) followed by placement of an everolimus-eluting

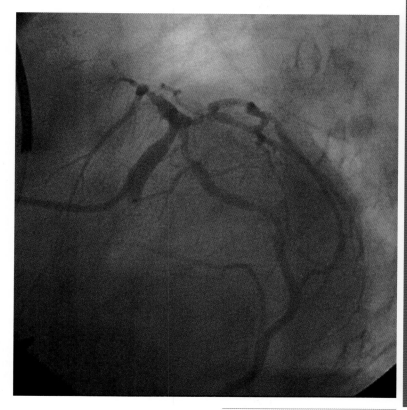

FIGURE 29-1. This is a left anterior oblique projection of the left coronary artery demonstrating severe disease in both the ramus intemedius and the left circumflex artery. Note the extreme angulation of the circumflex relative to the left main coronary artery.

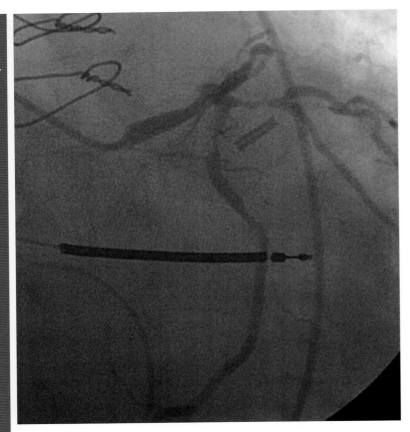

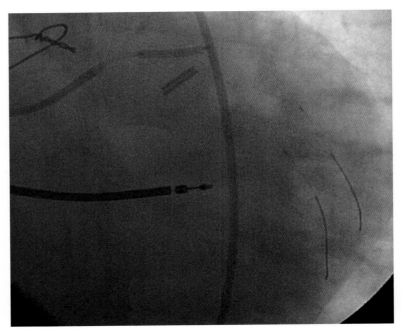

FIGURE 29-2. This is a right anterior oblique projection with caudal angulation demonstrating the ramus and circumflex lesions.

FIGURE 29-3. A balloon angioplasty followed by stenting of the ramus intermedius was performed with protection of a lower branch of the ramus.

stent (2.75 mm diameter by 18 mm long) (Figure 29-4 and Video 29-3).

Following the successful procedure on the ramus intermedius, the operator turned attention to the circumflex. Due to excessive angulation, the operator was unable to pass a 0.014 inch floppy-tipped conventional guidewire; a hydrophilic guidewire ultimately proved successful. The operator used a compliant balloon (2.5 mm diameter by 15 mm long) to predilate the lesion (Figures 29-5, 29-6 and Video 29-4) then removed the balloon catheter and attempted to pass an everolimus-eluting stent (3.0 mm diameter by 15 mm long). This was not successful because the stent would not advance around the acute angle. The guidewire was replaced with a stiffer shaft wire (Boston Scientific Mailman) and a shorter bare-metal stent was also attempted (3.0 mm

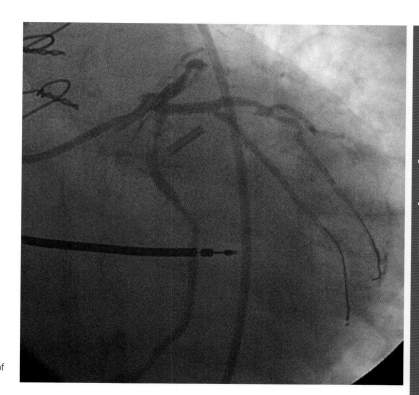

FIGURE 29-4. This angiogram depicts the result of intervention on the ramus intermedius branch.

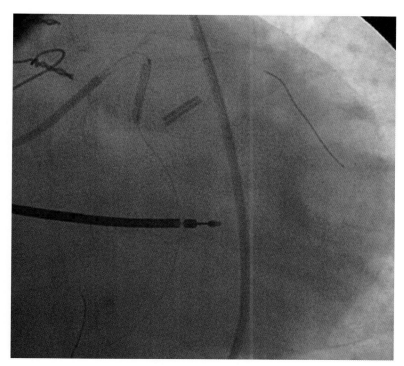

FIGURE 29-5. With great difficulty, a guidewire was advanced into the circumflex artery and balloon angioplasty performed.

diameter by 9 mm long) but failed to advance as well. During attempts to advance the stent, the guide catheter disengaged and distal wire access was lost. The guide was reengaged. Again, the operator had great difficulty advancing a 0.014 inch polymer-tipped guidewire and created a dissection resulting in vessel closure (Figures 29-7, 29-9 and Videos 29-5, 29-6). Attempts to regain the distal lumen using a variety of other guidewires failed. The patient reported chest pain but remained hemodynamically stable without arrhythmia. At this point, the procedure was stopped and the patient admitted to the coronary care unit.

POSTPROCEDURAL COURSE

After admission to the coronary care unit, she was placed on an intravenous infusion of nitroglycerin. She continued to report chest pain for several hours.

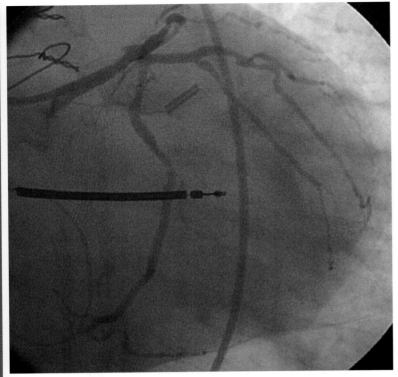

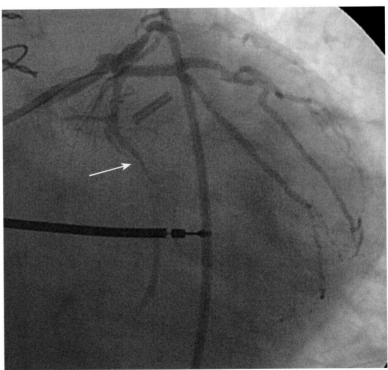

FIGURE 29-6. This is the angiographic appearance of the circumflex after balloon angioplasty. In retrospect, the operator would have settled for this result!

FIGURE 29-7. After losing access to the artery, attempts at recrossing the lesion resulted in extensive dissection of the artery as shown (arrow).

An admission electrocardiogram demonstrated lateral ST-segment depression and an initial troponin I was 0.04 ng/mL, peaking 20 hours after the intervention at 19.51 ng/mL. Transthoracic echocardiogram showed mild inferoposterior hypokinesis with preserved ejection fraction. She became free of chest pain, was observed in-hospital for several days, and was ultimately discharged on carvedilol, clopidogrel, aspirin, simvastatin, and lisinopril. She remained free of symptoms at 6-week follow-up.

DISCUSSION

Abrupt vessel closure after angioplasty is a serious complication associated with death, myocardial infarction, or need for emergency bypass surgery.[1] Most cases of abrupt vessel closure are due to extensive dissection of the artery with vessel occlusion caused by intimal flaps, intramural hematoma, or thrombus. During the balloon era, abrupt vessel closure complicated 2% to 8% of

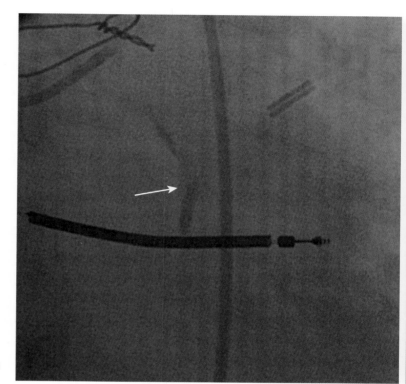

FIGURE 29-8. Contrast retention due to the extensive dissection is shown here (*arrow*).

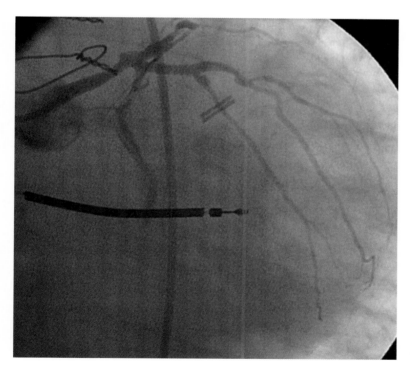

FIGURE 29-9. Final appearance of the artery with closure of the circumflex.

coronary interventions and the only definitive therapy consisted of emergency bypass surgery. Coronary stents offered the first effective percutaneous solution and dramatically reduced the need for emergency surgery.

Despite the advances in technology, abrupt closure remains an important risk in the current era. As demonstrated by this case, the inability to deliver a stent to a complex lesion or an extensively dissected segment leaves the operator few options in the event of vessel closure. Proximal vessel tortuosity, extreme angulation, heavy coronary calcification, and noncompliant vessels are all scenarios where a stent might not be deliverable. At this juncture, the operator is faced with the decision of emergency bypass surgery versus conservative medical management of the closed vessel and associated myocardial infarction. Emergency bypass surgery, still necessary in about 0.4% of percutaneous coronary interventions, is a fairly morbid event, associated with an in-hospital mortality of 8%, and is more likely to be justified when the occluded vessel supplies a large amount of myocardium.[2] In the case presented here, the benefit of revascularizing a small vascular territory was greatly outweighed by the risk of emergent surgery in a patient with significant comorbid conditions.

The difficult anatomy present in this case set the stage for this complication. Extreme angulation of the origin of the circumflex from the left main stem made it difficult to torque and advance guidewires, necessitating the use of a polymer-tipped wire. Although this allowed successful passage and enough support for balloon dilatation, a stent could not be delivered. The fateful event occurred when the operator lost guidewire access. There were probably numerous small intimal tears in the lesion caused by balloon angioplasty. Attempts to recross this complex lesion undoubtedly propagated these tears, leading to the extensive spiral dissection observed in this case. The complex labyrinth of intimal flaps thwarted the operator's attempts at finding the true distal lumen, especially given the extreme angulation and inability to precisely turn and advance the guidewire.

KEY CONCEPTS

1. Abrupt vessel closure remains a potential complication of coronary intervention, potentially resulting in serious morbidity including myocardial infarction, death, and emergency surgery.
2. In the current era, most cases are due to extensive vessel dissection and inability to repair with a stent.
3. Emergency surgery is still required in about 0.4% of coronary interventions.

Selected References

1. Klein LW: Coronary complications of percutaneous coronary intervention: A practical approach to the management of abrupt closure, *Catheter Cardiovasc Interv* 64:395–401, 2005.
2. Roy P, de labriolle A, Hanna N, Bonello L, Okabe T, Slottow TLP, Steinberg DH, Torguson R, Kaneshige K, Xue Z, Satler LF, Kent KM, Suddath WO, Pichard AD, Lindsay J, Waksman R: Requirement for emergent coronary artery bypass surgery following percutaneous coronary intervention in the stent era, *Am J Cardiol* 103:950–953, 2009.

Intracranial Hemorrhage After Coronary Intervention

Michael Ragosta, MD, FACC, FSCAI

CASE PRESENTATION

An active 73-year-old woman, who enjoyed good health with only a history of hypertension, hyperlipidemia, and osteoporosis, presented to the hospital emergency department on a Saturday night with a prolonged episode of rest angina. She became pain-free after administration of 325 mg of aspirin, subcutaneous enoxaparin, and sublingual nitrates. The initially-normal electrocardiogram evolved T-wave inversions on subsequent studies and troponin peaked at 0.52 ng/mL. She was diagnosed with a non-ST segment elevation myocardial infarction and remained pain-free on enoxaparin (1 mg/kg administered subcutaneously twice a day) and 325 mg of aspirin administered each day over the weekend with catheterization planned for Monday morning.

CATHETERIZATION

Left venticulography revealed mild anterior hypokinesis with preserved ejection fraction. Coronary angiography found no evidence of obstructive disease in the right or left circumflex coronary arteries. Severe atherosclerotic narrowing of the proximal segment of the left anterior descending artery was likely the explanation for her acute coronary syndrome (Figures 30-1, 30-2 and Videos 30-1, 30-2). Atherosclerosis also involved the first diagonal branch and the midsegment of the left anterior descending artery, but these lesions were felt to be nonobstructive. The lesion in the proximal segment of the left anterior descending artery was treated with balloon angioplasty followed by placement of a everolimus-eluting stent (2.5 mm diameter by 15 mm long) with an excellent angiographic result (Figure 30-3 and Video 30-3), and intravascular ultrasound confirmed stent apposition. The dose of enoxaparin planned for the morning of the procedure was held (last dose greater than 12 hours from catheterization) and procedural anticoagulation consisted of bivalirudin (33 mg intravenous bolus followed by an intravenous infusion of 1.7 mg/kg/hr) and 600 mg of clopidogrel administered orally at the time of the intervention. Hemostasis was achieved with a femoral artery closure device and she returned to a telemetry unit feeling well with no complaints.

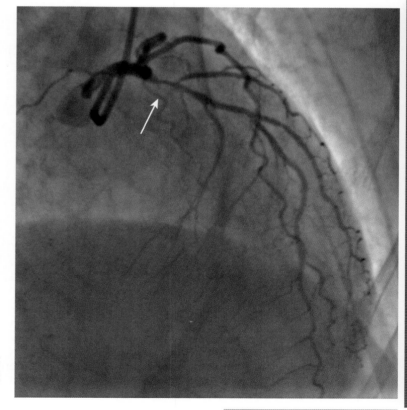

FIGURE 30-1. Coronary angiography performed in a right anterior oblique projection with cranial angulation showing a severe stenosis in the proximal left anterior descending artery (arrow).

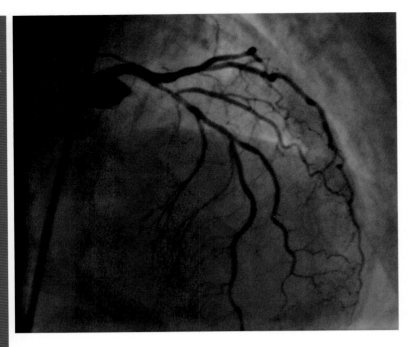

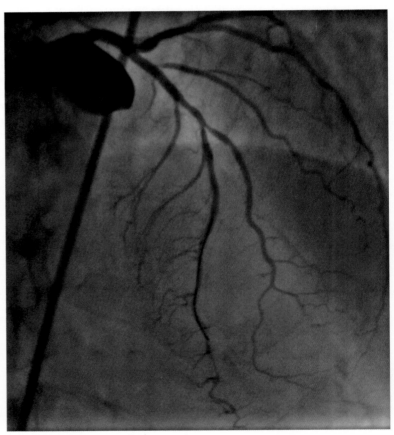

FIGURE 30-2. This is another view of the left anterior descending artery in the right anterior oblique view, showing the lesion in the proximal left anterior descending artery.

FIGURE 30-3. Angiogram obtained after placement of a stent in the proximal left anterior descending artery.

POSTPROCEDURAL COURSE

The patient remained symptom-free overnight, with discharge planned for the next day. However, the morning after her procedure, she reported the acute onset of headache, vertigo, and unsteady gait. An emergency noncontrast head CT scan was performed and showed a right cerebellar hemorrhage. She was transferred to the neuro intensive care unit for further evaluation and management. A brain magnetic resonance imaging study revealed an acute intraparenchymal hemorrhage centered in the right cerebellar hemisphere with mass effect upon the fourth ventricle and no evidence of hydrocephalus. In addition, there was no evidence of tumor or vascular malformation. Scattered, discrete small supratentorial white matter signal abnormalities were noted and were felt to represent chronic small vessel ischemic changes.

After consultation with cardiology, the aspirin and clopidogrel were held for 5 days, and the patient was monitored continuously in the intensive care unit. Fortunately, she remained neurologically stable with improvement in her vertigo and headache and no change in the size of the intracranial bleed on subsequent imaging. Blood pressure remained well-controlled on lisinopril and aspirin, and clopidogrel resumed on the fifth day. She remained stable for 3 additional days and was discharged with only mild gait instability.

DISCUSSION

Cerebrovascular accidents are a rare but dreaded complication of percutaneous cardiovascular procedures, occurring in 0.2% to 0.4% of procedures and associated with a high mortality.[1,2] Most of these events are caused by atheroembolism or clot. Despite the liberal use of procedural anticoagulation, intracranial hemorrhage is, fortunately, very rare. In large series of patients treated with bivalirudin, the risk of intracranial hemorrhage was exceedingly low (one event out of 2993 patients or 0.03%)[3]; the rate of intracranial hemorrhage when the more powerful glycoprotein IIb/IIIa inhibitors are used is similarly very small at only 0.07%.[3] Following intervention, anticoagulation is maintained using dual antiplatelet therapy with the risk of hemorrhagic stroke from the combination of aspirin and clopidogrel of only 0.1% with no difference from aspirin alone.[4]

Management of an intracranial bleed occurring soon after deployment of a coronary stent is a genuine medical catch-22. The same is true for any other major life-threatening bleed such as a serious gastrointestinal or genitourinary hemorrhage. On one hand, the anticoagulants must be stopped to staunch the life-threatening bleed; on the other hand, cessation of anticoagulants might cause acute stent thrombosis and a potentially fatal acute myocardial infarction. The decisions to stop, continue, or hold and reinstitute anticoagulants in the setting of a freshly-deployed stent should not be made in a cavalier fashion. Extensive discussions regarding the risks and benefits of each strategy should occur with the consultant expert as well as the patient and family, with a coherent plan in place to anticipate and treat any potential adverse outcome. In the present case, the serious nature of intracranial hemorrhage led to the wise decision to hold anticoagulation, thus preventing further bleeding and, fortunately, resulting in a favorable outcome.

KEY CONCEPTS

1. The risk of periprocedural cerebrovascular accident is very small and usually due to atheroembolic event; the risk of intracranial hemorrhage is exceedingly rare.
2. Non–access-related bleeding (gastrointestinal, genitourinary, intracranial) after stent placement provides a formidable challenge to the clinician. Cessation of antiplatelet agents, often necessary to prevent ongoing bleeding, may lead to acute stent thrombosis, and difficult decisions are necessary for optimal patient outcome. Careful collaboration with the appropriate specialists may help with these decisions.

Selected References

1. Hamon M, Baron JC, Viader F, Hamon M: Periprocedural stroke and cardiac catheterization, *Circulation* 118:678–683, 2008.
2. Aggarwal A, Dai D, Rumsfeld JS, Klein LW, Roe MT on behalf of the American College of Cardiology National Cardiovascular Data Registry: Incidence and predictors of stroke associated with percutaneous coronary intervention, *Am J Cardiol* 104:349–353, 2009.
3. Lincoff AM, Bittl JA, Harrington RA, for the REPLACE-2 Investigators: Bivalirudin and provisional glycoprotein IIb/IIIa blockade compared with heparin and planned glycoprotein IIb/IIIa blockade during percutaneous coronary intervention REPLACE-2 randomized trial, *JAMA* 289:853–863, 2003.
4. CURE Study Investigators: Effects of clopidogrel in addition to aspirin in patients with acute coronary syndromes without ST-segment elevation, *N Engl J Med* 345:494–502, 2001.

Coronary Artery Pseudoaneurysm After Stenting

Michael Ragosta, MD, FACC, FSCAI

CASE PRESENTATION

An actively smoking, 65-year-old woman with hypertension, hyperlipidemia, and carotid artery disease presented with dyspnea and chest discomfort radiating to her left arm, occurring at a low workload. A coronary angiogram found severe narrowing of a small caliber diagonal branch and at least moderate narrowing of a heavily calcified segment of the midportion of the left anterior descending artery (Figure 31-1). The circumflex and right coronary arteries appeared normal, and left ventricular function was preserved. Initially treated medically with aspirin, clopidogrel, beta-blockers, and statins, she continued to have persistent angina and was referred for intervention of the diagonal and possibly the left anterior descending artery several weeks later.

CARDIAC CATHETERIZATION

During the second procedure, the operator found it difficult to determine the significance of the disease in the midsegment of the left anterior descending artery and performed intravascular ultrasound. This showed extensive calcification and a minimal luminal area of 1.5 mm^2 (Figure 31-2). Based on this data, the operator planned to treat the disease in both the left anterior descending artery and diagonal branch. An 8 French 4.0 left Judkins guide was engaged into the left coronary ostium and 0.014 inch guidewires were positioned distally in both the left anterior descending artery and the diagonal branch; bivalirudin bolus and infusion were used as the procedural anticoagulant. The extensive calcification is shown in Figure 31-3. Balloon angioplasty of the diagonal using a 2.0 mm diameter by 20 mm long compliant

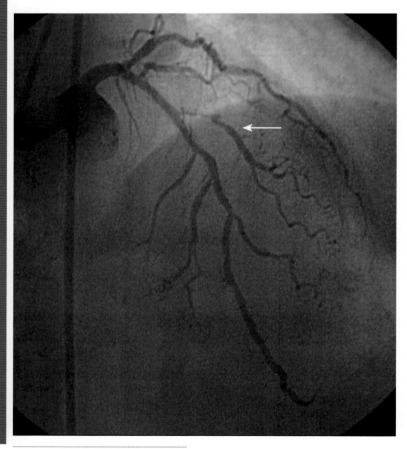

FIGURE 31-1. In this coronary angiogram, the first diagonal artery (*arrow*) is severely narrowed and the left anterior descending artery appears only moderately narrowed.

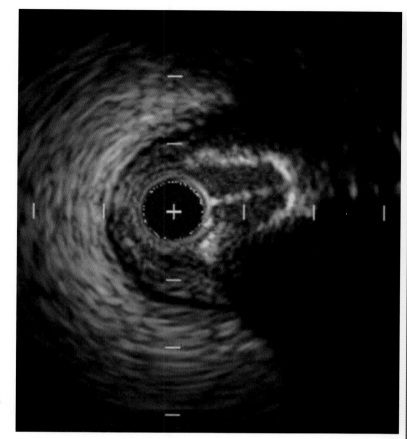

FIGURE 31-2. This intravascular ultrasound image was obtained in the mid-left anterior descending artery at the site of moderate narrowing. There is extensive calcification and severe luminal obstruction.

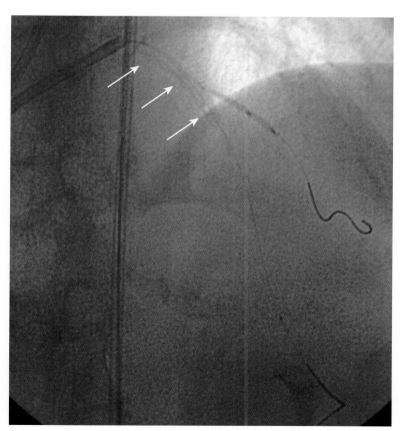

FIGURE 31-3. A guidewire was placed into both the diagonal and distal left anterior descending arteries and balloon angioplasty performed on the diagonal branch. Note the extensive calcification of the left anterior descending artery on fluoroscopy (arrows).

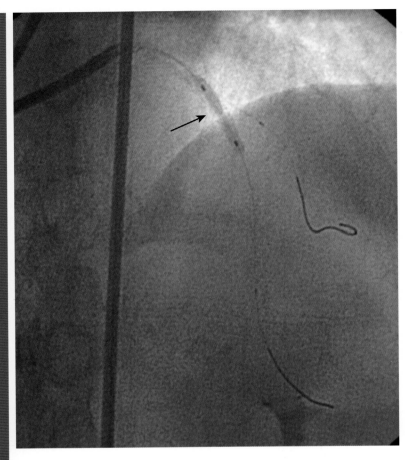

FIGURE 31-4. Balloon angioplasty of the left anterior descending artery was notable for persistence of a waist despite high pressure inflations (*arrow*).

balloon (see Figure 31-3) and the left anterior descending artery using a 2.5 mm diameter by 20 mm long compliant balloon (Figure 31-4) was performed. The operator noted that the balloon in the left anterior descending artery did not appear fully expanded at nominal inflation pressures, and, although the luminal appearance improved after angioplasty, a linear dissection in the left anterior descending artery and severe narrowing of the ostium of the diagonal branch were apparent (Figure 31-5 and Video 31-1). At this point, although the operator worried that a stent might not fully expand in the left anterior descending artery, the presence of a significant dissection led to a decision against rotational atherectomy. The operator chose a "crush stent" approach to preserve patency of the diagonal branch using a 2.25 mm diameter by 15 mm long bare-metal stent in the diagonal and a 2.5 mm diameter by 24 mm long paclitaxel-eluting stent in the left anterior descending artery (Figure 31-6). The diagonal stent expanded appropriately, but the operator noted a waist in the balloon used to deploy the left anterior descending artery stent, despite 14 atmospheres inflation pressure. The post-stent angiogram confirmed inadequate stent expansion at this site (Figure 31-7 and Video 31-2). A waist remained in the balloon at the site of persistent narrowing despite the use of a 2.5 mm diameter by 9 mm long noncompliant balloon inflated to 20 atmospheres pressure (Figure 31-8) and caused no change in the angiographic appearance of the lesion. The operator used a 3.0 mm diameter by 15 mm long noncompliant balloon,

slowly inflating the balloon until the waist suddenly resolved at 20 atmospheres. With the deflated balloon in place, an angiogram was performed, which revealed contrast extravasation outside of the wall of the artery consistent with a deep dissection or contained perforation (Figure 31-9 and Video 31-3). The bivalirudin infusion was stopped and the patient remained asymptomatic and hemodynamically stable. Five minutes later, another angiogram was performed and showed no evidence of contrast extravasation and an excellent luminal result in both the left anterior descending and diagonal arteries (Figure 31-10 and Video 31-4). She was observed an additional 10 minutes with no change in the angiogram. An echocardiogram showed no pericardial effusion. She was observed overnight and discharged the next morning.

POSTPROCEDURAL COURSE

She remained symptom-free for three months and then was admitted to the hospital after developing her typical anginal chest pain intermittently and occurring at rest, lasting up to 10 to 15 minutes and relieved by nitroglycerin. Electrocardiogram and serum biomarkers were negative and she underwent another coronary angiogram. This confirmed severe in-stent restenosis in the diagonal stent. Although the left anterior descending artery stent remained widely patent, the stent site appeared abnormal with contrast appearing outside the confines of the artery wall (Figure 31-11 and Video 31-5). This was felt

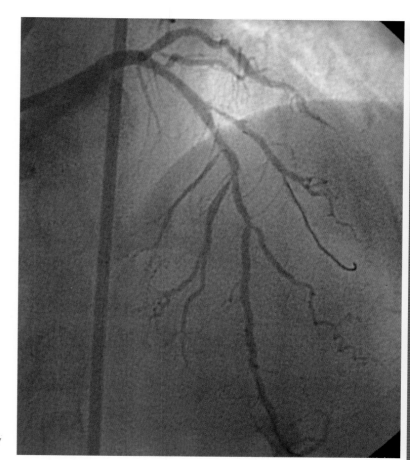

FIGURE 31-5. The angiographic result after balloon angioplasty is shown here.

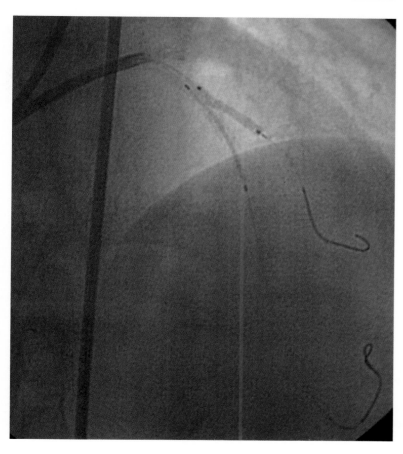

FIGURE 31-6. A "crush stent" procedure was used to treat the bifurcation.

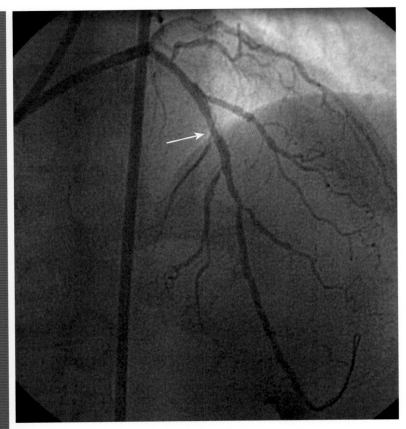

FIGURE 31-7. This is the angiographic result after stent deployment. Note the persistent narrowing in the stented segment of the left anterior descending artery (*arrow*).

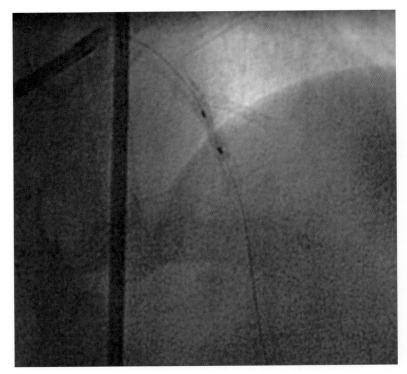

FIGURE 31-8. A waist remained even when a noncompliant balloon was inflated to high pressure.

to represent a pseudoaneurysm. After an extensive discussion regarding the options of medical therapy with close observation, surgery, or deployment of a covered stent, the patient and managing physician chose medical therapy with the plan to reimage the artery in 2 months.

She continued to have angina and, although the diagonal branch had now occluded, the repeat angiogram showed no change in the pseudoaneurysm 2 months later (Figure 31-12 and Videos 31-6, 31-7). Again, after extensive discussions, she was referred for surgery.

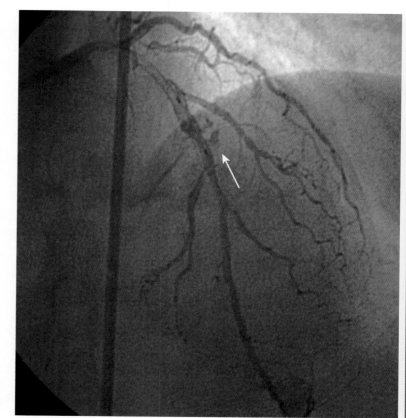

FIGURE 31-9. After fully expanding the stent, contrast extravasation was noted around the stent, consistent with a perforation (*arrow*).

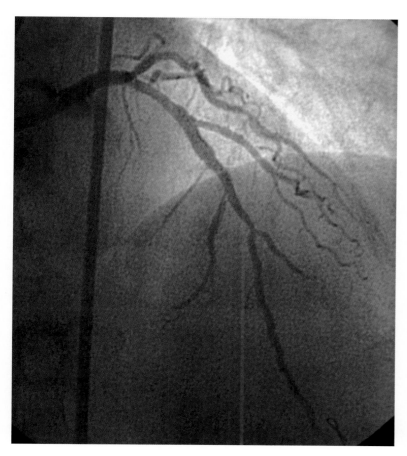

FIGURE 31-10. This is the final angiographic result, showing resolution of the perforation and no further evidence of contrast extravasation.

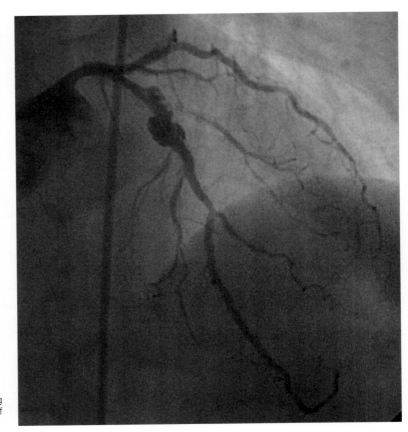

FIGURE 31-11. Angiogram obtained 3 months later showing a pseudoaneurysm at the stented site and near occlusion of the diagonal branch from in-stent restenosis.

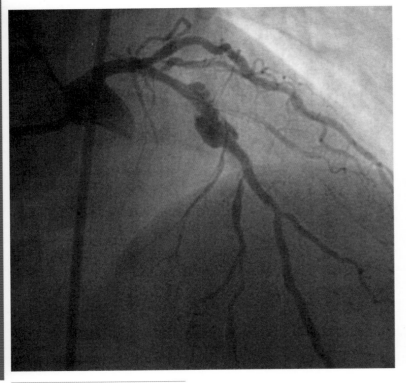

FIGURE 31-12. Angiogram obtained 2 months after the pseudoaneurysm was first identified (and 5 months after the intervention), showing occlusion of the diagonal and no change in the pseuodaneurysm.

The surgeon removed the stent and ligated and excluded the aneurysmal portion of the vessel using a left internal mammary artery graft to bypass the segment. She made an uneventful recovery and remained free of angina 1 year later.

DISCUSSION

This unusual case provides several valuable lessons. First, the initial perforation of the left anterior descending artery occurred because of the presence of extensive coronary calcification. Full stent deployment was not possible until the operator employed an oversized, noncompliant balloon inflated to very high pressures. Although this expanded the stent, it also deeply injured the artery causing a contained perforation. After the intravascular ultrasound confirmed the presence of a significant lesion and severe calcification was observed, an initial strategy of rotational atherectomy prior to balloon angioplasty might have prevented this complication. Very often, rotational atherectomy is not contemplated until the operator finds the predilatation balloon does not fully inflate despite high pressures. However, this strategy often causes arterial dissection at the site, a relative contraindication to high-speed rotational atherectomy.

The perforation observed in this case was likely "contained," meaning it most likely represented a very deep dissection confined by the adventia and did not communicate with the pericardial space. This type of perforation is very low risk for tamponade and often will seal spontaneously with cessation of procedural anticoagulation. In this case, bivalirudin was used and the operator stopped the infusion as soon as the perforation was identified. However, it should be noted that these perforations may result in delayed tamponade occurring several hours later from slow bleeding into the pericardial space, particularly if glycoprotein IIb/IIIa inhibitors are continued. Thus these agents should be stopped and the patient closely observed for hypotension in the early hours following the procedure.

Coronary aneurysms developing after percutaneous intervention are very rare. They were observed in 1.25% of patients in a recent study of 1197 patients undergoing routine angiography after drug-eluting stent implantation.[1] Aneurysms are most commonly caused after intervention from abnormal healing of a deep dissection, contained perforation, or vessel rupture, as observed in this case. Proper healing after these events may be further impaired by drug-eluting stents.[2]

The natural history of coronary aneurysms after intervention is not well-known. They may be incidental findings with no consequences, and many resolve spontaneously.[1,3] However, they have the potential for serious complications, including expansion and rupture of pseudoaneurysms, representing a potential source of coronary embolization; or acting as a nidus for stent thrombosis. Distinguishing a true aneurysm from a pseudoaneurysm can be accomplished by intravascular ultrasound and is based on the ability to identify an intact vessel wall in the case of true aneurysms, and

disruption of the vessel wall with damage to the adventia in the event of a pseudoaneurysm.[4]

There is no consensus on optimal management of coronary aneurysms and pseudoaneurysms. Individual case reports have described success with conservative management, PTFE-covered stents, and coil embolization.[5–7] Surgical options, as described in the present case, include ligation and resection of the aneurysm with distal bypass grafting.

KEY CONCEPTS

1. Extensive calcification may prevent full stent expansion. Aggressive post-stent balloon dilatation may cause vessel disruption and perforation. Pretreatment of the lesion with rotational atherectomy might avoid this potentially serious complication.
2. Contained perforations often resolve in the cardiac catheterization laboratory with cessation of procedural anticoagulation or with prolonged balloon inflations.
3. Although most contained perforations heal without sequelae, development of a coronary aneurysm at the site of the perforation may occur. Drug-eluting stents may increase this likelihood because of delayed healing.
4. Distinguishing a true aneurysm from a pseudoaneurysm after coronary intervention may be difficult. Many aneurysms appearing in the setting of a contained rupture represent pseudoaneurysms.
5. The treatment of coronary pseudoaneurysms includes: a) conservative therapy and follow-up with serial angiograms; b) deployment of a covered stent to exclude the aneurysm segment; and c) surgical repair and bypass grafting.

Selected References

1. Alfonso F, Perez-Vizcayno MJ, Ruiz M, Suarez A, Cazares M, Hernandez R, Escaned J, Banuelos C, Jiminez-Quevedo P, Macaya C: Coronary aneurysms after drug-eluting stent implantation. Clinical, angiographic, and intravascular ultrasound findings, *J Am Coll Cardiol* 53:2053–2060, 2009.
2. Aoki J, Kirtane A, Leon MB, Dangas G: Coronary artery aneurysm after drug eluting stent implantation, *J Am Coll Cardiol Interv* 1:14–21, 2008.
3. Mikhail B, Brewer RJ, Clark VL: Spontaneous closure of a perforation-induced coronary artery pseudoaneurysm, *J Interv Cardiol* 14:282–284, 2002.
4. Maehara A, Mintz GS, Ahmed JM, Fuchs S, Castagna MT, Pichard AD, Satler LF, Waksman R, Suddath WO, Kent KM, Weissman NJ: An intravascular ultrasound classification of angiographic coronary artery aneurysms, *Am J Cardiol* 88:365–370, 2001.
5. Szalat A, Durst R, Cohen A, Lotan C: Use of polytetrafluoroethylene-covered stent for treatment of coronary artery aneurysm, *Catheter Cardiovasc Interv* 66:203–208, 2005.
6. Maroo A, Rasmussen PA, Masaryk TJ, Ellis SG, Lincoff M, Kapadia S: Stent-assisted detachable coil embolization of pseudoaneurysms in the coronary circulation, *Catheter Cardiovasc Interv* 68:409–415, 2006.
7. Brasselet C, Perotin S, Fuzellier JF: Subacute development of a coronary artery pseudoaneurysm after primary angioplasty and stenting for acute myocardial infarction, *J Interv Cardiol* 15:168–170, 2003.

Coronary Air Embolism

Michael Ragosta, MD, FACC, FSCAI

CASE PRESENTATION

A 57-year-old woman, 7 years status post orthotopic heart transplantation for nonischemic cardiomyopathy, presents for her annual right and left heart catheterization, coronary angiogram, and endomyocardial biopsy. Her last routine coronary angiogram, performed 1 year earlier, demonstrated normal coronary arteries. She has been asymptomatic and feeling well.

CARDIAC CATHETERIZATION

The operator first measured right heart pressures; these were found to be normal with a right atrial pressure of 3 mmHg and preserved cardiac output. The right coronary artery was engaged with a right Judkins 4.0 catheter and appeared angiographically normal (Figure 32-1 and Video 32-1). Using a left Judkins 4.0 catheter, the operator engaged and imaged the left coronary artery; this also appeared angiographically normal (Figure 32-2). At this point, the patient remained symptom-free. Endomyocardial biopsy was performed from the right femoral vein using a 7 French, 98 cm, 40-degree curved sheath positioned into the right ventricle. Three samples were obtained, and while the operator was attempting a fourth sample, the patient developed hypotension and sinus bradycardia. Marked inferior ST-segment elevation appeared on the monitor screen.

The operator engaged a 6 French right Judkins 4.0 guide catheter into the right coronary artery. Angiography demonstrated occlusion of the right coronary artery in the midportion of the vessel (Figure 32-3 and Video 32-2). Another angiogram performed a few minutes later clearly showed air bubbles within the coronary (Figure 32-4 and Video 32-3). She was placed on nasal oxygen at 6 L/min, and heparin (70 U/kg) was administered by intravenous bolus. The operator placed a 0.014 inch floppy-tipped guidewire into the distal artery and aspirated the air bubbles using an aspiration catheter, with resolution of ST-segment elevation and restoration of TIMI-3 flow (Video 32-4). The left coronary was reimaged and showed no abnormalities; similarly, left ventriculography revealed normal ventricular function. The patient was transferred to the coronary care unit for further management.

POSTPROCEDURAL COURSE

Upon arrival in the coronary care unit, she remained hemodynamically stable and without chest pain and her admission electrocardiogram showed no evidence of ST-segment elevation. She reported no other symptoms and her physical examination, including a neurologic exam, was normal. Peak troponin I at 8 hours after the event was 2.65 ng/mL. She was discharged the following morning and was well at follow-up 6 weeks later.

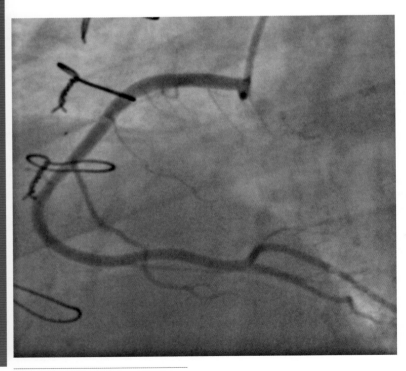

FIGURE 32-1. This is the patient's initial right coronary angiogram, revealing a normal artery 7 years after heart transplantation.

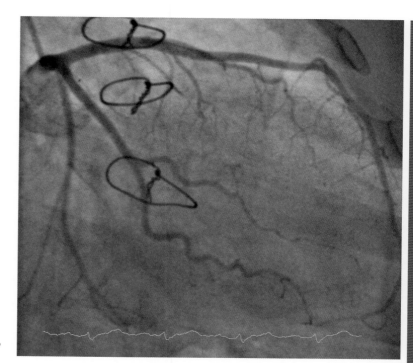

FIGURE 32-2. This is the patient's left coronary angiogram, revealing a normal artery 7 years after heart transplantation.

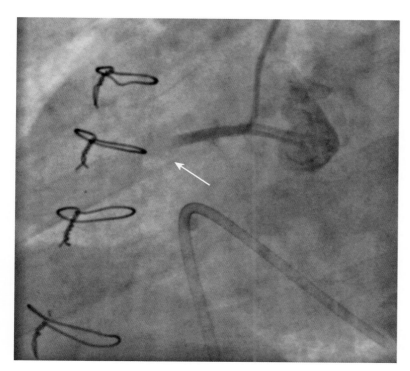

FIGURE 32-3. The angiogram obtained after performance of the right ventricular biopsy, with occlusion of the vessel. There is a vague cutoff of the vessel noted (*arrow*).

DISCUSSION

Air embolism into the coronary artery is a rare, but potentially serious, iatrogenic complication of cardiac catheterization and coronary intervention. During coronary angiography, coronary air embolism is most commonly due to operator error from failure to aspirate air after connecting the catheter to the manifold. During coronary interventional procedures, this problem may arise from catheter exchanges when the balloon catheter is removed and the hemostatic valve is left open, causing air to enter the guide into the potential space left by the balloon catheter. If the operator fails to purge the air from the guide catheter, coronary air embolism may result during subsequent coronary injections.

In the case presented here, coronary angiography proceeded without complication and thus it is unlikely that coronary air embolism originated from the coronary

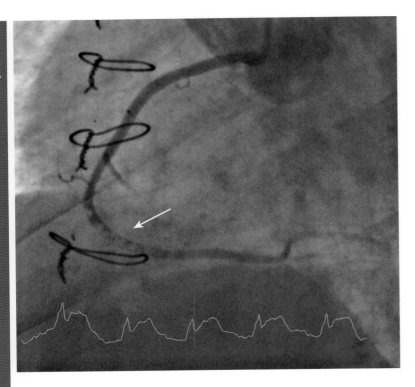

FIGURE 32-4. Air bubbles are seen in the coronary artery, confirming the diagnosis of air embolism (*arrow*).

catheters. The abrupt onset of bradycardia and ST-segment elevation began only after the fourth endomyocardial biopsy. It is likely that given the patient's very low right atrial pressure, air was introduced into the venous sheath during removal of the bioptome. Since the biopsy sheath was in the right ventricle, it was postulated that the cause of air embolism in this case was due to a small perforation of the septum created by the bioptome, allowing the tip of the biopsy sheath to enter the left ventricle. Air present within the sheath entered the left ventricle and migrated to the aorta, thus causing coronary air embolism.

The diagnosis of coronary air embolism is usually made angiographically. As exemplified by this case, air embolism may occlude the coronary, but the occluded site often appears vaguely defined rather than as the discrete vessel cutoff typically seen when occlusion is caused by a thrombus. The diagnosis is easily made when discrete bubbles are seen in the coronary artery. Air embolism may also result in the angiographic appearance of "no-reflow" or "slow flow."

Operators can prevent most cases by carefully aspirating catheters when performing exchanges and when connecting to the manifold. In the event that this complication occurs, several treatment options can be considered.[1] Small amounts of air may be tolerated without symptoms or adverse sequelae and usually dissipate spontaneously by dissolving into the blood, requiring no further therapy. Large amounts of air causing adverse clinical consequences require treatment. In addition to aspiration with a simple catheter, as performed in this case, the administration of high concentration oxygen helps dissipate the air bubbles.

KEY CONCEPTS

1. Coronary air embolism is a rare, but potentially serious, complication of coronary angiographic or interventional procedures.
2. Embolization of a small volume of air may be asymptomatic, while larger volumes of air may lead to serious adverse events including myocardial infarction and cardiogenic shock.
3. Conservative management is appropriate when the volume of air is small and there are no adverse clinical sequelae; larger volumes of air may be aspirated or treated with administration of high concentration oxygen.

Selected References

1. Dib J, Boyle AJ, Chan M, Resar JR: Coronary air embolism: A case report and review of the literature, *Catheter Cardiovasc Interv* 68:897–900, 2006.

Dissection of Both a Left Internal Mammary Graft and the Subclavian Artery

Michael Ragosta, MD, FACC, FSCAI

CASE PRESENTATION

A 73-year-old man with a long and complex coronary history presents with increasing angina pectoris over several months. His saga with coronary artery disease began 18 years earlier when he underwent single-vessel bypass graft surgery consisting of a left internal mammary artery to the left anterior descending artery. He developed recurrent angina 8 years ago and was found to have a severe stenosis of the left anterior descending artery distal to the left internal mammary artery anastomosis; the other arteries were without significant narrowing. This lesion was treated with a bare-metal stent with a good clinical result. Over the ensuing years he developed progressive coronary atherosclerotic narrowing of the circumflex and right coronary arteries associated with anginal chest pain, and these were treated with bare-metal stents with a satisfactory clinical result. His last catheterization and intervention occurred 3 years earlier, and he did well until several months ago when he again

developed severe angina with minimal exertion. He was referred for cardiac catheterization. In addition to coronary artery disease, he also has a history of diabetes, hypertension, and dyslipidemia.

CARDIAC CATHETERIZATION

An elective diagnostic coronary angiogram found no significant obstructive disease in the right coronary artery. The left internal mammary artery graft was widely patent but there was severe narrowing within the stent placed 8 years earlier (Figure 33-1 and Video 33-1). In addition, there was obstructive narrowing of the left circumflex artery proximal to an old stent (Figure 33-2) and chronic occlusion of the proximal left anterior descending artery. Based on these findings, the operator planned to treat the circumflex lesion and then the in-stent restenosis in the native left anterior descending artery, to be accessed via the left internal mammary artery graft using bivalirudin

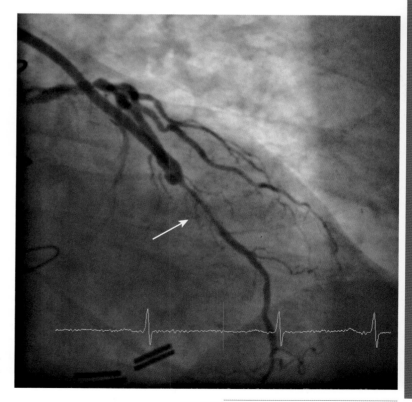

FIGURE 33-1. Selective angiography of the left internal mammary artery graft to the left anterior descending artery shows severe stenosis in the left anterior descending artery within an old bare-metal stent (*arrow*).

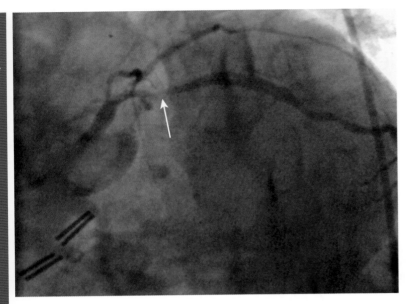

FIGURE 33-2. This left anterior oblique projection with caudal angulation of the left coronary artery shows occlusion of the left anterior descending artery and severe stenosis in the proximal left circumflex artery (*arrow*).

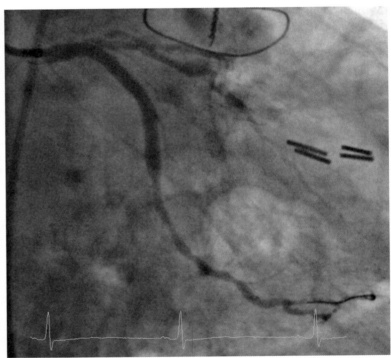

FIGURE 33-3. This angiogram was obtained after stenting the circumflex artery (right anterior oblique with caudal angulation).

as the procedural anticoagulant. The circumflex lesion responded well to balloon dilatation followed by placement of a 3.5 mm diameter by 23 mm long everolimus-eluting stent (Figure 33-3).

Once satisfied with the circumflex artery, the operator placed a 6 French left internal mammary guide catheter into the left subclavian, but noted contrast staining from the diagnostic angiogram still present in the proximal portion of the left internal mammary artery (Figure 33-4 and Video 33-2). A dissection of the proximal left internal mammary artery graft was suspected, and the guide catheter was cautiously engaged to allow further delineation of the dissection (Video 33-3). At this point, the subclavian artery did not appear to be involved, and the operator advanced a 0.014 inch floppy-tipped guidewire through the mammary artery and into the left anterior descending artery. With additional contrast injections, however, staining of the subclavian artery was noted, confirming that the dissection likely involved the ostium of the internal mammary artery, extending into the subclavian artery (Figure 33-5 and Video 33-4).

Despite the extensive dissection, the patient remained clinically stable and without chest pain. The operator planned to stent the dissection within the left internal mammary graft, but thought it wise to first treat the lesion in the left anterior descending artery as initially planned and thus deployed a 2.5 mm diameter by 28 mm long everolimus-eluting stent at the site.

Numerous bare-metal stents were deployed within the left internal mammary artery graft, ultimately requiring a

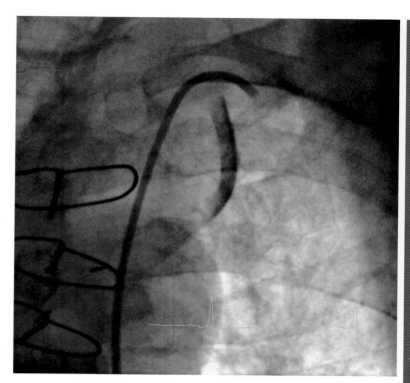

FIGURE 33-4. Before the planned intervention on the left anterior descending artery via the left internal mammary graft was begun, contrast staining was noted in the proximal segment of the left internal mammary artery graft.

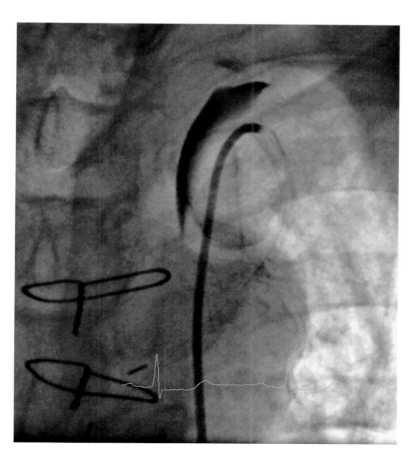

FIGURE 33-5. A dissection was also apparent in the subclavian artery.

total length of 118 mm to cover the entire dissected area (Figure 33-6 and Videos 33-4, 33-5). Once the operator was satisfied with the repair of the left internal mammary artery graft, attention was turned to the subclavian artery. Angiography confirmed a dissection flap, but this remained stable throughout the procedure, did not compromise the origin of the vertebral artery (Figures 33-7, 33-8 and Videos 33-6, 33-7), and did not result in a pressure gradient across the dissected segment. Because the entry site of the intimal flap was opposite the direction of blood flow, it was decided to treat this dissection conservatively and the procedure was halted.

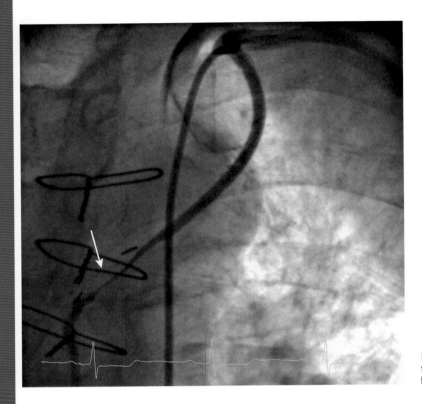

FIGURE 33-6. The dissection caused luminal compromise of the left internal mammary graft (*arrow*), likely from an intramural hematoma.

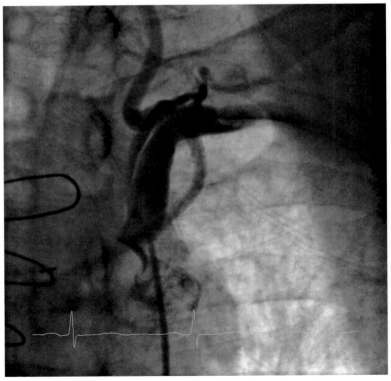

FIGURE 33-7. The extent of the intimal flap in the subclavian artery is shown here.

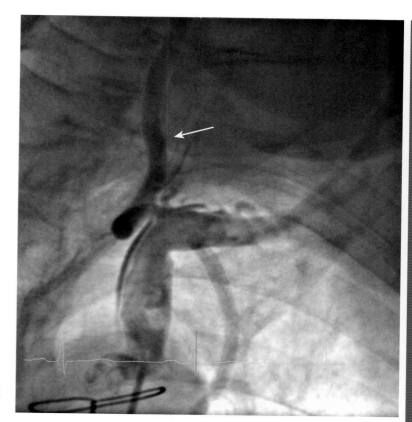

FIGURE 33-8. Another view of the intimal flap in the subclavian artery showed no involvement of the vertebral artery (*arrow*).

POSTPROCEDURAL COURSE

He was observed in the coronary care unit overnight and remained free of chest pain. Blood pressure in both arms remained equal overnight. He underwent a CT angiogram the next day that showed no evidence of a dissection flap at the site, suggesting that the intimal flap had sealed without extension or luminal compromise. He was discharged, and remained free of angina 2 months and one year later.

DISCUSSION

Selective angiography of left internal mammary artery grafts is routinely performed during diagnostic catheterization in patients who had prior surgery using this conduit. In most cases, the procedure is simple and is executed without complication. Due to the fact that the left internal mammary arises with an acute angle from the subclavian artery, a specially-shaped IMA catheter, characterized by a sharply-angled tip, is often used to successfully engage this vessel. In the case presented here, the sharply-angled tip of the catheter likely created a small intimal tear that may have been extended down the mammary artery with the injection of contrast. The injury was initially confined to the proximal segment of the mammary artery graft, and was not appreciated until the operator completed the circumflex intervention and passed a guide catheter to the subclavian to begin the intervention on the LAD. Subsequent manipulations, necessary to repair the dissection, initially worsened the extent of the dissection and, in fact, the dissection was propagated to the surrounding segment of the subclavian artery.

Luminal obstruction of the internal mammary artery in this case was due to both an extensive dissection flap and an intramural hematoma, and both of these aspects need to be addressed during repair of this problem. It is not enough to simply stent the entry site of the dissection; the intramural hematoma significantly compressed the lumen and this also required stenting, leading to a very long sequence of stents.

The subclavian dissection added further to the operator's quandary. This complication is very rare.[1] Although a stent could have been placed at the site of the subclavian tear,[2] the operator was concerned about the dissection's close proximity to both the vertebral and left internal mammary arteries and feared jeopardizing or "jailing" these important branches. The decision to treat the subclavian dissection conservatively was based on two important observations. First, there was no pressure gradient measurable across the subclavian dissection, indicating that the dissection did not create significant luminal obstruction. Second, the direction of blood flow was opposite the direction of the entry flap, thereby making it unlikely that the dissection would extend. This strategy proved successful, based on the imaging study performed the next day demonstrating no evidence of the subclavian dissection.

KEY CONCEPTS

1. While most selective angiograms of the left internal mammary artery graft are uncomplicated, the sharp hook of the IMA catheter may cause an intimal tear, leading to dissection of the internal mammary or subclavian artery.

2. Iatrogenic dissection of the subclavian artery is rare; careful delineation of the intimal flap and the proximity to the surrounding vessels is important to help determine the most appropriate therapy for this complication.

Selected References

1. Frohwein S, Ververis JJ, Marshall JJ: Subclavian artery dissection during diagnostic cardiac catheterization: The role of conservative management, *Catheter Cardiovasc Diagn* 34:313–317, 1995.
2. Galli M, Goldberg SL, Zerboni S, Almagor Y: Balloon expandable stent implantation after iatrogenic arterial dissection of the left subclavian artery, *Catheter Cardiovasc Diagn* 35:355–357, 1995.

Left Main Dissection During Intervention

Michael Ragosta, MD, FACC, FSCAI

CASE PRESENTATION

A 67-year-old woman with diabetes and chronic obstructive pulmonary disease previously underwent bare-metal stenting of her right coronary artery 1 year earlier, complicated by early restenosis and treated with brachytherapy. She remained symptom-free until the current admission, when she developed several days of increasing shortness of breath associated with chest pressure and diaphoresis. She presented to the emergency department when nitroglycerin no longer improved her discomfort and was diagnosed with unstable angina after the admission electrocardiogram showed no changes and serial troponin I assays remained normal. Her physician referred her for cardiac catheterization.

CARDIAC CATHETERIZATION

Coronary angiographic findings included moderate luminal narrowing in the right coronary artery, no significant obstructive disease of the left anterior descending artery, and severe disease in the circumflex involving the bifurcation of a large obtuse marginal branch (Figure 34-1 and Video 34-1). The operator anticipated difficulty with the proximal tortuosity of the circumflex and, after administration of bivalirudin, used an 8 French left Amplatz 2.0 guide catheter to engage the left coronary artery. Floppy-tipped guidewires were advanced into each branch of the circumflex and balloon angioplasty was performed (Figure 34-2). Following balloon angioplasty, angiography demonstrated persistent narrowing but no other angiographic complications (Video 34-2). The operator encountered difficulty advancing a 2.5 mm diameter by 18 mm sirolimus-eluting stent into the first obtuse marginal and achieved success by pushing the guide catheter deeply into the left main stem. After deploying the stent, angiography uncovered dissection of the left main stem (Figure 34-3 and Video 34-3). Several minutes after this angiogram, another coronary injection displayed dramatic worsening of the left main dissection (Figure 34-4 and Video 34-4) with near closure of the lumen and extensive contrast retention surrounding the left main stem. The patient reported severe chest pain but blood pressure and rhythm remained stable. A 3.5 mm diameter by 18 mm long sirolimus-eluting stent was deployed in the left main stem. This resolved her chest pain, restored luminal

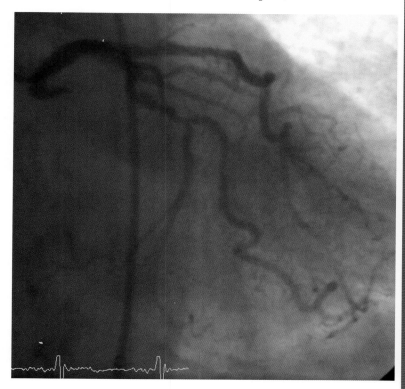

FIGURE 34-1. This is a right anterior oblique projection with caudal angulation of the left coronary artery, demonstrating the severe disease in the left circumflex at the bifurcation of the obtuse marginal artery. Note that the left main stem appears angiographically normal.

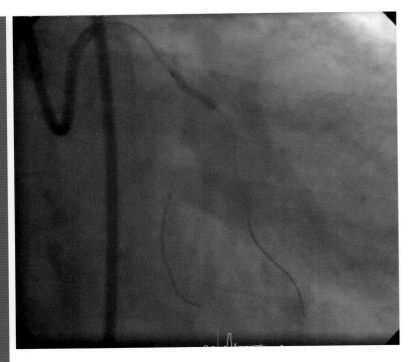

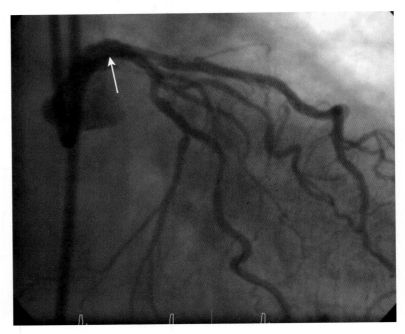

FIGURE 34-2. The operator used an 8 French Amplatz 2.0 guide catheter to achieve satisfactory back-up to perform the intervention.

FIGURE 34-3. After a stent was deployed in the obtuse marginal artery, angiography revealed a guide-related dissection of the left main stem (*arrow*).

patency, and eliminated evidence of contrast retention (Figure 34-5 and Video 34-5).

POSTPROCEDURAL COURSE

Following the procedure, she was admitted to the coronary care unit for observation. She had no further ischemic chest pain or electrocardiographic changes and troponin I assays did not rise. She was discharged from the hospital on the following day.

She was readmitted 2 months later with atypical chest pain, and another coronary angiogram was performed that showed no significant obstructive disease. One year

after the left main stent was placed, she again underwent angiography for recurrent atypical chest pain and an abnormal stress test. This again demonstrated wide patency of the left main and obtuse marginal stents (Figure 34-6 and Video 34-6).

DISCUSSION

Coronary artery dissections occurring during percutaneous coronary intervention are most commonly caused by balloon barotrauma at the site of the lesion; however, dissection may also arise from the guidewire or, as shown in this case, from the guide catheter. Although

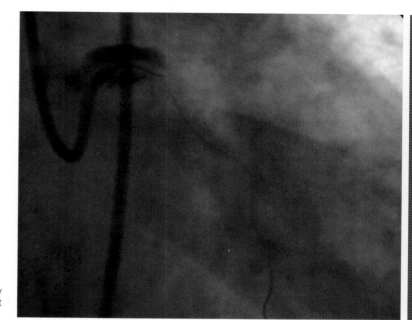

FIGURE 34-4. Within several minutes the dissection significantly worsened, causing luminal obstruction and extensive contrast retention outside of the left main stem.

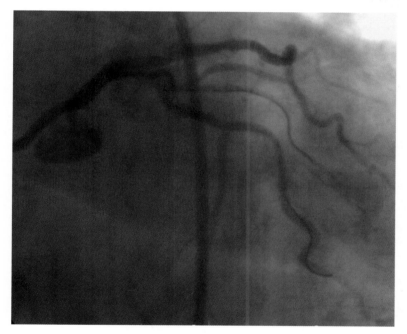

FIGURE 34-5. A stent placed in the left main stem repaired the dissection and restored luminal patency.

this complication occurs uncommonly, guide catheter dissection can result in serious problems including abrupt vessel closure, extension into major proximal branches or the aorta, and a need for additional and unplanned stents.[1] Several factors contribute to this complication, including the presence of ostial coronary disease, unusual vessel take-offs, and the use of aggressive guide catheters such as large bore (8 French or larger) or Amplatz catheters. The common practice of deep insertion of the guide catheter into the coronary artery in an effort to increase backup and allow passage of stents or balloons also leads to dissection, especially if the guide catheter is not coaxial to the artery. In the case shown here, left main dissection was likely caused by the large-bore Amplatz guide, chosen to support a circumflex intervention.

Management of a left main stem guide-related dissection depends on the extent of the dissection, its involvement with side branches or the aorta, and patient stability.[1,2] Small dissections that do not retain contrast or impair the lumen can be treated conservatively and will usually heal without sequelae. Large dissections causing symptoms or luminal compromise need more definite treatment. Stent repair is often successful, but can be challenging if the dissection extends beyond the bifurcation of the left main into the left anterior descending artery and circumflex vessels. Similarly, dissection might cause abrupt closure of the left main and hemodynamic collapse, creating less than ideal conditions for performance of a complex intervention. Surgery is indicated if a large dissection cannot be repaired percutaneously.

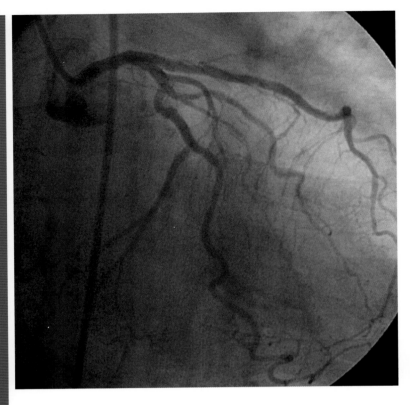

FIGURE 34-6. This angiogram obtained 1 year after the left main stent was placed shows continued patency of both the left main and obtuse marginal stents with no evidence of restenosis.

KEY CONCEPTS

1. Use of aggressive guide catheters to achieve suitable backup may lead to dissection of the proximal vessel.
2. Injury to the left main stem during coronary intervention of either the left circumflex or left anterior descending arteries may be lethal if not promptly recognized and treated.
3. Successful stenting of an injured left main stem often leads to a satisfactory long-term outcome.

Selected References

1. Mulvihill NT, Boccalatte M, Fajadet J, Marco J: Catheter-induced left main dissection: A treatment dilemma, *Catheter Cardiovasc Interv* 58:214–216, 2003.
2. Al-Saif SM, Lie MW, Al-Mubarak N, Agrawal S, Dean LS: Percutaneous treatment of catheter-induced dissection of the left main coronary artery and adjacent aortic wall: A case report, *Catheter Cardiovasc Interv* 49:86–89, 2000.

Left Main Dissection

Michael Ragosta, MD, FACC, FSCAI

CASE PRESENTATION

After presenting to the hospital with a 3-day history of intermittent chest pain and diaphoresis and found to have a non-ST segment elevation myocardial infarction, a healthy 49-year-old woman, with the coronary risk factors of tobacco abuse and dyslipidemia, underwent cardiac catheterization and was found to have a severe stenosis in the ramus intermedius branch (Figures 35-1, 35-2 and Video 35-1). Her other coronary arteries showed no angiographic evidence of significant athero-sclerotic disease. She was subsequently referred for percutaneous treatment of the ramus intermedius branch.

CARDIAC CATHETERIZATION

The patient received a 300 mg loading dose of clopido-grel the previous day and was administered 325 mg of aspirin. After receiving a bolus plus an infusion of bival-irudin, the left main coronary artery was engaged with a 6 French JCL 4 guide catheter without difficulty. The operator then attempted to pass a 0.014 inch floppy-tipped guidewire into the ramus intermedius branch but encountered resistance as soon as the wire tip exited the guide catheter. Gentle wire manipulations failed to

advance the guidewire beyond the tip of the guide. Although the guide catheter appeared coaxial to the left main stem, the operator withdrew the guide and re-engaged. This time, the guidewire easily advanced into the ramus intermedius. Throughout this period, the patient remained symptom-free.

After passing the wire successfully and predilating the ramus lesion with a 2.0 mm diameter by 12 mm long compliant balloon, the operator happened to note an unexpected narrowing of the distal left main stem and positioned another 0.014 inch floppy-tipped guidewire into the left anterior descending artery (Figure 35-3 and Video 35-2). Several intracoronary boluses of nitro-glycerin did not change the appearance of the distal left main narrowing. The physician proceeded with stenting of the ramus lesion using a 2.25 mm diameter by 16 mm long paclitaxel-eluting stent (Figure 35-4 and Videos 35-3, 35-4). The narrowing of the distal left main stem remained unchanged throughout the procedure on the ramus intermedius.

In order to determine both the mechanism and extent of the distal left main stem luminal narrowing, intra-vascular ultrasound was performed. The ultrasound catheter was pulled back from the ramus to the ostium

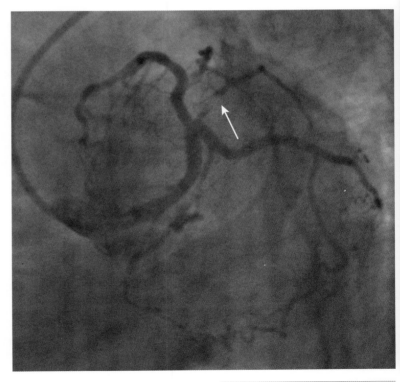

FIGURE 35-1. This is a left anterior oblique projection with caudal angulation of the left coronary artery demonstrating the focal severe stenosis of the ramus intermedius (*arrow*). Note the normal appearance of the distal left main stem.

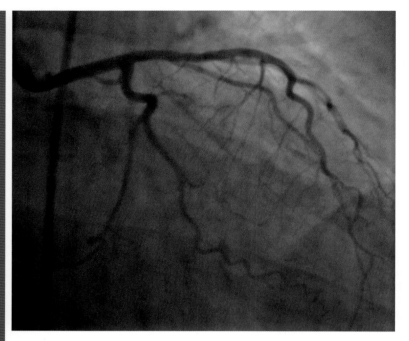

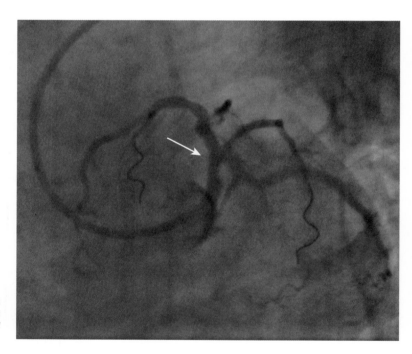

FIGURE 35-2. This angiogram of the left coronary artery in a right anterior oblique projection with caudal angulation shows the normal appearance of the left main artery and the apparent coaxial position of the guide catheter. The ramus lesion is obscured from view.

FIGURE 35-3. This angiogram was obtained after balloon angioplasty of the ramus intermedius and revealed an unexpected narrowing of the distal left main coronary artery (*arrow*).

of the left main (Video 35-5). At the distal end of the left main, an intramural hematoma was clearly apparent (Figure 35-5). More proximally, discrete intimal flaps were present and occupied almost 50% of the left main lumen (Figures 35-6, 35-7). Based on the ultrasound images, the operator decided to stent the injured segment of the left main stem with a 4.0 mm diameter by 12 mm long paclitaxel-eluting stent, thus restoring the vessel to a normal angiographic appearance (Figure 35-8 and Video 35-6). Repeat intravascular ultrasound assessment

confirmed excellent stent apposition and wide luminal patency of the left main stem.

POSTPROCEDURAL COURSE

Following the procedure, she remained free of chest pain. She was admitted to the coronary care unit for observation, and remained pain-free overnight. After ambulating without difficulty, she was discharged the next day on metoprolol, simvastatin, 325 mg of aspirin,

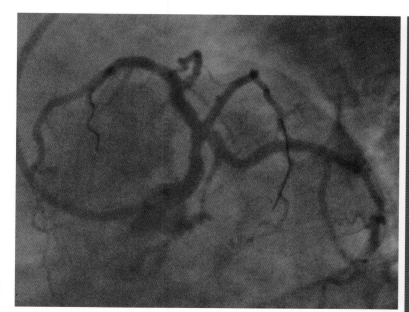

FIGURE 35-4. There is continued narrowing noted of the distal left main after stenting of the ramus intermedius and despite the generous administration of intracoronary nitroglycerin.

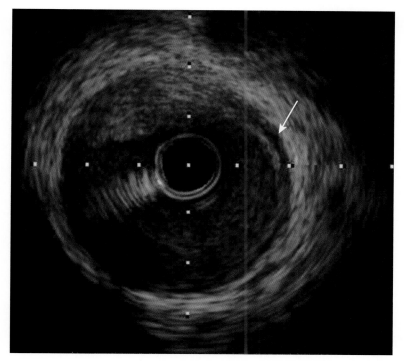

FIGURE 35-5. This is a representative intravascular ultrasound image of the distal left main, demonstrating an intramural hematoma and an intimal tear (*arrow*).

and 75 mg of clopidogrel indefinitely. At follow-up 6 weeks later, she felt well, remained tobacco-free, and was without recurrent chest pain.

DISCUSSION

This case validates the wisdom offered by experienced interventionalists that "there is no such thing as an easy angioplasty", but also emphasizes the importance of careful vigilance and scrutiny of the angiogram. The lesion in the ramus intermedius offered no particular challenges. The first clue that this case would not turn out to be "easy" occurred when the operator encountered

unexpected difficulty passing the guidewire out of the tip of the guide catheter. Although remedied by repositioning the guide catheter and wire, that event likely heightened the operator's awareness for the potential of a left main injury, focusing his attention on the subtle angiographic finding seen in the distal left main that was subsequently found to represent a dissection and intramural hematoma of the left main, with potentially serious consequences if untreated.

Guide-related injuries of the left main stem or proximal right coronary artery during percutaneous intervention are uncommon and usually caused by large-bore guide catheters with aggressive curves, lack of coaxial

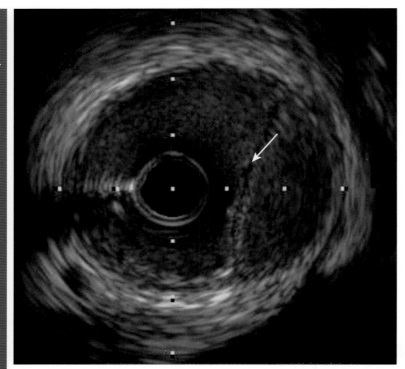

FIGURE 35-6. An intimal flap is prominent in this intravascular ultrasound image of the left main coronary artery (*arrow*).

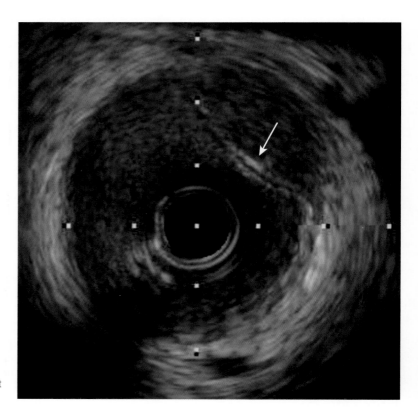

FIGURE 35-7. Another representative image of the prominent intimal flap in the left main coronary artery (*arrow*).

engagement, deep engagement in the coronary ostium to provide backup, and presence of underlying atherosclerosis.[1,2] Although possible, in this case, it does not appear that the guide catheter caused the intimal injury, as there was no evidence of a dissection by angiography. The major cause of this injury was likely due to the guidewire. The tip probably penetrated the intima and

entered the subintimal space, creating an intimal flap and an intramural hematoma.

The subtle luminal narrowing of a previously normal segment provided the most important clue to the presence of this complication. Usually, dissections create a visible flap and retention of contrast. In this case, these features were absent and only luminal narrowing was seen.

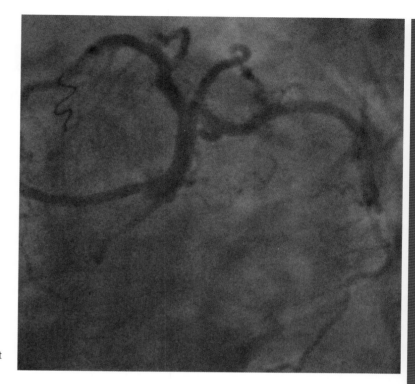

FIGURE 35-8. Final angiographic appearance of the left coronary artery following stenting of the left main stem.

Such a finding is either due to spasm or a dissection with an intramural hematoma. Failure to resolve with nitroglycerin convinced the operator that something more devious than spasm was at hand. Intravascular ultrasound was indispensible in this case. In addition to confirming the diagnosis, and demonstrating the intramural hematoma, the ultrasound images defined the extent of the injury and guided the stent repair.

Treatment of a guide- or wire-related injury depends on the extent of the injury and the presence of luminal compromise. Small tears without contrast retention or luminal compromise can be treated conservatively. Large dissections retaining contrast or causing luminal obstruction or intramural hematomas impinging upon the lumen need definite therapy with either stents or surgery.

Selected References

1. Mulvihill NT, Boccalatte M, Fajadet J, Marco J: Catheter-induced left main dissection: A treatment dilemma, *Catheter Cardiovasc Interv* 58:214–216, 2003.
2. Al-Saif SM, Lie MW, Al-Mubarak N, Agrawal S, Dean LS: Percutaneous treatment of catheter-induced dissection of the left main coronary artery and adjacent aortic wall: A case report, *Catheter Cardiovasc Interv* 49:86–89, 2000.

KEY CONCEPTS

1. The inability to advance a floppy-tipped guidewire out of the guide catheter might suggest lack of a coaxial position of the guide or possibly a subintimal position of the wire.
2. Guide- or wire-related dissections may result in subtle angiographic findings.
3. Narrowing of a previously normal arterial segment without evidence of the contrast retention or staining classically associated with a dissection suggests the presence of either spasm or an intramural hematoma. Failure to resolve with nitroglycerin suggests an intramural hematoma.
4. Intravascular ultrasound is an extremely helpful method to diagnose the etiology of unexplained angiographic abnormalities.
5. Although dissections may heal spontaneously, large dissection flaps or significant intramural hematomas should be treated with stents to ensure stability of the vessel.

Management Dilemmas and Controversies

Over the years, most common clinical questions in interventional cardiology have been addressed by at least one well-done, randomized, controlled trial. Based on these studies, professional societies regularly issue practice guidelines, and these form the basis for most decisions made in a clinical practice. As a result, the well-trained and knowledgeable interventional cardiologist is rarely stymied by a clinical problem.

Clinical trials have answered many important questions and have unequivocally defined the best practice for numerous commonly encountered clinical problems. For example, randomized controlled trials have clearly demonstrated the superiority of primary angioplasty over lytic therapy for acute ST-segment elevation myocardial infarction, the superiority of drug-eluting stents over bare-metal stents for reducing restenosis, the advantage of distal embolic protection for saphenous vein graft interventions, and the benefit of dual antiplatelet therapy at reducing rates of stent thrombosis. However, not all problems facing the interventional cardiologist have been unequivocally answered by a clinical trial. In addition, there remain many controversial topics and, in some areas, the available data are conflicting or of unclear relevance in the current era.

The cases in this section represent some of these undefined areas and controversial topics. It is expected that many of these dilemmas will be resolved by future research and clinical trials, only to be replaced by new, more challenging clinical problems. Finally, it should be clear that the management chosen for each case in this section represents one operator's opinion and it is not the author's intent to imply that it is the only way to handle the problem. Other approaches might have been just as effective or even better.

Multivessel Coronary Artery Disease: PCI Versus CABG?

Michael Ragosta, MD, FACC, FSCAI

CASE PRESENTATION

A 61-year-old woman with hypertension and a history of heavy tobacco abuse developed typical exertional angina 3 months prior to her presentation. Symptoms occurred during moderate exertion and resolved with rest. Medical therapy with beta-blockade and long-acting nitrates temporarily improved her symptoms, but she continued to report lifestyle-limiting angina and underwent an exercise stress test. During this test, she exercised for 7 minutes and developed chest discomfort associated with 1 to 2 mm downsloping ST-segment depression. Perfusion scintigraphy identified a moderate-sized inferolateral reversible defect. She was referred for catheterization.

CARDIAC CATHETERIZATION

Ventriculography demonstrated moderate hypokinesis of the inferior wall, but global function was normal with an estimated ejection fraction of 60%. The right coronary artery was completely occluded and the duration of the occlusion could not be precisely determined (Figure 36-1 and Video 36-1). In the left coronary artery, a severe stenosis was identified in the midsegment of the left circumflex artery (Figure 36-2 and Video 36-2), and a stenosis of at least moderate severity was seen in the midsegment of the left anterior descending artery (Figure 36-3 and Video 36-3). The presence of well-developed left to right collaterals and the duration of symptoms suggested that the right coronary artery was chronically occluded and at least 3 months old.

The patient remained on the catheterization table and the findings were explained to her. After a lengthy discussion regarding the options of bypass surgery versus multivessel percutaneous coronary intervention, the patient chose percutaneous revascularization with the understanding that, if the operator could not successfully treat the chronically occluded right coronary artery, surgical revascularization would be necessary.

With this strategy in mind, the operator began with the right coronary artery. Procedural anticoagulation

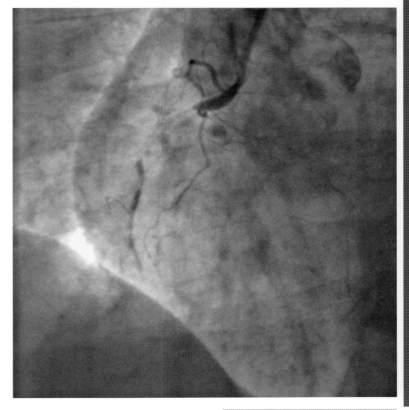

FIGURE 36-1. This is an LAO image of the right coronary artery demonstrating total occlusion.

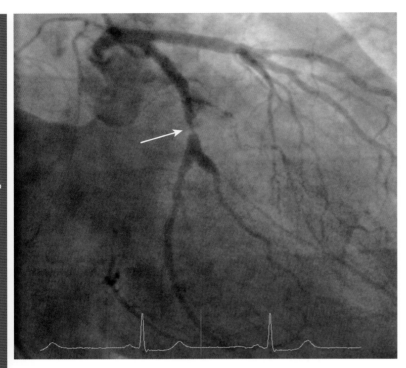

FIGURE 36-2. A severe stenosis was present in the left circumflex artery (*arrow*).

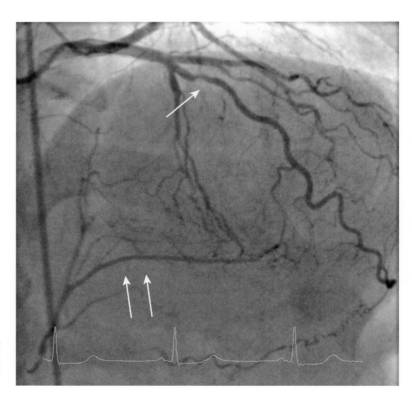

FIGURE 36-3. This is an RAO image with cranial angulation of the left coronary artery demonstrating a moderate stenosis of the LAD (*arrow*) and extensive collateral circulation to the distal right coronary artery (*double arrow*).

was accomplished with bivalirudin; the patient had already received pretreatment with 300 mg of clopidogrel the night before the procedure. After engaging a 6 French right Judkins guide catheter, the operator loaded a stiff-tipped 0.014 inch guidewire (Miracle Bros, 3, Asahi) into the lumen of a 2.5 mm diameter by 15 mm long, "over-the-wire," compliant balloon catheter. The stiff-tipped guidewire easily crossed the occlusion and was advanced into the distal right coronary artery (Figure 36-4). The "over-the-wire" balloon was advanced distally and the stiff-tipped wire was removed and replaced by a floppy-tipped guidewire. Patency was restored after performing balloon angioplasty with the 2.5 mm balloon; however, the artery appeared diffusely diseased distally with an

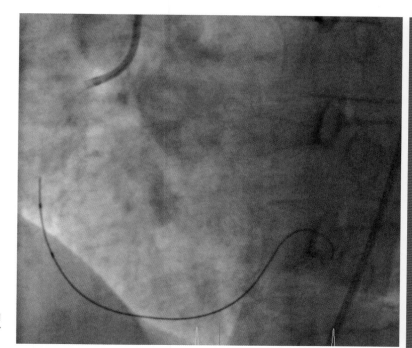

FIGURE 36-4. A stiff-tipped angioplasty guidewire was used to cross the totally occluded segment of the right coronary artery.

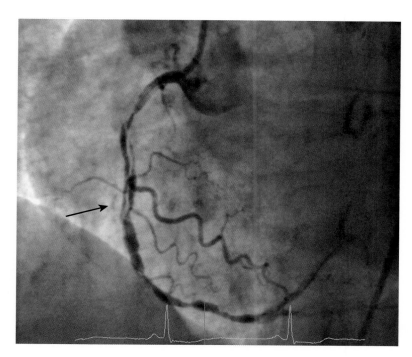

FIGURE 36-5. Result after balloon angioplasty; there is extensive dissection and distal disease observed (*arrow*).

extensive dissection in the midsection (Figure 36-5 and Video 36-4). Multiple everolimus-eluting stents were placed, ranging in diameter from 2.5 mm distally to 3.5 mm proximally, covering 98 mm of length. The proximal and midsegments were postdilated with a 4.0 mm non-compliant balloon and an excellent final angiographic result was obtained (Figure 36-6 and Video 36-5).

The procedure was stopped in order to conserve contrast volume and limit radiation exposure. The following day, the operator treated the circumflex artery with a 3.5 mm diameter everolimus-eluting stent without difficulty (Figure 36-7 and Video 36-6). Because the left anterior descending artery stenosis was of unclear significance, this lesion was assessed with a pressure wire to determine fractional flow reserve (Figure 36-8). Maximum vasodilation was achieved with an injection of 200 mcg of intracoronary adenosine and the fractional flow reserve was calculated to be 0.86, indicating that the lesion in the LAD was not hemodynamically significant; thus stenting was not performed (Figure 36-9).

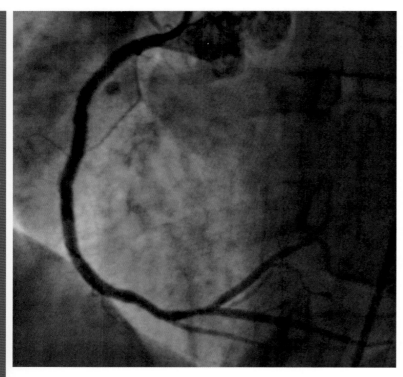

FIGURE 36-6. Final angiographic result after extensive stenting performed in the right coronary artery.

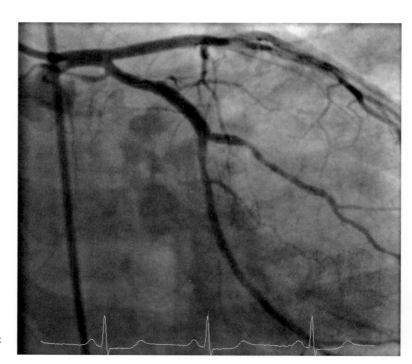

FIGURE 36-7. Post-stent result in the left circumflex artery.

POSTPROCEDURAL COURSE

After an overnight observation without complication, she was discharged on lisinopril, aspirin, clopidogrel, and simvastatin. At a follow-up visit 2 months later, she reported no further angina.

DISCUSSION

The management of multivessel coronary disease is controversial and challenging. First, the physician must decide whether to recommend bypass surgery or multivessel PCI. This often depends on numerous factors,

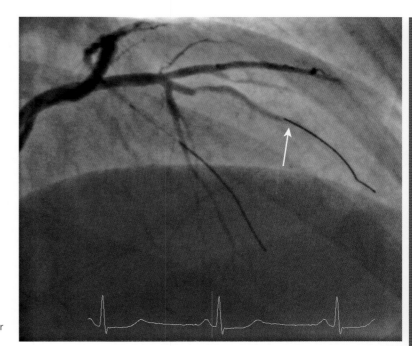

FIGURE 36-8. Location of the pressure wire transducer (*arrow*) in the left anterior descending artery.

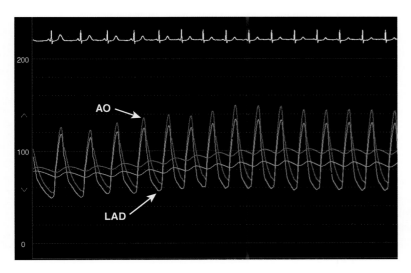

FIGURE 36-9. These pressure tracings were recorded from the catheter tip **(AO)** and from the pressure transducer distal to a coronary stenosis in the left anterior descending artery **(LAD)** after maximal hyperemia created by an intracoronary injection of adenosine. Fractional flow reserve is defined as the ratio of mean distal coronary pressure to mean aortic pressure during maximal hyperemia, which in this case was 86 mmHg/100 mmHg or 0.86.

including coronary anatomy, the technical feasibility of bypass surgery or PCI, completeness of revascularization, the presence of comorbid illness, and patient preference. If multivessel PCI is chosen, the physician is also faced with the problem of determining exactly which lesions require intervention.

This case is a good example of a typical patient with multivessel disease facing a decision regarding optimal revascularization strategy. Often, at least one lesion is complex, such as the chronic occlusion of the right coronary artery present in this case. The decision to proceed with surgery or multivessel PCI is often predicated on the complexity of the lesions. The presence of a chronic occlusion or a complex bifurcation lesion may be a "deal breaker" and push the physician to recommend surgery. On the other hand, comorbid illnesses that increase the risk of surgery or the presence

of poor distal targets or nonviable myocardium usually cause the physician to lean toward percutaneous revascularization.

The decision regarding which vessels to revascularize is typically made by a visual assessment of the angiogram. While this approach is certainly acceptable for lesions that are severely stenotic, treatment of a lesion that is ambiguous or moderately narrowed but not actually flow-limiting exposes the patient to increased risk without providing any benefit. Recently, the strategy of fractional flow reserve guided revascularization has been shown to be superior to angiographic guided therapy in patients with multivessel coronary disease undergoing stenting.[1] In the case presented here, fractional flow reserve was very helpful and determined that the left anterior descending artery was non–flow-limiting and thus did not require treatment with a stent.

The controversy regarding multivessel intervention versus coronary bypass surgery has been debated for many years. In the balloon angioplasty era, numerous randomized controlled studies were performed comparing balloon angioplasty to bypass surgery; the largest study with the longest follow-up was the BARI trial.[2] Similar to other related trials, the BARI study found no difference in death or myocardial infarction between patients treated with balloon angioplasty versus those undergoing bypass surgery. The main difference, also observed in earlier trials, was that patients undergoing balloon angioplasty had a higher rate of repeat revascularization procedures compared to patients undergoing bypass surgery.

Additional randomized controlled trials were repeated in the bare-metal stent era[3–6] and the drug-eluting stent era.[7,8] Again, the rate of death or MI was similar for groups treated with bare-metal stents compared to those treated with bypass surgery. Although stents reduced the rate of restenosis compared to balloon angioplasty, and drug-eluting stents reduced restenosis rates compared to bare-metal stents, the stent-treated groups continued to have higher rates of repeat revascularization compared to the groups treated with bypass surgery. Of interest, in the large-scale, randomized SYNTAX trial, a higher rate of stroke was observed for patients treated with coronary bypass surgery compared to PCI (2.2% vs. 0.6%).[8]

In the end, the decision whether to revascularize a patient with multivessel coronary disease surgically or by a percutaneous approach is complex and depends on multiple factors, including coronary anatomy, the nature of the ischemic syndrome, compliance with medications (particularly long-term, dual antiplatelet therapy), comorbid illness, patient preference, and operator skill. This controversy will likely continue long into the future.

KEY CONCEPTS

1. Revascularization decisions in patients with multivessel coronary disease are often complex and are based on coronary anatomy, comorbid illness, and patient preference.
2. In the setting of multivessel coronary disease, fractional flow reserve can be helpful in determining which lesions require revascularization.
3. For patients with multivessel coronary disease amenable to both surgery and percutaneous approaches, there is no difference between these two strategies in terms of death or myocardial infarction; however, patients treated percutaneously have a higher rate of repeat revascularization procedures despite the use of drug-eluting stents.

Selected References

1. Tonino PAL, De Bruyne B, Pijls NHJ, Siebert U, Ikeno F, van't Veer M, Klauss V, Manoharan G, Engstrom T, Oldroyd KG, Ver Lee PN, MacCarthy PA, Fearon WF, for the FAME Study Investigators: Fractional flow reserve versus angiography for guiding percutaneous coronary intervention, *N Engl J Med* 360:213–224, 2009.
2. The Bypass Angioplasty Revascularization Investigation (BARI) Investigators: Comparison of coronary bypass surgery with angioplasty in patients with multivessel disease, *N Engl J Med* 335:217–225, 1996.
3. Serruys PW, Unger F, Sousa JE, Jatene A, Bonnier HJRM, Schonbergern JPAM, Buller N, Bonser R, van den Brand MJB, van Herwerden LA, Morel MAM, van Hout BA, for the Arterial Revascularization Therapies Study Group, *N Engl J Med* 344:1117–1124, 2001.
4. Serruys PW, Ong ATL, van Herwerden LA, Sousa JE, Jatene A, Monnier JJRM, Schonberger JPMA, Buller N, Bonser R, Disco C, Backx B, Hugenholtz PG, Firth BG, Unger F: Five-year outcomes after coronary stenting versus bypass surgery for the treatment of multivessel disease. The final analysis of the Arterial Revascularization Therapies Study (ARTS) randomized trail, *J Am Coll Cardiol* 46:575–581, 2005.
5. Morrison DA, Sethi G, Sacks J, et al, for the Investigators of the Department of Veterans Affairs Cooperative Study #385: The Angina with Extremely Serious Operative Mortality Evaluation (AWESOME). *J Am Coll Cardiol* 38:143–149, 2001.
6. The SOS Investigators: Coronary artery bypass surgery versus percutaneous coronary intervention with stent implantation in patients with multivessel coronary artery disease (the Stent or Surgery trial): a randomized controlled trial, *Lancet* 360:965–970, 2002.
7. Park DW, Yun SC, Lee SW, Kim YH, Lee CW, Hong MK, Kim JJ, Choo SJ, Song H, Chung CH, Lee JW, Park SW, Park SJ: Long-term mortality after percutaneous coronary intervention with drug-eluting stent implantation versus coronary artery bypass surgery for treatment of multivessel coronary artery disease, *Circulation* 117:2079–2086, 2008.
8. Serruys PW, Morice MC, Kappetein AP, Colombo A, Holmes DR, Mack MJ, Stahle E, Feldman TE, van den Brand M, Bass EJ, Van Dyck N, Leadley K, Dawkins KD, Mohr FW: for the SYNTAX Investigators. Percutaneous coronary intervention versus coronary artery bypass grafting for severe coronary artery disease, *N Engl J Med* 360:961–972, 2009.

Inability to Stent in the Face of a Large Dissection

Michael Ragosta, MD, FACC, FSCAI

CASE PRESENTATION

An active 60-year-old man with a history of tobacco abuse, prostate cancer, hypertension, and several prior myocardial infarctions in the remote past presented with chest pain. He underwent coronary bypass surgery 16 years earlier consisting of a left internal mammary graft to the left anterior descending artery (LAD). He was in his usual state of health until midnight prior to admission when he awoke with severe substernal chest pain radiating to both shoulders and accompanied by dyspnea and diaphoresis. Sublingual nitroglycerin tablets alleviated the pain temporarily, only for it to recur. He drove himself to the emergency department at 5:00 AM, where he was noted to have ST-segment depressions in the anterolateral leads on his ECG; the first troponin was negative. He was admitted and treated with unfractionated heparin, aspirin, clopidogrel, nitroglycerin, and a beta blocker and became pain-free. He was referred for catheterization the next day.

CARDIAC CATHETERIZATION

The left internal mammary graft to the LAD was intact and the LAD supplied collaterals to the circumflex (Video 37-1). The native LAD and circumflex were both occluded. Heavy calcification affected the right coronary artery and severe disease was present in the midsegment of this artery (Figures 37-1, 37-2 and Videos 37-2, 37-3). Because of extensive calcification, rotational atherectomy was planned. This was performed with a 1.5 mm burr through an 8 French right Judkins guide catheter after a temporary pacemaker was placed and procedural anticoagulation was achieved with unfractionated heparin and eptifibatide. Following rotational atherectomy, balloon angioplasty using a compliant, 2.5 mm diameter by 20 mm long balloon was accomplished at several locations within the mid-right coronary, and full inflation of the balloon was noted at nominal inflation pressures (Figure 37-3). The angiogram obtained after rotational atherectomy and balloon angioplasty is shown in

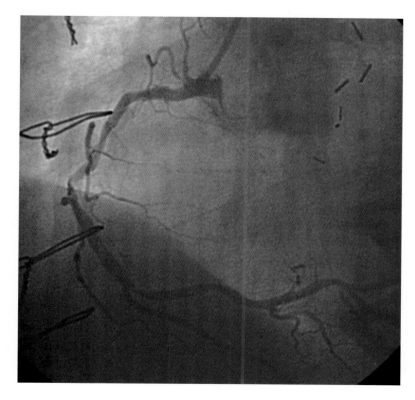

FIGURE 37-1. This is the left anterior oblique projection of the right coronary angiogram showing a severe stenosis in the mid portion of the artery.

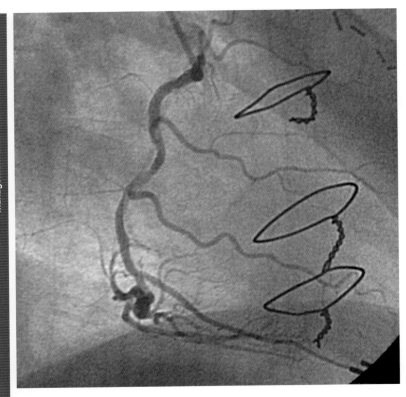

FIGURE 37-2. This is the right anterior oblique projection of the right coronary artery showing the severe stenosis of the midsegment of the right coronary artery and extensive calcification.

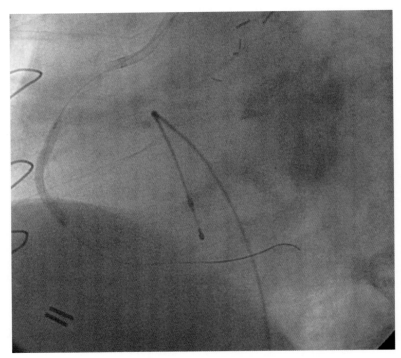

FIGURE 37-3. The balloon was fully expanded after performance of rotational atherectomy.

Figures 37-4 and 37-5 and Videos 37-4 and 37-5. While the left anterior oblique projections appeared acceptable, the right anterior oblique projection revealed a large dissection in the midsection.

The operator then attempted to advance a stent (3.0 mm diameter by 20 mm long paclitaxel-eluting stent) to the mid-right coronary lesion with the goal of covering the entire dissection. However, the stent would not advance to the desired location. The operator decided to withdraw this stent and try a shorter, bare-metal stent; however, the first stent was firmly embedded in the lesion and would not withdraw to the guide. The operator feared that the stent might come off the balloon if additional force was applied and deployed the stent at

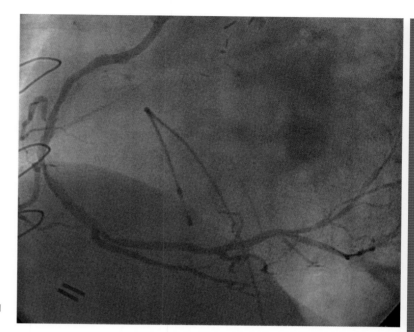

FIGURE 37-4. Angiographic appearance following rotational atherectomy and balloon angioplasty.

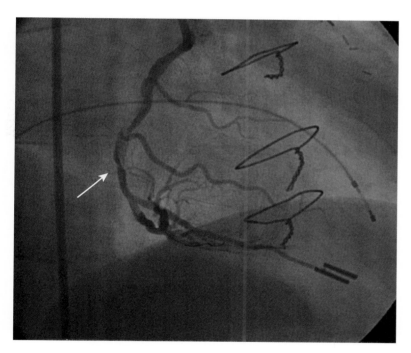

FIGURE 37-5. An extensive dissection is apparent in the right anterior oblique projection (*arrow*).

the location, it became trapped (Figure 37-6). The angiogram obtained after this stent was deployed proximal to the desired location is shown in Figure 37-7. This stent was then aggressively postdilated with a noncompliant balloon and the unstented lesion in the midportion of the artery aggressively ballooned with a noncompliant balloon to high pressures after an additional and more supportive guidewire was placed as a "buddy" wire to facilitate another attempt at stent placement. The operator then chose a 3.0 mm diameter by 8 mm long bare-metal stent. With great difficulty, this stent was advanced distally, covering the distal part of the dissection

(Figure 37-8 and Video 37-6); however, there remained a prominent dissection proximal to this in the midsegment of the artery. Again, the operator aggressively ballooned this area with noncompliant balloons. While the angiographic result appeared acceptable in the left anterior oblique projection (Video 37-7), the prominent dissection was most apparent in the right anterior oblique projection and narrowed the lumen significantly (Figure 37-9 and Video 37-8). One additional 3.0 mm diameter by 8 mm long bare-metal stent was advanced through the proximal stent and covered an additional portion of the dissection, but the operator could not pass this

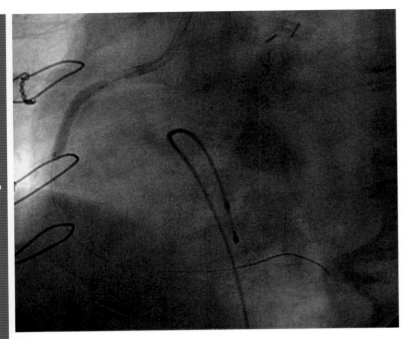

FIGURE 37-6. This figure shows the location of the first stent deployment. This stent could not be advanced beyond the curve in the midportion of the artery and could not be withdrawn into the guide catheter, so it was deployed at this location.

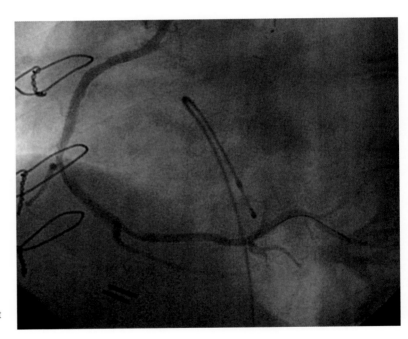

FIGURE 37-7. Angiographic appearance after first stent deployment.

third stent far enough to cover the dissection completely. Despite aggressive ballooning, additional attempts to completely cover the dissection by inserting yet another stent failed. The operator decided to stop the procedure after watching the patient for 15 minutes on the catheterization table and after observing no deterioration in the angiogram or the patient's clinical status, or any change in the electrocardiogram. The final angiographic results are shown in Figures 37-10 through 37-12 and Videos 37-9 and 37-10.

POSTPROCEDURAL COURSE

He remained free of chest pain overnight and was discharged the next afternoon after ambulating without symptoms on clopidogrel, aspirin, atenolol, amlodipine, simvastatin, and lisinopril. He remained free of symptoms at follow-up 1 month later but was subsequently lost to follow-up.

DISCUSSION

Coronary dissections are a common complication of percutaneous coronary intervention and, if untreated, can lead to serious sequelae including abrupt vessel closure, periprocedural myocardial infarction, closure of major side branches, emergency bypass surgery, and even death. Coronary stents successfully treat most dissections such that, in the current era, the risk of sustained

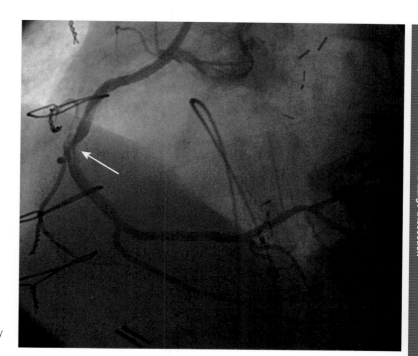

FIGURE 37-8. Uncovered dissection in the mid-right coronary artery, LAO view (*arrow*).

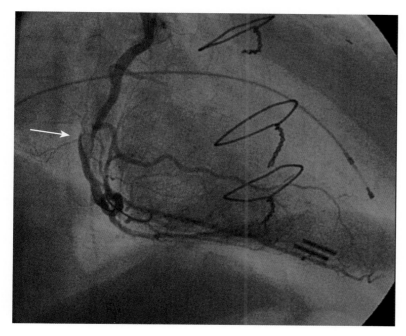

FIGURE 37-9. Uncovered dissection in the mid-right coronary artery, RAO view (*arrow*).

vessel closure or the need for emergency bypass surgery due to a coronary dissection is very rare. However, as demonstrated by this case, the modern-day interventionalist is sometimes faced with the predicament of a coronary dissection that cannot be stented. The current generation stents are highly deliverable but occasionally, due to the presence of excessive tortuosity, heavy calcification, the presence of prior stents, or inadequate guide catheter backup, a stent may not be deliverable. In such cases, the only options available are either to leave the dissection alone and treat medically or to perform emergency bypass surgery.

The decision to leave a dissection alone depends upon the anticipated risk of vessel closure or other adverse event. The angiographic appearance of coronary dissections can be classified according to the system described by the National Heart, Lung, and Blood Institutes (Table 37-1). Using this classification scheme, the outcomes of 691 coronary dissections from the balloon era (1987-1990) were determined.[1] Type A dissections are of no clinical consequence and were not studied. The incidence of adverse events such as emergency bypass surgery and abrupt vessel closure were very low for Type B dissections. However, Type C through F dissections had a substantially higher incidence of adverse events. The risk of abrupt vessel closure and emergency bypass surgery was nearly 10% for Type C dissections and was between 30% and 60% for the more

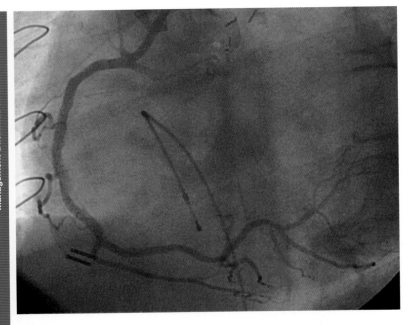

FIGURE 37-10. Final angiographic appearance, LAO view.

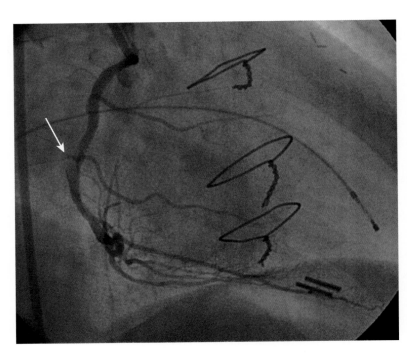

FIGURE 37-11. Final angiographic appearance, RAO view. Residual dissection is shown (arrow).

serious Type D, E, and F dissections.[1] Overall procedural success in this series was 93.7% for Type B dissections (similar to patients without angiographically evident dissections), and was only 38% for patients with Type C through F dissections. Although this information is derived from the balloon angioplasty era and may have little relevance in predicting outcomes in the current era with its advances in pharmacology, this information assists the operator in predicting the risk of vessel closure in cases of a dissection that cannot be stented.

In this case, the angulation and excess calcium led to the dissection. The operator was surprised by the difficulty in passing the stent since a balloon easily passed and fully expanded. Deploying the stent proximal to the

lesion only made it more difficult to subsequently pass a stent to the dissected area; however, the operator had no choice, as the stent became firmly lodged in the lesion and there was a risk of stent embolization if excessive force was used to withdraw the stent back into the guide.

Medical therapy for a large dissection is limited, but most advocate the use of a platelet glycoprotein IIb/IIIa inhibitor as an adjunct to prevent thrombotic occlusion. An intraaortic balloon pump may be helpful in the presence of ongoing ischemic symptoms or if the patient is referred for emergency bypass surgery. In many cases, abrupt vessel closure as a consequence of a serious dissection develops in the catheterization laboratory within a few minutes to hours of the procedure. Thus,

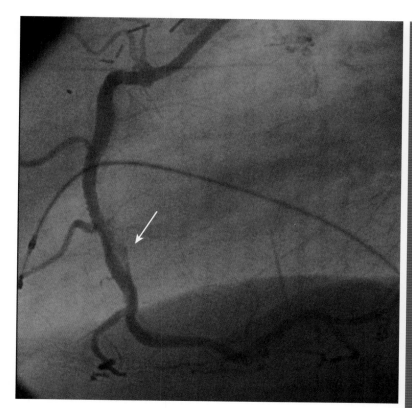

FIGURE 37-12. Final angiographic appearance, lateral view. Residual dissection is shown (*arrow*).

TABLE 37-1 NHLBI Classification of Coronary Dissection

Type	Angiographic Description
A	Radiolucency within lumen during contrast injection with minimal or no persistent contrast staining
B	Parallel tracts or double lumen separated by radiolucency during injection with minimal or no persistent contrast staining
C	Contrast outside the lumen with persistent staining after clearance of dye injection
D	Spiral luminal filling defects with extensive contrast staining
E	Intraluminal filling defects with > 50% luminal obstruction
F	Dissection with closure

many clinicians wisely keep the patient on the catheterization laboratory table when they are managing a dissection that cannot be stented and reimage the artery at intervals to assess for deterioration in the lumen or in blood flow. Also, maintaining the arterial access sheath in place for a few hours is good practice to facilitate a prompt return to the catheterization laboratory if necessary. Coronary bypass surgery is indicated when the artery supplies a significant vascular territory and there is abrupt closure that cannot be reopened or there is a dissection with luminal compromise and ongoing symptoms, electrocardiographic changes, or hemodynamic instability.

The dissection noted in this case would be classified as a Type E dissection with a high likelihood of closure if left untreated. Despite the presence of an unstented dissection, the patient actually did very well, but this is likely because stents were successfully delivered on either side of the dissection and because glycoprotein

IIb/IIIa inhibitors were used, both of which might have altered the natural history of this type of dissection. Although the patient had a favorable acute outcome, the presence of an unstented dissection adjacent to successfully deployed coronary stents is a risk factor for stent thrombosis.[2,3] Whether this concern justifies a more aggressive approach and is an indication for surgery is unclear.

KEY CONCEPTS

1. Although most dissections are treatable with coronary stents, there remain occasional cases in which stents cannot be delivered.
2. A classification system developed during the balloon era is useful in predicting the risk of a serious adverse event from an unstentable dissection.
3. Management of an unstented dissection includes medical therapy with glycoprotein IIb/IIIa inhibitors and close observation or emergency bypass surgery.

Selected References

1. Huber MS, Mooney JF, Madison J, Mooney MR: Use of a morphologic classification to predict clinical outcome after dissection from coronary angioplasty, *Am J Cardiol* 68:467–471, 1991.
2. Lemeslea G, Delhaye C, Bonello L, de Labriolle A, Waksman R, Pichard A: Stent thrombosis in 2008: Definition, predictors, prognosis and treatment, *Arch Cardiovasc Dis* 101:769–777, 2008.
3. Cheneau E, Leborgne L, Mintz GS, et al: Predictors of subacute stent thrombosis: Results of a systematic intravascular ultrasound study, *Circulation* 108:43–47, 2003.

How to Assess Lesions of Intermediate Severity: FFR or IVUS?

Michael Ragosta, MD, FACC, FSCAI

CASE PRESENTATION

A 66-year-old man without prior cardiac history developed progressive dyspnea on exertion, culminating in rest chest pain. In the emergency department, the electrocardiogram was normal, but he was found to have an elevated troponin I (5.77 ng/mL), and he was admitted with the diagnosis of a non-ST segment elevation myocardial infarction. He became pain-free on nitrates, beta-blockers, low-molecular-weight heparin, aspirin, and clopidogrel. Past medical history was notable for hypertension, dyslipidemia, prior tobacco abuse, adenomatous colon polyps, benign prostatic hypertrophy, and hypothyroidism. Troponin I subsequently rose to 16.5 ng/mL and he was referred for cardiac catheterization the next day.

CARDIAC CATHETERIZATION

There was a severe stenosis of a small, distal branch of the right coronary artery, which appeared to represent the culprit lesion (Figure 38-1 and Video 38-1). The operator considered this artery too small and the lesion too distal for intervention. Atherosclerotic plaque without significant narrowing was seen in the mid-right

coronary artery and the first obtuse marginal artery. A long, moderate stenosis affected the proximal to mid-segment of the left anterior descending (LAD) artery at a bifurcation with a large diagonal branch (Figure 38-2 and Video 38-2). The left ventriculogram revealed normal function and no specific wall motion abnormalities. Concerned about the lesion of intermediate severity seen in the left anterior descending artery, the physician decided to assess the lesion's significance by measuring fractional flow reserve, or FFR. Thus, a guide catheter was engaged in the left coronary artery and, after administering a bolus of 50 U/kg of unfractionated heparin, the operator advanced a pressure wire to the distal LAD. The wire transducer was placed distal to the LAD lesion and simultaneous distal coronary pressure and aortic pressure from the guide catheter tip were sampled after maximum coronary vasodilatation was achieved with 100 mcg of intracoronary adenosine (Figure 38-3). Fractional flow reserve was calculated as the ratio of the mean coronary pressure distal to the stenosis (62 mmHg) to mean pressure of the aorta at the guide catheter (76 mmHg) during maximal hyperemia. This ratio calculated to an FFR of 0.82. Thus, the lesion was

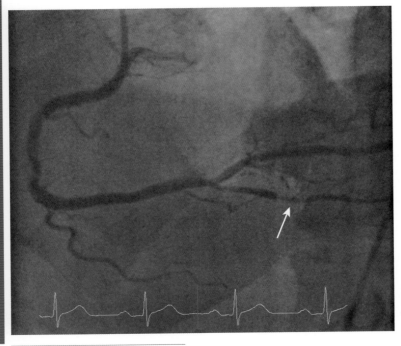

FIGURE 38-1. This is a left anterior oblique projection of the right coronary artery. There is a severe stenosis in a distal branch of the right coronary artery (*arrow*). Although this likely represents the culprit lesion, the vessel is of very small caliber and the lesion is very distal and would not be ideally suited to percutaneous intervention.

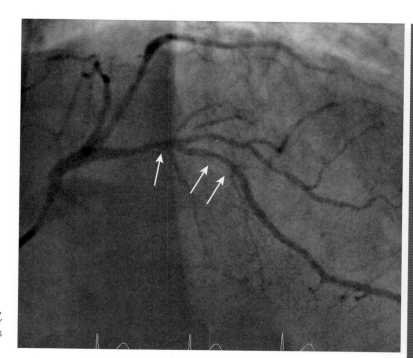

FIGURE 38-2. The left coronary angiogram revealed a long, moderate stenosis in the proximal to midsegment (*arrows*) near a bifurcation of a large diagonal branch. The significance of this intermediate stenosis is not clear from the angiogram.

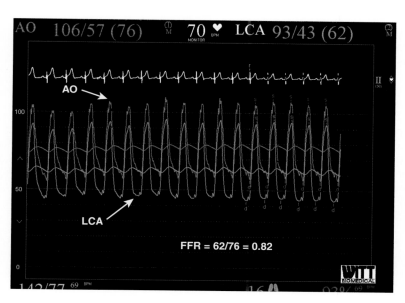

FIGURE 38-3. Simultaneous pressure measured from the aorta **(AO)** and left coronary artery **(LCA)** distal to the moderate disease in the LAD during maximal hyperemia achieved with 100 mcg of intracoronary adenosine. Fractional flow reserve, or FFR is determined as the ratio of the mean distal pressure in the LCA (62 mmHg) to mean AO pressure (76 mmHg) during maximal hyperemia and calculates to 0.82. An FFR less than 0.75 represents a hemodynamically significant stenosis.

determined to be a non–flow-limiting stenosis. Based on the results of the angiogram and the FFR determination, it was decided to treat him medically.

POSTPROCEDURAL COURSE

The patient had no further symptoms. He was discharged on metoprolol, isosorbide mononitrate, aspirin, clopidogrel, valsartan, and Synthroid. During a stress test performed one month later, he exercised for a total of 12 minutes using the standard Bruce exercise protocol, achieving stage 4 and a maximum of 12.9 METs. Gated SPECT myocardial perfusion revealed normal left ventricular function with a calculated ejection fraction of 66% and a small zone of reduced uptake in the mid- to basal inferolateral segment, which was partly reversible

and appeared to represent an infarct with peri-infarct ischemia. This zone corresponded to the distal right coronary disease observed on the angiogram. There was no ischemia in the LAD or diagonal territories. Over 2 years of follow-up, he remains free of symptoms and cardiac events.

DISCUSSION

Coronary angiography forms the basis for revascularization decisions in patients with coronary artery disease. When an artery appears normal or minimally diseased or if there is an obvious, severe stenosis, interpretation is easy and decision-making straightforward. However, angiography has well-known limitations, particularly for lesions of moderate or intermediate severity, arbitrarily defined as a 40% to 70% stenosis.[1] In addition, lesions are often eccentric or may be within segments difficult to visualize clearly, leaving the physician with doubt as to the stenosis severity. In such circumstances, adjunctive testing helps the physician decide the significance of a lesion with greater confidence.

Currently, there are two adjunctive techniques commonly used to assess lesion significance: intravascular ultrasound and fractional flow reserve. Intravascular ultrasound, or IVUS, is an anatomically-based technique to precisely measure the arterial lumen. Fractional flow reserve, or FFR, is physiologically based and takes into consideration the multiple, complex variables impacting coronary flow, including lesion severity and length and collateral flow.

Assessment of an ambiguous lesion with intravascular ultrasound requires the identification of a "worse" segment (minimal luminal diameter) and quantification of the lumen. It is not appropriate to make a decision based on the observation that the IVUS "looks bad," as it is the degree of anatomic lumen compromise that determines lesion significance, not the atherosclerotic plaque burden. In patients with intermediate stenoses of major epicardial arteries (excluding the left main stem), the following IVUS parameters are associated with "significant" lesions": 1) minimal luminal cross-sectional area narrowing less than 4.0 mm^2; 2) minimal luminal diameter less than 1.8 to 2.0 mm; and 3) percentage of area stenosis greater than 70%.[2,3] Left main stem lesions are deemed significant if the minimal luminal area is less than 6 mm^2 in one study[4] and less than 7.5 mm^2 in another.[5] There are several important caveats to the use of IVUS for determination of lesion significance. First, IVUS parameters have been validated only in large, proximal arteries (average 3.0 mm). The absolute lumen values noted above do not apply to small or distal arteries. Second, disease involving a long segment or tandem proximal lesions may not narrow the lumen below the threshold diameter at any given slice, yet may still compromise flow. Finally, the IVUS catheter may cause spasm, leading to an artifactually small lumen.

Fractional flow reserve describes the ratio of the maximum achievable flow in the presence of a stenosis to the theoretical maximum flow in the same vessel in the absence of a stenosis. It is simple to perform, requiring the measurement of simultaneous aortic and distal coronary pressures using a special angioplasty guidewire outfitted with a micromanometer during maximal hyperemia. The mathematics, experimental basis, technique, limitations, and validation of FFR have been well-described.[6–11] It can be calculated simply by the formula:

$$FFR = \frac{\text{mean hyperemic distal intracoronary pressure}}{\text{mean hyperemic aortic pressure}}$$

The unequivocal normal value of 1.0 is well accepted and has been firmly established in humans. The value below which a stenosis is deemed "significant" is of some debate. Multiple studies confirmed that lesions associated with ischemia have FFR <0.75. Lesions with FFR between 0.75 and 0.80 are generally recognized as "borderline" and may, in fact, represent significant

lesions. In such cases, decisions regarding revascularization require clinical judgment. Importantly, there are numerous studies demonstrating that revascularization of lesions with FFR greater than 0.75 to 0.80 can safely be deferred, thereby establishing FFR as a valuable tool and important adjunct to angiography in clinical decision making.[12–14]

In the case presented here, the culprit vessel was clearly a distal branch of the right coronary artery and FFR was used to assess a lesion found incidentally on angiography. This scenario is very commonly encountered. Importantly, FFR was recently found to be superior to an angiography-guided strategy in determining which vessels need revascularization in patients with multivessel coronary disease.[15] Recently published practice guidelines have established measurement of FFR as a Class IIa indication to determine whether PCI of a specific lesion is warranted and as an alternative to noninvasive functional testing such as stress testing for assessment of the effects of intermediate stenoses (30% to 70%) in patients with anginal syndromes.[16]

KEY CONCEPTS

1. Angiography has well-known limitations. The clinical significance of coronary lesions of moderate severity (30% to 70%) is unclear based on angiography alone, and often requires adjunctive techniques for further delineation.

2. Intravascular ultrasound (IVUS) and fractional flow reserve (FFR) are commonly used adjunctive techniques to determine the significance of ambiguous coronary lesions.

3. IVUS is an anatomically-based method requiring quantification. For proximal epicardial coronary arteries, a minimal luminal cross-sectional area narrowing of less than 4.0 mm^2 is associated with ischemia; for the left main stem the threshold is below either 6.0 mm^2 or 7.5 mm^2, depending on the study.

4. FFR is physiologically based using coronary pressures. A normal value is 1.0, and values less than 0.75 are associated with ischemia. Deferral of intervention in patients with FFR greater than 0.75 is safe based on several long-term outcome trials.

Selected References

1. Fischer JJ, Samady H, McPherson JA, Sarembock IJ, Powers ER, Gimple LW, Ragosta M: Comparison between visual assessment and quantitative angiography versus fractional flow reserve for native coronary narrowings of moderate severity, *Am J Cardiol* 90:210–215, 2002.

2. Briguori C, Anzuini A, Airoldi F, Gimelli G, Nishida T, Adamian M, Corvaja N, DiMario C, Colombo A: Intravascular ultrasound criteria for the assessment of the functional significance of intermediate coronary artery stenoses and comparison with fractional flow reserve, *Am J Cardiol* 87:136–141, 2001.

3. Abizaid A, Mintz GS, Pichard AD, Kent KM, Satler LF, Walsh CL, Popma JJ, Leon MB: Clinical, intravascular ultrasound, and quantitative angiographic determinants of the coronary flow reserve

before and after percutaneous transluminal coronary angioplasty, *Am J Cardiol* 82:423–428, 1998.

4. Vasti V, Ivan E, Yalamanchili V, Wongpraparut N, Leesar MA: Correlations between fractional flow reserve and intravascular ultrasound in patients with an ambiguous left main coronary artery stenosis, *Circulation* 110:2831–2836, 2004.

5. Fassa AA, Wagatsuma K, Higano ST, Mathew V, Barsness GW, Lennon RJ, Holmes DR, Lerman A: Intravascular ultrasound guided treatment for angiographically indeterminate left main coronary artery disease. A long term follow-up study, *J Am Coll Cardiol* 45:204–211, 2005.

6. Pijls NHJ, van Son JAM, Kirkeeide RL, De Bruyne B, Gould KL: Experimental basis of determining maximum coronary, myocardial, and collateral blood flow by pressure measurements for assessing functional stenosis severity before and after percutaneous transluminal coronary angioplasty, *Circulation* 87:1354–1367, 1993.

7. Pijls NHJ, Van Gelder B, Van der Voort P, Peels K, Bracke FALE, Bonnier HJRM, El Gamal MIH: Fractional flow reserve: a useful index to evaluate the influence of an epicardial coronary stenosis on myocardial blood flow, *Circulation* 92:3183–3193, 1995.

8. De Bruyne B, Baudhuin T, Melin JA, Pijls NH, Sys SU, Bol A, Paulus WJ, Heyndrickx GR, Wijns W: Coronary flow reserve calculated from pressure measurements in humans: validation with positron emission tomography, *Circulation* 89:1013–1022, 1994.

9. De Bruyne B, Bartunek J, Sys SU, Heyndrickx GR: Relation between myocardial fractional flow reserve calculated from coronary pressure measurements and exercise-induced myocardial ischemia, *Circulation* 92:39–46, 1995.

10. Pijls NHJ, De Bruyne B, Peels K, van der Voort PH, Bonnier HJRM, Bartunek J, Koolen JJ: Measurement of fractional flow reserve to assess the functional severity of coronary-artery stenoses, *N Engl J Med* 334:1703–1708, 1996.

11. Bishop AH, Samady H: Fractional flow reserve: critical review of an important physiologic adjunct to angiography, *Am Heart J* 147:792–802, 2004.

12. Bech GJW, DeBruyne B, Bonnier HJRM, Bartunek J, Wijns W, Peels K, Heyndrickx GR, Koolen JJ, Pijls NHJ: Long-term follow-up after deferral of percutaneous transluminal coronary angioplasty of intermediate stenosis on the basis of coronary pressure measurement, *J Am Coll Cardiol* 31:841–847, 1998.

13. Bech GJ, DeBruyne B, Pijls NH, deMuinck ED, Hoorntje JC, Escaned J, Stella PR, Boersma E, Bartunek J, Koolen JJ, Wijns W: Fractional flow reserve to determine the appropriateness of angioplasty in moderate coronary stenosis: a randomized trial, *Circulation* 103:2928–2934, 2001.

14. Pijls NHJ, van Schaardenburgh P, Manoharan G, Boersma E, Bech JW, van't Veer M, Bar F, Hoorntje J, Koolen J, Wijns W, De Bruyne B: Percutaneous coronary intervention of functionally non-significant stenosis. 5 year follow-up of the DEFER study, *J Am Coll Cardiol* 49:2105–2111, 2007.

15. Tonino PAL, DeBruyne B, Pijls NHJ, Siebert U, Ikeno F, van't Veer M, Klauss V, Manoharan G, Engstrom T, Oldroyd KG, Ver Lee PN, MacCarthy PA, Fearon WF, for the FAME Study Investigators: Fractional flow reserve versus angiography for guiding percutaneous coronary intervention, *N Engl J Med* 360:213–224, 2009.

16. Kushner FG, Hand M, Smith SC Jr, King SB 3rd, Anderson JL, Antman EM, Bailey SR, Bates ER, Blankenship JC, Casey DE Jr, Green LA, Hochman JS, Jacobs AK, Krumholz HM, Morrison DA, Ornato JP, Pearle DL, Peterson ED, Sloan MA, Whitlow PL, Williams DO: 2009 focused updates: ACC/AHA guidelines for the management of patients with ST-elevation myocardial infarction (updating the 2004 guideline and 2007 focused update) and ACC/AHA/SCAI guidelines on percutaneous coronary intervention (updating the 2005 guideline and 2007 focused update): a report of the American College of Cardiology Foundation/American Heart Association Task Force on Practice Guidelines, *J Am Coll Cardiol* 54:2205–2241, 2009.

PCI Versus Medical Therapy for Stable Angina

Angela M. Taylor, MD, MS

CASE PRESENTATION

A 73-year-old woman with a past medical history of poorly controlled hypertension, hyperlipidemia, hypothyroidism, and gastroesophageal reflux disease and a family history of coronary artery disease presented with exertional chest and arm discomfort and shortness of breath. She underwent an exercise stress thallium test during which she exercised 6 minutes in a standard Bruce protocol, achieved 73% of her age-predicted heart rate, and reached a maximum blood pressure of 200/90 mmHg. The test was terminated secondary to fatigue. Nuclear imaging revealed no convincing evidence of ischemia. Due to continued symptoms, she underwent cardiac catheterization. The right coronary artery was dominant, with minimal disease (Figure 39-1). The left coronary showed minimal disease of the left anterior descending artery and a severe stenosis in the mid-circumflex artery (Figures 39-2, 39-3 and Video 39-1). After her physician discussed the risks and benefits of percutaneous intervention versus optimal medical therapy, she chose medical management. Her medical regimen was maximized and included an angiotensin-receptor blocker, a calcium-channel blocker, aspirin, a beta-blocker, long-acting nitrates, and a statin. However, despite this therapy, she continued to experience exertional chest pressure and shortness of breath that significantly limited her physical activity. Thus, 3 months later she decided to pursue percutaneous intervention of the circumflex artery.

CARDIAC CATHETERIZATION

The lesion appeared unchanged by angiography. Anticoagulation was achieved with a bolus and infusion of bivalirudin. A 0.014 inch floppy-tipped guidewire was advanced into the circumflex artery beyond the lesion. The lesion was successfully predilated with a 2.0 mm diameter by 20 mm long compliant balloon. A 2.5 mm diameter by 24 mm long drug-eluting stent was then deployed (Figure 39-4 and Video 39-2). Hemostasis was achieved with a vascular closure device and she was discharged the next morning after an uncomplicated overnight stay.

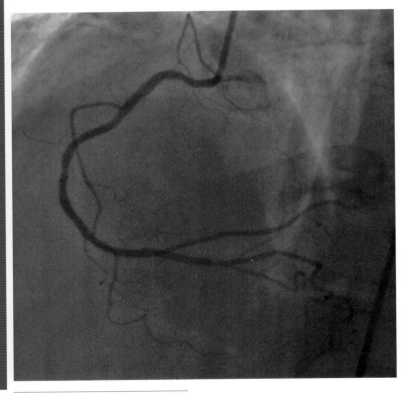

FIGURE 39-1. Right coronary angiogram, demonstrating a dominant right coronary artery with minimal disease.

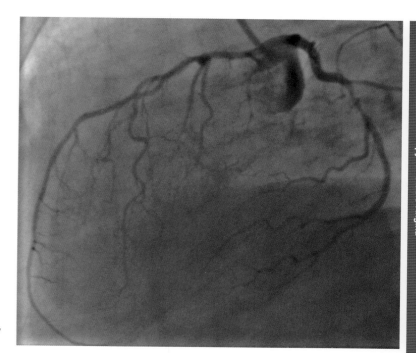

FIGURE 39-2. This lateral projection of the left coronary artery demonstrated minimal disease in the LAD.

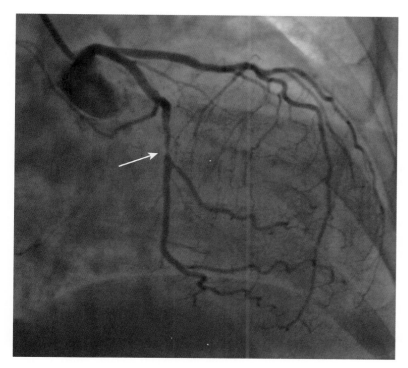

FIGURE 39-3. The AP caudal projection of the left coronary artery showed a severe lesion in the circumflex artery (*arrow*).

POSTPROCEDURAL COURSE

The patient improved remarkably following PCI and immediately returned to her previous level of activity. She remained angina-free at 2-year follow-up.

DISCUSSION

In the United States, over 1 million coronary interventions are performed annually. The majority of percutaneous coronary interventions (PCI) are performed electively in patients with stable coronary artery disease, with only about 15% being performed in the setting of an acute coronary syndrome.[1,2] It has been clearly demonstrated that PCI in the setting of an acute coronary syndrome can provide benefit in terms of death and myocardial infarction.[3,4] This same benefit, however, does not appear to be present when PCI is performed for stable coronary disease.[5,6] Until recently, however, little was known about the benefits of PCI for stable syndromes in patients receiving optimal medical therapy. The COURAGE trial is the largest and most recent trial investigating whether PCI in addition to

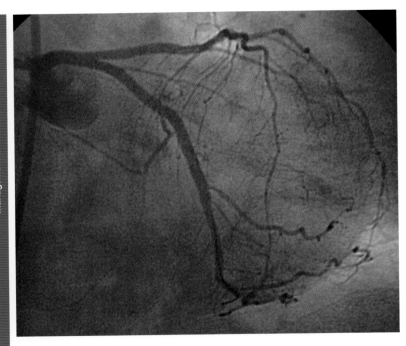

FIGURE 39-4. Angiographic appearance of the left circumflex artery after successful PCI.

optimal medical therapy can reduce cardiovascular events compared to optimal medical therapy alone in this lower-risk population. Similar to previous trials, the addition of PCI added no benefit in terms of death, myocardial infarction, or stroke over an average follow-up of 4.6 years. However, similar to the case shown here, there was significant crossover of the medical therapy group to PCI because of ongoing symptoms despite medical therapy; in addition, the PCI group demonstrated a greater freedom from angina throughout most of the follow-up period.[7]

Current ACC/AHA guidelines recommend an initial approach of optimal medical therapy, lifestyle intervention, and risk factor reduction in the population with stable coronary artery disease. PCI is advocated only with failure of this strategy.[8,9] Much debate, however, still exists as to the proper management of this population. Argument can certainly be made for both strategies. Initial medical therapy mitigates the risk of a potentially unnecessary procedure. However, for many medically treated patients, symptoms may not improve significantly, or, they may note significant side effects from the medications, including fatigue from beta blockers or headaches from long-acting nitrates. In patients with ongoing angina, lifestyle strategies such as exercise, may be difficult, if not impossible to achieve. Further, clinical depression may coexist in patients who are significantly limited in daily activities. A strategy of initial PCI may return patients to routine activities and work more quickly than medical therapy alone. Therefore, while PCI provides no benefit in terms of death or myocardial infarction in a stable population, a better understanding of the psychosocial outcomes of the two strategies is needed.

The dilemma of the best strategy for treating stable patients with angina is well-demonstrated in the patient presented in this case. The current guidelines were followed in the management of this patient and she did undergo a trial of optimal medical management prior to PCI. Unfortunately, she experienced 3 additional months of activity-limiting angina before an intervention promptly resolved her symptoms. Fortunately, she had no complications associated with her procedure and is now going about her daily activities free of angina.

KEY CONCEPTS

1. PCI in the setting of an acute coronary syndrome reduces death and myocardial infarction.
2. PCI in the setting of stable angina does not reduce death or myocardial infarction; however, there is significant improvement in symptoms of angina.
3. Current ACC/AHA guidelines recommend a trial of optimal medical therapy for stable coronary artery disease prior to performing PCI.

Selected References

1. Lloyd-Jones D, Adams R, Carnethon M, et al: Heart disease and stroke statistics – 2009 update. A report from the American Heart Association Statistics Committee and Stroke Statistics Committee, *Circulation* 119:e1–e161, 2009.
2. Feldman DN, Gade CL, Slotwiner AJ, et al: Comparison of outcomes of percutaneous coronary interventions in patients of three age groups, *Am J Cardiol* 98:1334–1339, 2006.
3. Keeley EC, Boura JA, Grines CL: Primary angioplasty versus intravenous thrombolytic therapy for acute myocardial infarction: a quantitative review of 23 randomized trials, *Lancet* 361:13–20, 2003.
4. Mehta SR, Cannon CP, Fox KA, et al: Routine versus selective invasive strategies in patients with acute coronary syndromes: a collaborative meta-analysis of randomized trials, *J Am Med Assoc* 293:2908–2917, 2005.
5. Pitt B, Waters D, Brown WV, et al: Aggressive lipid lowering therapy compared with angioplasty in stable coronary artery disease, *N Engl J Med* 341:70–76, 1999.

6. Henderson RA, Pocock SJ, Clayton TC, et al: Seven-year outcomes in the RITA-2 trial: coronary angioplasty versus medical therapy, *J Am Coll Cardiol* 42:1161–1170, 2003.
7. Boden WE, O'Rourke RA, Teo KK, et al: Optimal medical therapy with or without PCI for stable coronary disease, *N Engl J Med* 356:1–14, 2007.
8. Smith SC Jr, Feldman TE, Hirshfeld JW Jr, et al: ACC/AHA/SCAI 2005 guideline update for percutaneous coronary intervention, *Circulation* 113:156–175, 2006.
9. King SB, Smith SC, Hirshfeld JW, et al: 2007 Focused Update of the ACC/AHA/SCAI 2005 guideline update for percutaneous coronary intervention, *Circulation* 117:261–295, 2008.

PCI Versus Medical Therapy for Stable Angina

Should a Nonculprit Artery Undergo PCI in the Setting of Acute STEMI?

Angela M. Taylor, MD, MS

CASE PRESENTATION

A previously active 56-year-old man with past medical history of type 2 diabetes and dyslipidemia presented with 2 days of intermittent substernal chest pain that had become gradually more severe. On presentation to the emergency department, he was tachycardic, with a heart rate of 100 bpm, and his blood pressure was 95/60 mmHg. His presenting electrocardiogram revealed ST elevation in V1 and V2 with ST depressions in V3 through V6. Chest x-ray demonstrated mild pulmonary edema. He was taken emergently to the cardiac catheterization laboratory for presumed occlusion of the left anterior descending (LAD) artery.

CARDIAC CATHETERIZATION

Hemodynamics obtained prior to coronary angiography revealed an elevated pulmonary capillary wedge pressure at 30 mmHg, elevated left ventricular end-diastolic pressure at 35 mmHg, a narrowed aortic pulse pressure, and tachycardia, consistent with the early phase of cardiogenic shock. Thus, the operator placed an intraaortic balloon pump for hemodynamic support. Angiography found a widely patent right coronary artery with mild luminal irregularities (Figure 40-1). Two consecutive severely narrowed tubular stenoses were present in a large, bifurcating, obtuse marginal branch of the circumflex artery. The LAD was occluded in its proximal portion just after the takeoff of a large septal branch (Figure 40-2 and Video 40-1). Anticoagulation was achieved with heparin and eptifibatide, and a 0.014 inch guidewire was easily advanced distally in the LAD. The lesion was predilated with a 2.5 mm diameter by 15 mm long compliant balloon with full balloon expansion and return of flow to the artery (Figure 40-3 and Video 40-2). Subsequently, a 3.0 mm diameter by 23 mm long sirolimus-eluting stent was placed successfully in the LAD with resultant TIMI-2 flow (Figure 40-4 and Video 40-3). His blood pressure remained low and he required

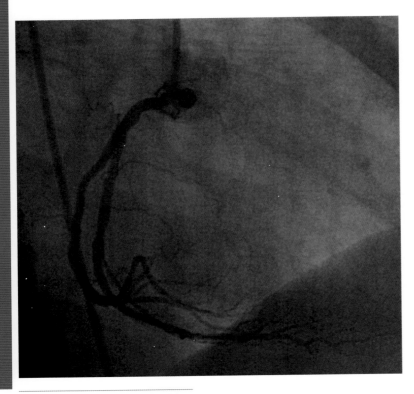

FIGURE 40-1. Luminal irregularities in the right coronary artery.

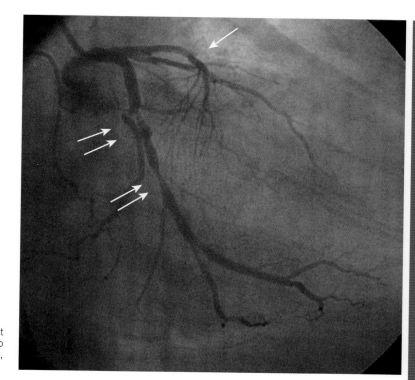

FIGURE 40-2. The LAD is occluded in its proximal portion just after the takeoff of a large septal branch (*arrows*). There are two consecutive severe tubular stenoses in a large, bifurcating, obtuse marginal branch of the circumflex artery (*double arrows*).

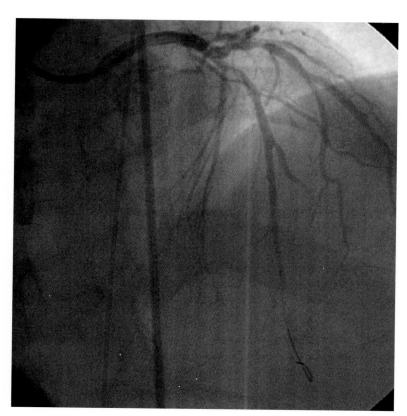

FIGURE 40-3. Angiography of the LAD after predilation shows return of flow to the artery.

a dopamine infusion (10 mcg/kg/min) for hemodynamic support. Given the patient's deteriorating hemodynamic status, the operator was concerned about ongoing ischemia from the severe stenosis in the large circumflex artery and decided to perform percutaneous intervention on this vessel also. The 0.014 inch guidewire

was removed from the LAD and advanced into the obtuse marginal. The sequential lesions were predilated with a 2.5 mm diameter by 15 mm long balloon with full balloon expansion. The distal lesion was treated with a 2.5 mm diameter by 13 mm long sirolimus-eluting stent, and a 3.0 mm diameter by 13 mm long sirolimus-eluting

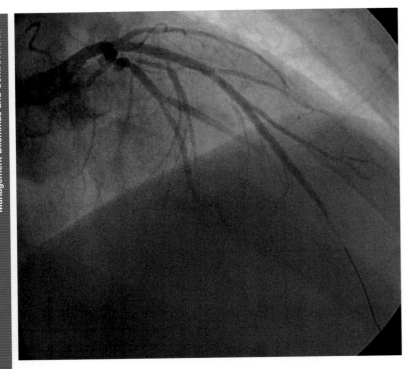

stent was deployed across the proximal lesion so there was overlap of the two stents. The final angiogram shows TIMI-3 flow in both the circumflex and LAD (Figure 40-5, and Video 40-4).

POSTPROCEDURAL COURSE

Intraaortic balloon pump support was continued for 24 hours following the PCI. Inotropic support was successfully weaned and he was discharged on optimal medical therapy 4 days after presentation, including aspirin, clopidogrel, and a statin, a beta-blocker, and an ACE inhibitor. The patient experienced some atypical chest pain approximately 5 months after the procedure and underwent exercise stress testing with nuclear imaging. He was able to complete 11 METs on a treadmill. Perfusion imaging demonstrated a fixed defect in the distal LAD territory with a left ventricular ejection fraction of 52%. He successfully completed cardiac rehabilitation and was walking one to two miles daily at home without any symptoms of angina or heart failure.

DISCUSSION

In patients with ST-elevation myocardial infarction (STEMI), the initial goal of cardiac catheterization is to identify and open the infarct-related artery (IRA). A secondary goal is to image and evaluate the remaining coronary arteries for the presence of additional obstructive disease allowing for further risk stratification and management. In the current era, 40% to 50% of patients presenting with STEMI are found to have significant multivessel coronary disease.[1-3] It is well-accepted that patients with multivessel disease in the setting of STEMI are at higher risk for both early and late cardiac events than patients with single-vessel disease.[1-3] Several

mechanisms may account for this. Disease in a non-IRA may prevent or impair collateral formation and function, creating more extensive ischemia and infarction during the acute occlusion. Additionally, previous infarctions may have lowered the ejection fraction, placing the patient at higher risk for heart failure or shock in the acute setting. And, finally, it has been shown that, in the setting of an acute myocardial infarction, plaques in non-IRAs have a higher frequency of rupture and vulnerable characteristics and non–infarct-related arteries have impairments in flow and flow reserve, suggesting a more global effect on the coronary circulation during an acute coronary syndrome.[4-7]

Given the increased risk in these patients, physicians are faced with the dilemma of how best to manage multivessel disease during catheterization for acute myocardial infarction. There is no definitive evidence to guide the physician in the proper management of the non-IRA, specifically whether the artery should be treated at the initial presentation, treated in a staged fashion, or if further risk stratification should be performed. Arguments can be made both for and against treatment of the non–infarct-related artery at initial presentation. The possibility of abrupt vessel closure or stent thrombosis in the non-IRA during intervention may lead to additional infarction and potentially devastating consequences. An equally compelling argument can be made that intervention on the non-IRA would decrease ischemic risk and improve collateral formation, thus resulting in decreased infarct size. Retrospective studies, prior to extensive use of drug-eluting stents and glycoprotein IIb/IIIa inhibitors, have suggested higher rates of reinfarction and target vessel revascularization if PCI of the non-IRA is performed during the initial presentation for STEMI.[8,9] No large prospective trials address this dilemma. Accordingly, current practice guidelines do

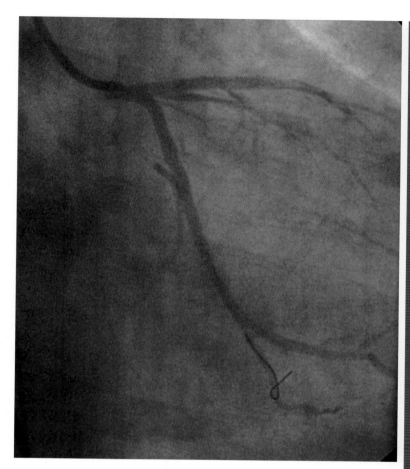

FIGURE 40-5. Angiography of the circumflex artery after stenting.

not recommend performance of an intervention on obstructive lesions in a non-IRA at the time of acute infarct angioplasty, with the exception of patients having hemodynamic compromise, where it might be considered reasonable.[10]

There are even fewer data addressing non-IRA PCI in patients with hemodynamic compromise. It is clear from prospective trials that PCI of the infarct-related artery is beneficial.[11] However, retrospective data suggest higher in-hospital mortality in patients with cardiogenic shock undergoing multivessel PCI during primary PCI for STEMI.[12] Definitive prospective studies need to be performed to better address this issue.

In the case presented here, the patient did well with the operator's chosen strategy of multivessel PCI and had no PCI-related complications. Further, he incurred the risk of only one procedure in terms of vascular access and was not inconvenienced by having to return for repeat PCI. However, it is unclear if there were any benefits in terms of infarct size or mortality and the outcome may have been similarly favorable if PCI had been deferred.

KEY CONCEPTS

1. The current ACC/AHA guidelines do not recommend routine non-IRA PCI in hemodynamically stable patients with STEMI.
2. In patients with hemodynamic compromise, non-IRA PCI may be considered.

Selected References

1. Muller DW, Topol EJ, Ellis SG, et al: Multivessel coronary artery disease: a key predictor of short-term prognosis after reperfusion therapy for acute myocardial infarction. Thrombolysis and Angioplasty in Myocardial Infarction (TAMI) Study Group, *Am Heart J* 121(4 Pt 1):1042–1049, 1991.
2. Jaski BE, Cohen JD, Trausch J, et al: Outcome of urgent percutaneous transluminal coronary angioplasty in acute myocardial infarction: comparison of single-vessel versus multivessel coronary artery disease, *Am Heart J* 124:1427–1433, 1992.
3. Kahn JK, Rutherford BD, McConahay DR, et al: Results of primary angioplasty for acute myocardial infarction in patients with multivessel coronary artery disease, *J Am Coll Cardiol* 16:1089–1096, 1990.
4. Rioufol G, Finet G, Ginon I, et al: Multiple atherosclerotic plaque rupture in acute coronary syndromes: three-vessel intravascular ultrasound study, *Circulation* 106:804–808, 2002.
5. Kotani J, Mintz GS, Castagna MT, et al: Intravascular ultrasound analysis of infarct-related and non-infarct-related arteries in patients who presented with an acute myocardial infarction, *Circulation* 107:2889–2893, 2003.
6. Goldstein JA, Demetriou D, Grines CL, Pica M, Shoukfeh M, O'Neill WW: Multiple complex coronary plaques in patients with acute myocardial infarction, *N Engl J Med* 343:915–922, 2000.
7. Gibson CM, Ryan KA, Murphy SA, et al: Impaired coronary blood flow in nonculprit arteries in the setting of acute myocardial infarction. The TIMI Study Group. Thrombolysis in myocardial infarction, *J Am Coll Cardiol* 34:974–982, 1999.
8. Roe MT, Cura FA, Joski PS, et al: Initial experience with multivessel percutaneous coronary intervention during mechanical reperfusion for acute myocardial infarction, *Am J Card* 88:170–173, 2001.
9. Corpus RA, House JA, Marso SP, et al: Multivessel percutaneous coronary intervention in patients with multivessel disease and acute myocardial infarction, *Am Heart J* 148:493–500, 2004.

10. 2009 Focused updates: ACC/AHA guidelines for the management of patients with ST-elevation myocardial infarction and ACC/AHA/SCAI guidelines on percutaneous coronary intervention, *JACC* 54:2205–2241, 2009.

11. Webb JG, Lowe AM, Sanborn TA, et al: Percutaneous coronary intervention for cardiogenic shock in the SHOCK trial, *JACC* 42:1380–1386, 2003.

12. Cavender MA, Milford-Beland S, Roe MT, et al: Prevalence, predictors, and in-hospital outcomes of non-infarct artery intervention during primary percutaneous intervention for ST-segment elevation myocardial infarction, *Am J Cardiol* 104(4): 507–513, 2009.

Postoperative Acute STEMI

Angela M. Taylor, MD, MS

CASE PRESENTATION

A 69-year-old man with a history of coronary artery disease presented for a left nephroureterectomy for transitional cell carcinoma. Two years prior to presentation, he underwent percutaneous coronary intervention with placement of a 3.0 mm diameter by 18 mm long sirolimus-eluting stent in the proximal circumflex and a 2.5 mm diameter by 18 mm long sirolimus-eluting stent in the mid-left anterior descending artery. He was treated for 6 months with dual antiplatelet therapy consisting of aspirin and clopidogrel, after which he was continued on low-dose aspirin. Aspirin was discontinued 3 weeks prior to surgery. The nephroureterectomy was performed laparoscopically under general anesthesia and the patient tolerated the procedure with no complications. Following transfer to the postanesthesia care unit, the patient developed marked ST depressions in leads V2 through V5, followed by ventricular fibrillation requiring multiple defibrillations with subsequent intubation. One dose of amiodarone was given and a lidocaine drip was started. After consultation with the surgeons, a heparin bolus was given and he was transferred to the cardiac catheterization laboratory for emergent angiography.

CARDIAC CATHETERIZATION

The right coronary artery was small and nondominant, with luminal irregularities (Figure 41-1). The left anterior descending artery (LAD) was patent with a long tubular stenosis of mild severity just prior to the previously placed stent. The stent itself was widely patent. The circumflex artery was occluded at the ostium within the previously placed stent, consistent with late stent thrombosis (Figure 41-2 and Video 41-1). Anticoagulation was achieved with heparin and abciximab, and a 0.014 inch guidewire was advanced easily through the thrombosed stent and into the distal circumflex. The lesion was dilated with a 3.0 mm diameter by 15 mm long compliant balloon with return of flow to the artery, but with residual thrombus (Figure 41-3 and Video 41-2). The operator felt there was residual stenosis and attempted to dilate the lesion with a 3.0 mm diameter by 15 mm long noncompliant balloon. However, the balloon would not advance into the stented segment. A 2.5 mm diameter by 15 mm long noncompliant balloon was advanced easily into the lesion and inflated to high pressure. Subsequently, the 3.0 mm diameter noncompliant balloon passed easily and the lesion was dilated multiple times with high-pressure inflations. The final angiogram revealed minimal thrombus

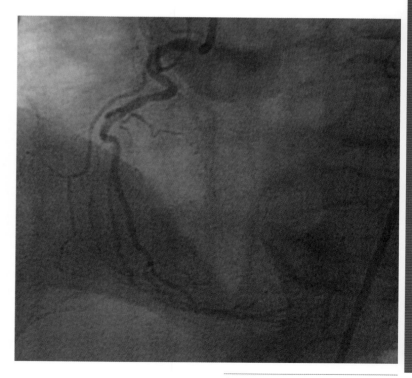

FIGURE 41-1. Right coronary angiography revealed a small, nondominant right coronary artery with luminal irregularities.

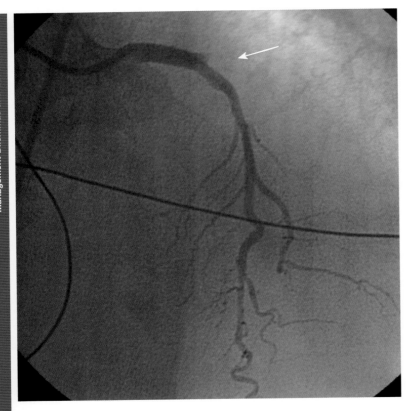

FIGURE 41-2. There was occlusion of the left circumflex artery within the previously placed stent (*arrow*).

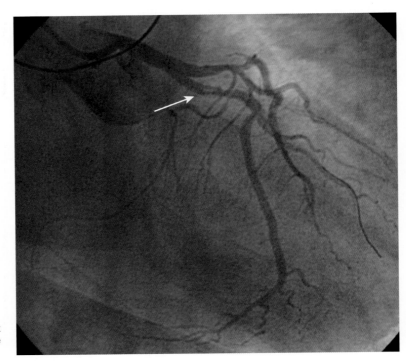

FIGURE 41-3. This is the angiogram of the left circumflex artery after balloon dilation, demonstrating return of flow to the artery but significant residual thrombus (arrow).

within the stented segment and the artery had TIMI-3 flow (Figure 41-4 and Video 41-3).

POSTPROCEDURAL COURSE

The patient was treated for mild heart failure with diuretics and was easily extubated the day following the procedure. His postoperative course was complicated by aspiration pneumonia, and he was discharged 9 days after admission with mild fatigue but no cardiac symptoms. He suffered no increase in surgical bleeding from the procedural anticoagulation. Five months after discharge, the patient had no angina or heart failure symptoms and had no evidence of residual cancer.

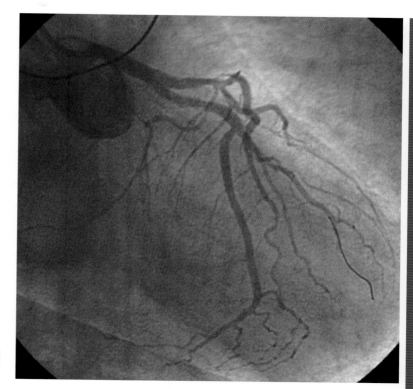

FIGURE 41-4. This is the final angiogram of the left circumflex artery, demonstrating a patent artery with minimal residual thrombus.

DISCUSSION

The frequency of stent thrombosis after placement of bare-metal or drug-eluting stents is rare if there is no interruption in antiplatelet therapy. Although the proper duration of dual antiplatelet therapy following bare-metal stents is fairly well defined, this is not the case for drug-eluting stents. Late stent thrombosis has been seen as far as 2 years post drug-eluting stent implantation and often occurs when antiplatelet therapy is discontinued, particularly in the setting of noncardiac surgery. Perioperative stent thrombosis generally presents as an ST-elevation myocardial infarction and can be a devastating event. The recent surgery greatly complicates management of stent thrombosis, since anticoagulants needed for the procedure may cause dangerous perioperative bleeding complications.

Approximately 5% of patients undergoing stent placement require noncardiac surgery within the following year.[1] The current guidelines recommend postponement of noncardiac surgery for at least 6 months following bare-metal stent placement and for at least 1 year following drug-eluting stent placement.[2,3] However, there appears to be some degree of later risk with cessation of antiplatelet therapy and/or with surgery that has not been well defined. Several retrospective studies have now addressed the risk of stent thrombosis at several time points after stent implantation. With increasing time from implantation, risk of thrombosis decreases; however, the incidence of stent thrombosis was still significant beyond 3 months for bare-metal stents and beyond 12 months for drug-eluting stents. Over half of the patients experiencing an event were on single or dual antiplatelet therapy up to the time of the procedure, demonstrating that many events may not be preventable even with continuation of antiplatelet therapy.[4,5] Several factors have been found to correlate with adverse events, including stent thrombosis, in the perioperative period, including: myocardial infarction within 30 days of surgery, preoperative heparin use, emergency surgery, longer treated lesion length, lower preoperative ejection fraction, shorter time following stenting, and use of aspirin or clopidogrel 24 hours prior to surgery.

Stent thrombosis in the perioperative period also presents challenges in terms of anticoagulation strategies.[6] Use of antithrombotic agents during the procedure in combination with antiplatelet agents following the procedure significantly increases the risk of major bleeding.

Due to the devastating implications of stent thrombosis, the possible need for surgery in the upcoming year should be clearly ascertained by the operator when determining the type of stent to be implanted, or whether revascularization is even necessary prior to surgery. In the absence of high-risk features, such as left main disease, unstable angina, or severe cardiomyopathy, the incidence of perioperative myocardial infarction is not changed by preoperative revascularization. Thus, in stable patients, revascularization can generally be safely delayed until after the perioperative period.[7]

Fortunately, in the case presented here, the patient was successfully resuscitated and flow was restored to the stented artery. Also, it was fortunate that the patient did not also thrombose the stent in the LAD. Despite the use of heparin, abciximab, aspirin, and clopidogrel, the patient had no significant surgical site bleeding. Following this event, it was recommended that the patient remain indefinitely on clopidogrel and low-dose aspirin in order to help prevent future episodes of stent thrombosis.

KEY CONCEPTS

1. Approximately 5% of patients undergoing coronary stenting require noncardiac surgery within the following year.
2. Perioperative stent thrombosis generally presents as an ST-elevation myocardial infarction.
3. The time from stent implantation to surgery is inversely proportional to the risk of stent thrombosis.
4. Many postoperative stent thromboses occur despite continuation of dual antiplatelet therapy, suggesting there are other factors at play.

Selected References

1. Vicenzi MN, Ribitsch D, Luha O, et al: Coronary artery stenting before noncardiac surgery: more threat than safety? *Anesthesiology* 94:367–368, 2001.
2. Fleisher LA, Beckman JA, Brown KA, et al: ACC/AHA 2007 guidelines on perioperative cardiovascular evaluation and care for noncardiac surgery: a report of the ACC/AHA task force on practice guidelines, *J Am Coll Cardiol* 50e:e159–e241, 2007.
3. Grines Cl, Bonow RO, Casey DE, Jr , et al: Prevention of premature discontinuation of antiplatelet therapy in patients with coronary artery stents: a scientific advisory form the AHA, ACC, SCAI, and ACS, and ADA, with representation from the ACP, *J Am Coll Cardiol* 49:734–739, 2007.
4. van Kujik JP, Flu WJ, Schouten O, et al: Timing of surgery after coronary artery stenting with bare metal or drug-eluting stents, *Am J Cardiol* 104:1229–1234, 2009.
5. Brilakis ES, Banerjee S, Berger PB: Perioperative management of patients with coronary stents, *J Am Coll Cardiol* 49:2145–2150, 2007.
6. Anwaruddin S, Askari AT, Saudye H, et al: Characterization of post-operative risk associated with prior drug-eluting stent use, *J Am Coll Cardiol Interv* 2:542–549, 2009.
7. Poldermans D, Schouten O, Vidakovic R, et al: A clinical randomized trial to evaluate the safety of a noninvasive approach in high-risk patients undergoing major vascular surgery: the DECREASE-V pilot study, *J Am Coll Cardiol* 49:1763–1769, 2007.

Coronary Cavernous Fistula

Michael Ragosta, MD, FACC, FSCAI

CASE PRESENTATION

A 55-year-old man presented for management of a coronary cavernous fistula. One year prior to presentation, this otherwise healthy and active man with a history of hypertension, dyslipidemia, and obstructive sleep apnea developed progressive shortness of breath with exertion. This ultimately progressed to rest dyspnea and he presented to a local hospital with congestive heart failure requiring hospitalization. An echocardiogram found normal systolic function and no valvular abnormalities. Suspicious of coronary artery disease, his physician referred him for cardiac catheterization. To the operator's surprise, the angiogram revealed a massive right coronary artery to right atrial fistula (Figure 42-1 and Video 42-1) and several fistulous connections from the left circumflex to the right atrium (Figure 42-2 and Video 42-2). The left anterior descending artery appeared normal, with no fistulae identified, and ventricular function was normal.

Diagnosed with high-output heart failure, he was referred to a surgeon for correction of the fistulae. Surgery consisted of ligation of the right coronary artery with placement of a vein graft to the distal right coronary and ligation of the circumflex fistulae near the atrium. After an uneventful recovery, he did well for several months but then noted increasing dyspnea with fairly minimal exertion; he did not report any chest pain or angina. His symptoms interfered with his ability to work and he was referred for a diagnostic cardiac catheterization.

CARDIAC CATHETERIZATION

Right heart catheterization found fairly normal right sided pressures (mean right atrial pressure of 8 mmHg and pulmonary artery pressure of 27/5 mmHg). The oxygen saturation of blood sampled from the pulmonary artery was 67% with no evidence of a significant left-to-right shunt by oximetry. Cardiac output by the Fick method was 5.07 L/min. Angiography revealed wide patency of the vein graft to the right coronary (Figure 42-3) and continued exclusion of the fistula with no evidence of the fistula from the right coronary (Figure 42-4 and Video 42-3). The left coronary artery demonstrated a single fistulous connection to the right atrium (Figure 42-5 and Video 42-4) representing the distal fistula; the more proximal fistula previously noted was no longer evident.

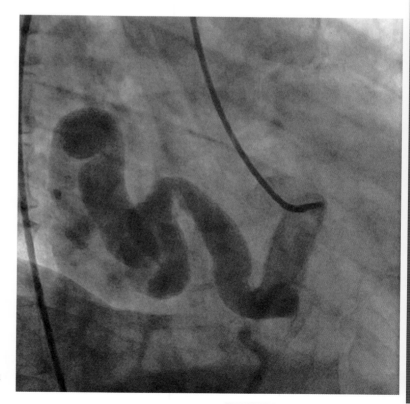

FIGURE 42-1. This is a right coronary angiogram, showing a large fistula to the right atrium.

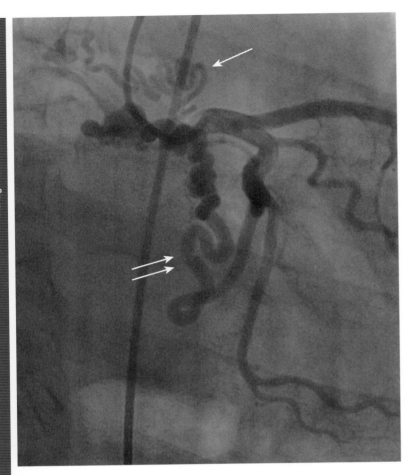

FIGURE 42-2. This is a left coronary angiogram showing two discrete fistulae, one proximal (*arrow*) and one more distal (*double arrow*), to the right atrium.

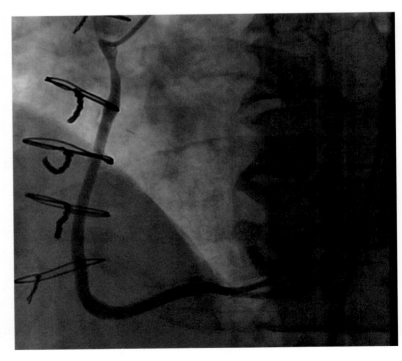

FIGURE 42-3. This is an angiogram of the patent vein graft to the distal right coronary artery.

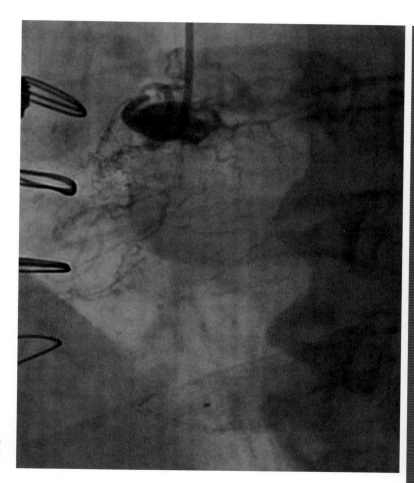

FIGURE 42-4. After surgical correction of the fistula, the native right coronary artery remains occluded with no evidence of the previously noted fistula to the right atrium.

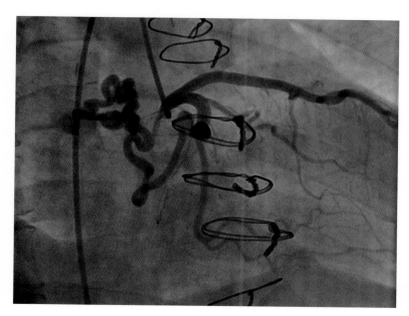

FIGURE 42-5. Postoperative angiogram of the left coronary demonstrating the presence of a large, persistent fistula; the smaller, more proximal fistula is no longer present.

His physician decided to pursue percutaneous closure of the remaining fistula, based on the presence of the patient's ongoing symptoms, which were thought to possibly represent ischemia from "steal." There was also concern regarding the size of the fistula and the possibility of its further enlargement.

A 6 French 4.5 C-shaped guide catheter was inserted in the left coronary artery, and 50 U/kg of unfractionated heparin was administered. A 300 cm 0.014 inch floppy-tipped guidewire was advanced into the distal circumflex and a second, 300 cm 0.014 inch floppy-tipped guidewire placed into the fistula (Figure 42-6

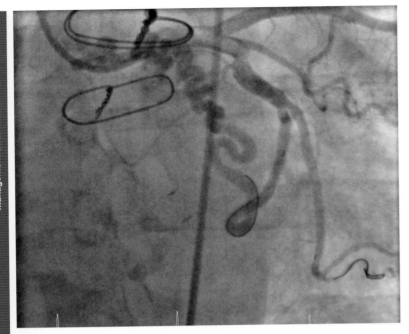

FIGURE 42-6. FIGURE 42-6. With a guide catheter engaged in the left coronary artery, one guidewire was placed in the distal circumflex and a second wire in the fistula.

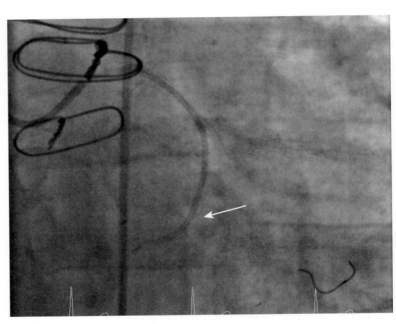

FIGURE 42-7. A 4 French JB1 catheter (*arrow*) was advanced into the fistula to allow positioning of the embolization coils.

and Video 42-5). A 4 French JB1 catheter was then advanced over this latter wire and positioned into the fistula and the 0.014 inch guidewire was removed (Figure 42-7). Contrast injected through the JB1 catheter confirmed an acceptable position in the fistula (Video 42-6). A Cook stainless-steel embolization coil (38-4-3) was then advanced through the catheter using a 0.038 inch Cook Newton wire, and positioned into the fistula (Video 42-7). This did not completely occlude the fistula. Thus, a second coil was placed, successfully occluding flow (Figure 42-8 and Video 42-8). The guidewire and catheter were removed from the circumflex artery and a final angiogram was obtained, showing no residual flow in the fistula (Video 42-9).

POSTPROCEDURAL COURSE

His postprocedural course was uncomplicated, and he was discharged after an overnight stay. At follow-up 1 month later, he remained free of symptoms.

DISCUSSION

Coronary cavernous fistulae are abnormal, usually congenital, direct connections between one or more coronary arteries and a cardiac chamber. They are rare, seen in less than 0.5% of angiograms, and are often incidentally found on a coronary angiogram performed for another reason. Coronary fistulae vary greatly in terms of their size, location, and clinical significance. Many

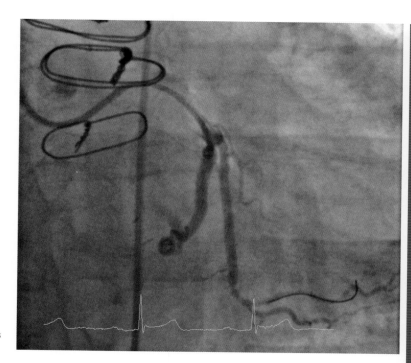

FIGURE 42-8. Two coils successfully occluded the fistulous connection.

fistulae are small and do not result in a measurable shunt; however, very large fistulae may occur, as in this case involving the right coronary artery. They may arise from any of the coronary arteries, but originate most commonly from the right coronary, followed by the left anterior descending artery. Most commonly, they terminate in a right-sided chamber such as the right atrium, right ventricle, coronary sinus, or pulmonary artery. Rarely, they may terminate in the superior vena cava, left atrium, or left ventricle.

Many fistulae are asymptomatic. If symptoms are present, they include angina, dyspnea, and heart failure and are usually caused by a large left-to-right shunt, high cardiac output, or coronary steal and associated ischemia.[1,2] In addition, a fistula may become aneurysmal and rupture, causing hemopericardium, or may become a nidus for infective endocarditis.

The treatment of coronary fistulae depends on their size and complexity and the presence of symptoms. Small fistulae are usually asymptomatic and are often left untreated. Large and symptomatic fistulae are usually closed. Optimal management of asymptomatic but large fistula remains controversial. Some experts advocate their closure in order to prevent late consequences such as aneurysmal dilatation, rupture, and endocarditis.

Surgical techniques are highly effective but are limited by the morbidity associated with major heart surgery. In this case, surgery was highly effective at closing the very large right coronary artery fistula but was less effective at resolving the fistulae originating from the left circumflex artery. This was likely due to the fact that the surgeon approached the circumflex fistulae by attempting to ligate the fistula's termination in the right atrium and was unable to completely identify all of the connections by this method.

A variety of percutaneous methods to close coronary fistulae have been described, including coils, vascular occlusion plugs, covered stents, and umbrella devices.[3–5] These procedures may be very challenging technically depending on the anatomy, and are effective at closing the fistula in 80% to 85% of cases.[3] Complications include device embolization, coronary artery dissection, myocardial infarction, and arrhythmia. Surgery may be preferred in the presence of extreme tortuosity, multiple drainage sites, or the presence of significant coronary artery branches at the site of device delivery.

KEY CONCEPTS

1. Coronary fistulae represent abnormal connections between the coronary circulation and an adjacent (and usually right-sided) cardiac chamber.
2. Fistulae vary greatly in terms of size, location, and clinical significance.
3. Many are asymptomatic. Symptoms may be caused by large shunts, high output, or ischemia from steal. Other adverse sequelae include aneurysmal dilatation, rupture, and infective endocarditis.
4. Treatment includes conservative therapy with observation, surgical exclusion, and a variety of percutaneous closure techniques.

Selected References

1. Liberthson RR, Sagar K, Berkoben JP, Weintraub RM, Levine FH: Congenital coronary arteriovenous fistula. Report of 13 patients, review of the literature and delineation of management, *Circulation* 59:849–854, 1979.

2. Brueck M, Bandorski D, Vogt PR, Kramer W, Heidt MC: Myocardial ischemia due to an isolated coronary fistula, *Clin Res Cardiol* 95:550–553, 2006.
3. Armsby LR, Keane JF, Sherwood MC, Forbess JM, Perry SB, Lock JE: Management of coronary artery fistulae. Patient selection and results of transcatheter closure, *J Am Coll Cardiol* 39:1026–1032, 2002.
4. Collins N, Mehta R, Benson L, Horlick E: Percutaneous coronary artery fistula closure in adults: Technical and procedural aspects, *Catheter Cardiovasc Interv* 69:872–880, 2007.
5. Olivotti L, Moshiri S, Santoro G, Nicolino A, Chiarella F: Percutaneous closure of a giant coronary arteriovenous fistula using free embolization coils in an adult patient, *J Cardiovasc Med* 9:733–736, 2008.

Slow Reflow After PCI for Acute ST-Segment Elevation Myocardial Infarction

Lawrence W. Gimple, MD, FACC, FSCAI

CASE PRESENTATION

A 37-year-old woman with multiple atherosclerotic risk factors was in her usual state of health until approximately 1:00 PM on the day of admission, when she developed the acute onset of substernal chest pain. She presented to the emergency department approximately 4½ hours later. The initial electrocardiogram revealed anterior ST-segment elevation. She was promptly treated with aspirin, clopidogrel, unfractionated heparin, sublingual nitroglycerin, morphine sulfate, and metoprolol, and was referred promptly to the cardiac catheterization laboratory.

Significant past medical history included lupus nephritis with stage 4 chronic kidney disease and proteinuria, hypertension, obesity, type 2 diabetes mellitus (poorly controlled), and dyslipidemia. She had never smoked, and denied use of alcohol or illicit drugs. Her medications on admission included glipizide, pioglitazone, atenolol, amlodipine, sodium bicarbonate, hydrochlorothiazide, omeprazole, and candesartan. On admission, her blood pressure was 159/91 mmHg, her heart rate was 86 bpm, and the rest of her physical exam was unremarkable. Admission laboratory values were notable for hyperglycemia (glucose 325 mg/dL), and renal insufficiency (serum creatinine 2.2 mg/dL).

CARDIAC CATHETERIZATION

The initial coronary angiogram showed occlusion of the left anterior descending (LAD) coronary artery with the appearance of intraluminal thrombus (Figure 43-1 and Video 43-1). The circumflex and right coronary arteries were without significant obstruction. The operator decided to proceed with immediate PCI of the LAD. The ACT was adjusted with additional boluses of unfractionated heparin to maintain an ACT between 250 and 300 seconds, and eptifibatide was administered as adjunctive therapy (two intravenous boluses, each of 180 mcg/kg, and an infusion of 2.0 mcg/kg per minute continued for 14 hours). The left coronary artery was engaged with a JL4 guide, and the lesion was easily crossed with a 0.014 inch floppy-tipped guidewire. In this case, a thrombus extraction catheter was not used. The operator centered a 2.5 mm diameter by 15 mm long compliant balloon on the lesion and inflated it to 6 atmospheres of pressure (Figure 43-2). Following balloon angioplasty, there was a good angiographic result with resolution of the stenosis and thrombus, but "slow reflow" was noted in the LAD, with significantly slower filling of the distal LAD compared with the circumflex artery (Figure 43-3 and Video 43-2). To treat the slow flow, the operator administered boluses of intracoronary

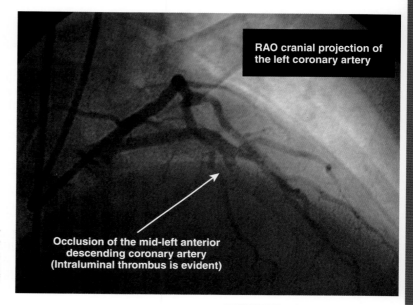

RAO cranial projection of the left coronary artery

Occlusion of the mid-left anterior descending coronary artery (Intraluminal thrombus is evident)

FIGURE 43-1. This left coronary angiogram in the right anterior oblique cranial view shows acute occlusion of the mid-left anterior descending coronary artery. Intraluminal thrombus is seen as a persistent space-filling defect with contrast surrounding the thrombus on three sides. This is a typical appearance of an acutely occluded coronary artery.

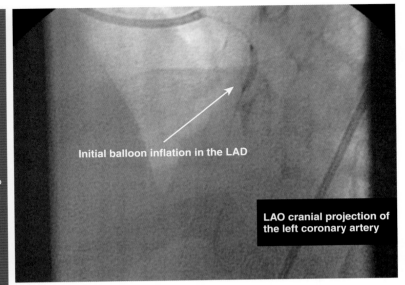

Initial balloon inflation in the LAD

LAO cranial projection of the left coronary artery

FIGURE 43-2. This left anterior oblique cranial view shows an inflated angioplasty balloon in the midportion of the left anterior descending coronary artery.

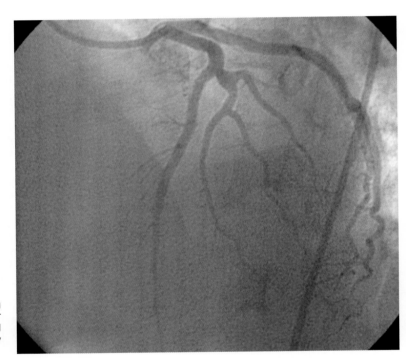

FIGURE 43-3. This left anterior oblique cranial view following balloon angioplasty shows patency of the left anterior descending coronary artery. The video images show slow distal coronary blood flow despite multiple doses of intracoronary adenosine.

adenosine via the guiding catheter, beginning with boluses of 50 mcg and increasing to 80 mcg as tolerated. Flow improved, although it remained abnormal. At this point, the operator treated the lesion with a 3.0 mm diameter by 18 mm long paclitaxel-eluting stent and further dilated it with 16 atmospheres inflation pressure using a 3.5 mm diameter by 15 mm long noncompliant balloon. Flow worsened after stenting (Figures 43-4, 43-5 and Videos 43-3, 43-4). Again, the operator administered multiple intracoronary boluses of adenosine via the guiding catheter, beginning with boluses of 50 mcg and increasing to 80 mcg as tolerated, until a total of 700 mcg had been administered. At the conclusion of the case, LAD flow was improved, although it had not returned to normal. The patient reported resolution of chest pain and remained hemodynamically stable,

although persistent ST elevation was noted on the monitor and on a subsequent 12-lead ECG. The right femoral access sheath was removed with manual compression after 4 hours when the ACT measured less than 180 seconds but while the eptifibatide infusion was continuing.

POSTPROCEDURAL COURSE

Following the catheterization, she was admitted to the coronary care unit. A 12-lead ECG demonstrated persistent ST-segment elevation. She remained hemodynamically stable and free of symptoms. Because of her renal insufficiency and exposure to contrast, she was treated with N-acetylcysteine. Over the next 48 hours, her renal function deteriorated, with the serum creatinine peaking at 3.1 mg/dL before returning to baseline in 5 days.

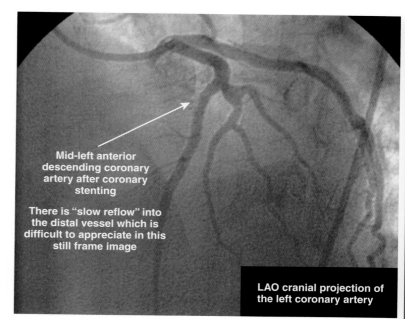

FIGURE 43-4. This left anterior oblique cranial view following coronary stenting using a long paclitaxel drug-eluting stent shows patency of the left anterior descending coronary artery. The video images show slow distal coronary blood flow despite multiple doses of intracoronary adenosine.

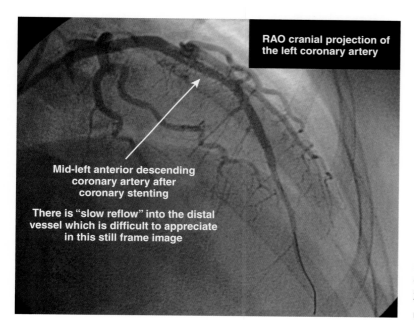

FIGURE 43-5. This right anterior oblique cranial view following coronary stenting using a long paclitaxel drug-eluting stent shows patency of the left anterior descending coronary artery. The video images show slow distal coronary blood flow despite multiple doses of intracoronary adenosine.

An echocardiogram showed anterior hypokinesis and apical akinesis with an ejection fraction of 35% to 40%. She was discharged on aspirin, clopidogrel, atorvastatin, niacin, carvedilol, and candesartan along with her diabetic medications.

She had no further cardiac symptoms during follow-up. Two years later, she developed end-stage renal failure from lupus nephropathy and required long-term dialysis. After the onset of end-stage renal failure, she began to report shortness of breath, and her left ventricular function appeared worse, with an estimated ejection fraction of 25%. Repeat cardiac catheterization showed total occlusion of the LAD at the site of the previous drug-eluting stent and severe left ventricular dysfunction (Figures 43-6, 43-7 and Videos 43-5, 43-6).

She was treated with an implantable defibrillator for primary prevention of ventricular arrhythmias and her medications for congestive heart failure were optimized.

DISCUSSION

The terms "no-reflow" or "slow-reflow" describe the phenomenon when there is an apparent reduction in coronary blood flow seen by angiography following a percutaneous coronary revascularization procedure, despite the presence of a widely patent lumen and in the absence of a mechanical complication such as a dissection.[1] As seen in this case, no-reflow can initially occur immediately after balloon angioplasty but is often

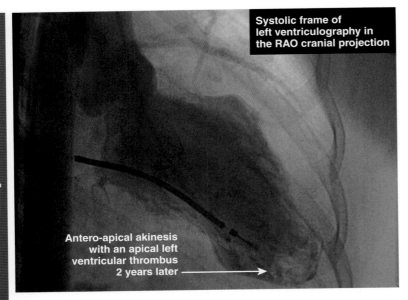

Systolic frame of left ventriculography in the RAO cranial projection

Antero-apical akinesis with an apical left ventricular thrombus 2 years later

FIGURE 43-6. This right anterior oblique cranial left ventriculogram was taken 2 years later when the patient re-presented with congestive heart failure. There is severe anterior and apical akinesis with a filling defect in the left ventricular apex consistent with left ventricular apical thrombus.

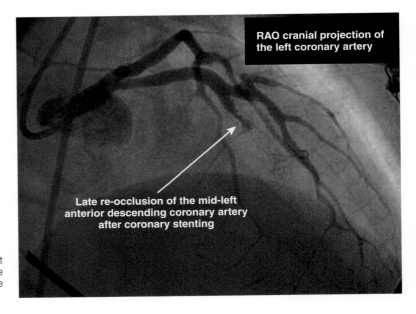

RAO cranial projection of the left coronary artery

Late re-occlusion of the mid-left anterior descending coronary artery after coronary stenting

FIGURE 43-7. This left coronary angiogram in the right anterior oblique cranial view shows chronic reocclusion of the mid-left anterior descending coronary artery 2 years later at the site of the previous stent.

exacerbated by stenting, presumably due at least in part to distal embolization of atherothrombotic material during stent expansion ("cheese-grater effect"). No-reflow can occur in up to 5% of PCI procedures and is more commonly seen with acute coronary syndromes, during rotational atherectomy, and in saphenous vein bypass graft interventions. In the last, distal protection devices can significantly reduce the frequency of no-reflow. No-reflow is more commonly seen during acute PCI for acute ST-elevation MI as in this case.[2,3] Other predictors of the no-reflow phenomenon include the presence of bulky and large plaque burden, intracoronary thrombus, lipid pools (seen on intravascular ultrasound), and total coronary occlusion on the presenting angiogram. In a study comparing coronary aspirates from patients with normal flow to those with no-reflow, the latter contained more atheromatous plaque, more platelets and thrombotic material, more macrophages, and more cholesterol crystals.[4]

In addition to distal embolization, presumed mechanisms of the no-reflow phenomenon include myocardial necrosis, reperfusion injury, macrovascular and microvascular vasoconstriction, local increase in angiotension II receptor density, and neutrophil activation with plugging and endothelial interaction. Diminished microvascular flow can be determined clinically in a qualitative manner by observing slower filling of the infarct artery compared to the opposite artery. Semiquantitative methods include TIMI frame count, TIMI blush score, contrast echocardiography, intracoronary Doppler measurement, and advanced imaging techniques using MRI.

The no-reflow phenomenon is a clinically important finding, as it is associated with significantly worse outcomes. No-reflow is associated with increased mortality, which reaches as high as 27% in some series. It is associated with greater microvascular damage, persistent elevation of the ST segments by ECG, and worse left ventricular function. Patients with no-reflow phenomenon and poor left ventricular function with microvascular damage are at increased risk for late stent closure, as was observed in this case.

Once it develops, no-reflow has been treated in the cardiac catheterization laboratory with mixed success, using intracoronary adenosine, nitroprusside, or verapamil. Other medications have also been reported as effective including abciximab and eptifibatide; however, none of these agents have been well-studied in a randomized, controlled fashion and definitive proof regarding their efficacy is lacking. In addition, none of these agents is specifically approved for this indication. While most operators administer these drugs through the guide catheter, some operators have proposed selective delivery directly into the distal coronary bed using subselective catheters positioned distally in the coronary artery. This approach has, anecdotally, been found effective when injection into the guide showed no improvement in flow.

The initial approach to primary PCI reperfusion for acute ST-elevation myocardial infarction has been an evolving field. Based on recent randomized controlled trials, there is increasingly compelling data to suggest that routine performance of thrombus extraction with a simple aspiration catheter improves clinical outcomes prior to stenting for acute ST-elevation MI.[4,5] The procedure in the case presented here was performed prior to the routine use of these devices and this may have contributed to the no-reflow that complicated her intervention.

KEY CONCEPTS

1. No-reflow can occur in up to 5% of PCI procedures and is more commonly seen when PCI is performed in the setting of acute coronary syndromes, during rotational atherectomy, or in saphenous vein bypass graft interventions.

2. Predictors of the no-reflow phenomenon include large plaque burden, intracoronary thrombus, lipid pools by IVUS, and total occlusion on the presenting angiogram.

3. No-reflow is associated with increased mortality, greater microvascular damage, persistent ST-segment elevation on ECG, and worse left ventricular function.

4. No-reflow has been treated in the cardiac catheterization laboratory, with mixed success, using intracoronary adenosine, nitroprusside, or verapamil. The glycoprotein IIb/IIIa receptor antagonists (particularly abciximab), have also been shown to be helpful, but definitive proof is lacking.

5. There is increasingly compelling data to suggest that thrombus extraction with an aspiration catheter improves clinical outcomes prior to stenting for acute ST-elevation MI.

Selected References

1. Kloner RA, Ganote CE, Jennings RB: The 'no-reflow' phenomenon after temporary coronary occlusion in the dog, *J Clin Invest* 54:1496–1508, 1974.
2. Ito H, Tomooka T, Sakai N, et al: Lack of myocardial perfusion immediately after successful thrombolysis: a predictor of poor recovery of left ventricular function in anterior myocardial infarction, *Circulation* 85:1699–1705, 1992.
3. Neumann FJ, Blasini R, Schmitt C, et al: Effect of glycoprotein IIb/IIIa receptor blockade on recovery of coronary flow and left ventricular function after the placement of coronary artery stents in acute myocardial infarction, *Circulation* 98:2695–2701, 1998.
4. Svilaas T, Vlaar, PJ, van der Horst, IC, et al: Thrombus aspiration during primary percutaneous coronary intervention – The TAPAS Trial, *N Engl J Med* 358:557–567, 2008.
5. Sardella G, Mancone M, Bucciarelli-Ducci C, et al: Percutaneous coronary intervention improves myocardial reperfusion and reduces infarct size. The EXPIRA (thrombectomy with export catheter in infarct-related artery during primary percutaneous coronary intervention) Prospective, Randomized Trial, *J Am Coll Cardiol* 53:309–315, 2009.

Crush Stent or Provisional Stenting for Bifurcation Lesion?

Michael Ragosta, MD, FACC, FSCAI

CASE PRESENTATION

A 52-year-old man with end-stage renal disease, on dialysis for 5 months, developed ventricular tachycardia during vascular access surgery for dialysis. Past history was notable for longstanding and poorly controlled hypertension leading to end-stage kidney disease and a history of systolic heart failure, with an echocardiogram showing global left ventricular dysfunction and ejection fraction of 35% to 40%. He underwent cardiac catheterization 5 months earlier when he first presented with heart failure in the setting of renal failure, and was found to have a normal right coronary artery (Figure 44-1), a normal circumflex system, and moderate disease in the left anterior descending (LAD) artery just after the first septal perforator, but he also had a severe stenosis of the ostium of a large diagonal branch (Figures 44-2 through 44-4 and Video 44-1). Based on this evaluation, his heart failure and systolic dysfunction were thought to be secondary to the renal failure and hypertensive heart disease, with coexisting coronary artery disease. He was treated medically with lisinopril, metoprolol, aspirin, and amlodipine and did well until he developed sustained polymorphic ventricular tachycardia and chest pain during AV fistula graft placement for dialysis. This episode required resuscitation with cardioversion and intubation. Sinus rhythm was restored and subsequent electrocardiograms showed no acute changes but serial troponin I assays were elevated, consistent with a non-ST segment elevation myocardial infarction. He was loaded with clopidogrel and referred for repeat coronary angiography with the plan to treat the diagonal lesion previously observed.

CARDIAC CATHETERIZATION

The angiographic appearance of the coronary arteries had not changed since the prior catheterization. Because the diagonal artery was very large in caliber and vascular distribution and the disease involved the ostium of this vessel, and because there was also disease involving the left anterior descending artery at the bifurcation, the operator planned to use a "crush" stent technique to treat the complex disease of the

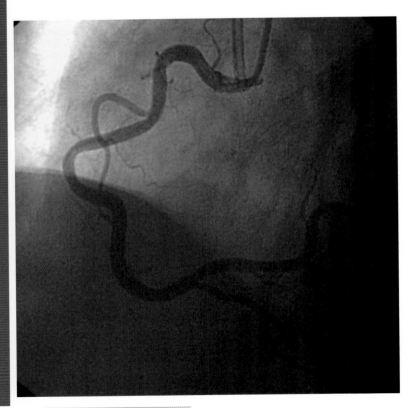

FIGURE 44-1. The right coronary artery was normal.

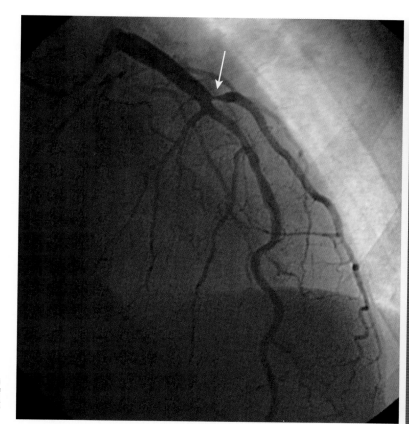

FIGURE 44-2. This is the left coronary angiogram obtained in the right anterior oblique projection, showing severe disease of the ostium of the diagonal and moderate disease of the left anterior descending artery (arrow).

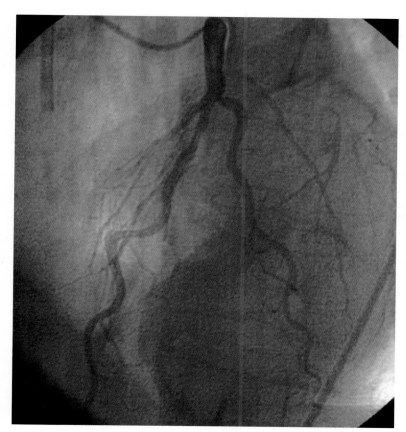

FIGURE 44-3. This is a left anterior oblique projection with cranial angulation of the left coronary artery showing the extent of the diagonal artery. The lesions are not well visualized in this view.

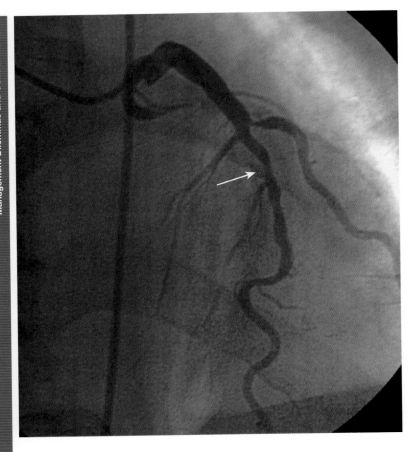

FIGURE 44-4. Another view of the left coronary angiogram obtained in the right anterior oblique projection, showing severe disease of the ostium of the diagonal and moderate disease of the left anterior descending artery (arrow).

LAD/diagonal bifurcation. After achieving therapeutic anticoagulation with unfractionated heparin, an 8 French, "C" left 4.5 guide catheter was engaged in the left coronary artery and floppy-tipped guidewires were placed in the diagonal and the LAD. A 3.5 mm diameter by 12 mm long paclitaxel-eluting stent was positioned in the diagonal at the ostium and a 3.5 mm diameter by 28 mm long paclitaxel-eluting stent was positioned in the LAD with the LAD stent spanning the ostium of the diagonal artery (Figure 44-5). With the LAD stent in place, the operator first deployed the diagonal stent (Figure 44-6). The catheter and guidewire were removed from the diagonal branch and the LAD stent was deployed (Figure 44-7). A floppy guidewire was then passed into the diagonal through the side of the LAD stent struts and both the LAD and diagonal stents were postdilated using a "kissing" balloon strategy (3.5 mm diameter by 15 mm long noncompliant balloon in the LAD and 3.5 mm diameter by 6 mm long noncompliant balloon in the diagonal) (Figure 44-8). The final angiographic result is shown in Figure 44-9 and Video 44-2.

POSTPROCEDURAL COURSE

He had no complications and was discharged the next day on clopidogrel and aspirin in addition to his usual medications. No further events occurred during follow-up and he remained without cardiac symptoms.

DISCUSSION

Bifurcation lesions remain a significant challenge. Ischemic complications from loss or compromise of the side branch as well as high restenosis and stent thrombosis rates with complex stenting strategies limit the utility of percutaneous approaches.[1,2] Bifurcation lesions vary depending on the size of the involved vessels, the location of the plaque relative to these branches, the angle at which the side branch originates from the parent vessel, and the area of myocardium supplied by the side branch. The heterogeneous nature of bifurcation lesions complicates their management since few studies control for these important factors, leaving the operator unsure as to the optimal strategy for any individual patient.

Recent randomized controlled trials suggest that bifurcation lesions can initially be managed simply by stenting the main vessel with the use of provisional stenting of the side branch only if an inadequate result is obtained.[3,4] When this strategy is adopted, a second stent is necessary in the side branch in only one third of cases.[5] However, this strategy does not necessarily apply to all bifurcation lesions. For example, if the side branch is very large in caliber and vascular distribution, and if access to the side branch is not predictably achievable after a stent is placed in the main vessel, then the operator may chose a more complex stenting procedure that reliably provides an acceptable acute result. In the case presented here, the bifurcation was characterized by severe disease primarily of the ostium of a very large diagonal side branch. The disease of the main branch

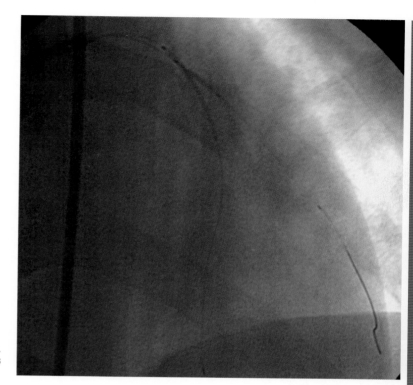

FIGURE 44-5. The first step in the crush stent technique. Stents are positioned in both branches. The LAD stent has been placed across the diagonal branch.

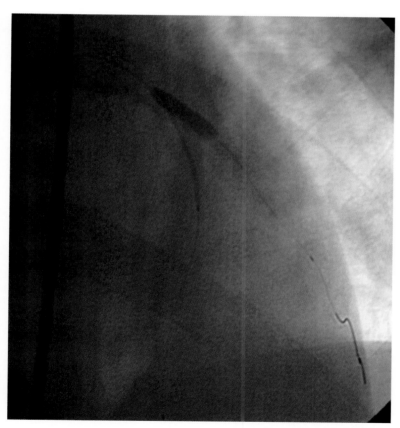

FIGURE 44-6. The diagonal stent was inflated first.

(the left anterior descending artery) appeared to be more modest in severity. However, stenting the diagonal branch alone might have shifted plaque into the LAD, potentially worsening the stenosis severity in that vessel or even closing it. Furthermore, if the operator chose to treat just the diagonal ostium, adequate treatment of this area would have required that the stent protrude into the LAD. This might have impaired future access to the LAD beyond the stent, and, in the event of luminal compromise of the LAD after diagonal stenting or if

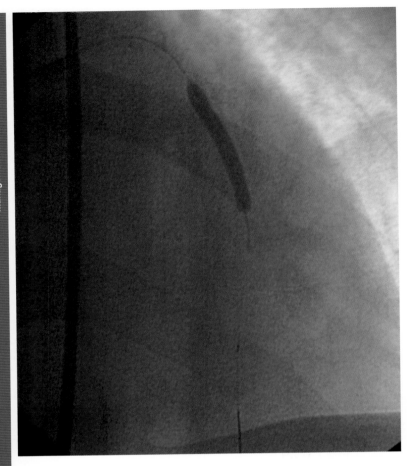

FIGURE 44-7. After the stent catheter and guidewire were removed from the diagonal branch, the LAD stent was deployed, crushing the back end of the diagonal stent.

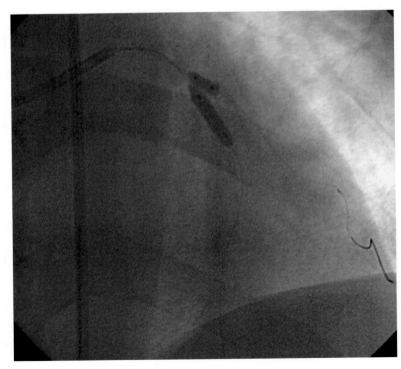

FIGURE 44-8. A guidewire was reinserted into the diagonal artery and final kissing balloons were performed.

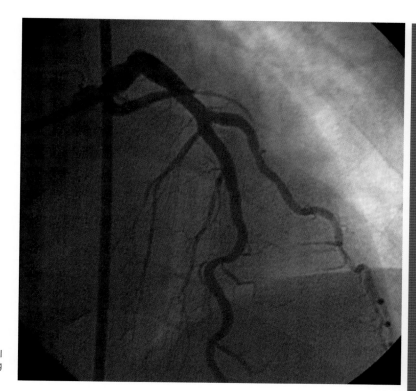

FIGURE 44-9. Final angiographic result of the LAD/diagonal bifurcation after the crush stent technique and final kissing balloon.

the LAD disease progressed and required intervention, the presence of a stent protruding out of the diagonal ostium might have made a percutaneous approach difficult or even impossible. With this in mind, the operator chose a more predictable strategy of using a crush stent technique to treat this bifurcation.

The crush stent technique remains a controversial management strategy for bifurcations. Although it leads to a highly predictable acute outcome, it has been associated with stent thrombosis rates of 2% to 4%.[5,6] Furthermore, the best outcomes with this technique depend upon performance of final "kissing balloon" angioplasty. When final kissing-balloon angioplasty of the bifurcation is performed, the restenosis rates of the main branch and side branch are 6% and 10% respectively.[6] If kissing-balloon angioplasty is not performed, the restenosis rates of the main branch and side branch are 12% and 41%, respectively.[6] Clearly, novel techniques and, possibly, dedicated bifurcation stents are necessary to improve the outcomes in this complex lesion subset.

KEY CONCEPTS

1. PCI of bifurcation lesions is associated with increased risk of periprocedural infarction from side-branch closure and a higher rate of stent thrombosis and restenosis.
2. Although a simple strategy of stenting only the main vessel and provisional stenting of the side branch may represent optimal management for most bifurcation lesions, unique anatomical features may favor more complex strategies in order to more predictably preserve side branches.

Selected References

1. Al Suwaidi J, Yeh W, Cohen HA, Detre KM, Williams DO, Holmes DR Jr: Immediate and one year outcome in patients with coronary bifurcation lesions in the modern era (NHLBI dynamic registry), *Am J Cardiol* 87:1139–1144, 2001.
2. Yamashita T, Nishida T, Adamian MG, Briguori C, Vaghetti M, Corvaja N, Albiero R, Finci L, DiMario C, Tobis JM, Colombo A: Bifurcation lesions: two stents versus one stent: immediate and follow-up results, *J Am Coll Cardiol* 35:1145–1151, 2000.
3. Steigen TK, Maeng M, Wiseth R, et al: Nordic PCI Study Group Randomized study on simple versus complex stenting of coronary artery bifurcation lesions: the Nordic Bifurcation Study, *Circulation* 114:1955–1961, 2006.
4. Colombo A, Bramucci E, Sacca S, Violini R, Lettieri C, Zanini R, Sheiban I, Paloscia L, Grube E, Schofer J, Bolognese L, Orlandi M, Niccoli G, Latib A, Airoldi F: Randomized study of the crush technique versus provisional side-branch stenting in true coronary bifurcations. The CACTUS (Coronary Bifurcations: Application of the Crushing Technique Using Sirolimus Eluting Stents) Study, *Circulation* 119:71–78, 2009.
5. Moussa I, Costa RA, Leon MB, Lansky AJ, Lasic Z, Cristea E, Trubelja N, Carlier SG, Mehran R, Dangas GD, Weisz G, Kreps EM, Collins M, Stone GW, Moses JW: A prospective registry to evaluate sirolimus eluting stents implanted at coronary bifurcation lesions using the "crush technique", *Am J Cardiol* 97:1317–1321, 2006.
6. Hoye A, Iakovou I, Ge L, van Mieghem CAG, Ong ATL, Cosgrave J, Sangiorgi GM, Airoldi F, Montorfano M, Michev I, Chieffo A, Carlino M, Corvaja N, Aoki J, Rodriguez Granillo GA, Valgimigli M, Sianos G, van der Giessen WJ, de Feyter PJ, van Domburg RT, Serruys PW, Colombo A: Long-term outcomes after stenting of bifurcation lesions with the "crush" technique: Predictors of an adverse outcome, *J Am Coll Cardiol* 47:1949–1958, 2006.

Is Open-Heart Surgical Backup Necessary for PCI?

Michael Ragosta, MD, FACC, FSCAI

CASE PRESENTATION

A healthy 58-year-old man with several risk factors for coronary disease, including hypertension and dysplipidemia, developed severe left-sided substernal chest pain while walking down his driveway to get the mail. The pain migrated to his left arm and was associated with diaphoresis and dyspnea. The discomfort continued all night and he presented to a community hospital the next morning with ongoing residual chest pain. His initial electrocardiogram showed T-wave inversion inferiorly and his initial troponin was already elevated at 2.7 ng/mL. He was admitted to the hospital with a diagnosis of non-ST segment elevation myocardial infarction and was treated with 300 mg clopidogrel, aspirin, unfractionated heparin, beta-blocker, and nitrates. He quickly became pain-free, and the cardiology consultant recommended urgent cardiac catheterization. The patient was at a facility that offered cardiac catheterization, had recently begun a percutaneous coronary interventional program, but did not have an open-heart surgery program; the nearest hospital offering open-heart surgery was 30 miles away.

CARDIAC CATHETERIZATION

The patient stayed at the community hospital and the procedure was scheduled with an experienced interventional cardiologist (who performed more than 200 interventions each year), whose primary practice was at a large university hospital with surgical backup. Left ventricular function appeared normal with no wall motion abnormalities. The right coronary artery had a severe stenosis in the proximal segment; this lesion appeared hazy, but there was normal TIMI flow in the artery (Figure 45-1 and Video 45-1). The left coronary angiogram was notable for a normal appearing circumflex artery and a moderate lesion in the midsegment of the left anterior descending (LAD) artery (Figures 45-2, 45-3). To further assess the hemodynamic significance of the LAD stenosis, the operator measured fractional flow reserve (FFR); this calculated to 0.84 and was therefore deemed not significant.

Based on the patient's clinical syndrome and the angiogram, the disease in the right coronary artery appeared to represent the culprit lesion responsible for the acute coronary syndrome. The interventional cardiologist thought the lesion appeared fairly straightforward, without high-risk features that would necessarily preclude performance of a stenting procedure at a facility without surgical backup.

Thus, the interventionalist proceeded with PCI and placed a 6 French right Judkins guide catheter in the right coronary artery after procedural anticoagulation was achieved with bivalirudin. The operator first dilated the lesion with a 3.0 mm diameter by 20 mm long

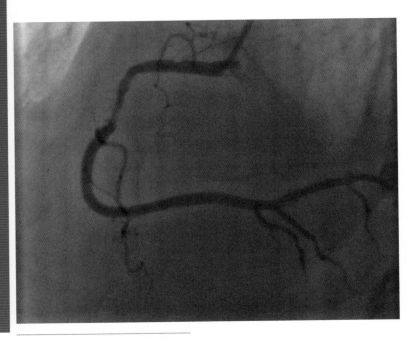

FIGURE 45-1. This is a left anterior oblique angiogram of the right coronary artery, showing the severe lesion with a hazy appearance in the proximal right coronary artery.

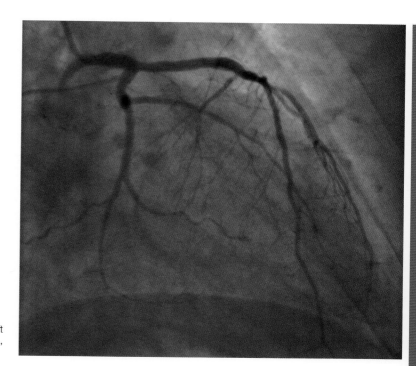

FIGURE 45-2. This is a representative image of the left coronary artery in the right anterior oblique caudal projection, showing no significant disease of the left circumflex artery.

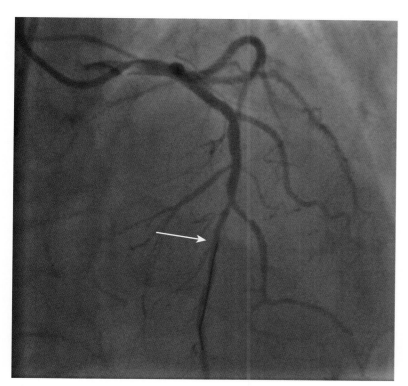

FIGURE 45-3. There was a moderate stenosis noted in the mid-segment of the left anterior descending artery. This lesion was assessed by fractional flow reserve (FFR) using a pressure wire (arrow shows position of the pressure transducer); FFR was 0.84 and thus was not considered a significant lesion.

compliant balloon and then placed a 4.0 mm diameter by 28 mm long drug-eluting stent. As the operator was satisfied with the angiographic result in several views (Figures 45-4, 45-5 and Videos 45-2, 45-3), intravascular ultrasound was not performed and the case was terminated. The patient felt well with no chest pain or discomfort. Hemostasis was easily accomplished with a vascular closure device.

The patient had been moved off the cardiac catheterization laboratory table and onto a stretcher awaiting transfer to his hospital bed when he reported chest pain, diaphoresis, and nausea. The monitor leads showed marked ST-segment elevation and sinus bradycardia. Fearing acute stent thrombosis, the patient was immediately returned to the cardiac catheterization laboratory and the physician quickly regained arterial access and imaged the right coronary artery. The right coronary

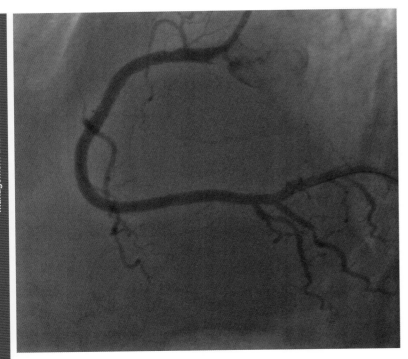

FIGURE 45-4. The left anterior oblique projection of the right coronary artery following stenting showed an excellent angiographic result.

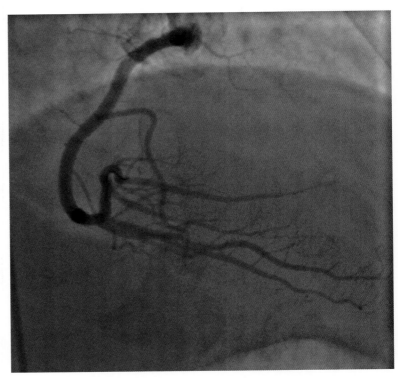

FIGURE 45-5. The right anterior oblique projection of the right coronary artery following stenting showed an excellent angiographic result.

was completely occluded distal to the stent and there appeared to be a linear dissection beyond the distal end of the stent that was not apparent on the post-PCI films (Figure 45-6). At this point, the patient had ongoing severe chest pain and bradycardia but maintained an adequate arterial pressure.

The operator administered atropine, unfractionated heparin, and eptifibatide, and attempted to open the artery. Gaining the true lumen proved extremely difficult, but finally the operator was able to insert floppy-tipped guidewires into both the posterior descending and the posterolateral branches (Figure 45-7). The angiogram revealed an extensive spiral dissection originating at the distal end of the stent and progressing to the bifurcation of the posterior descending and posterolateral branches. The operator placed bare-metal stents at the origin of both the posterolateral artery (Figure 45-8 and Video 45-5) and the posterior descending artery (Figure 45-9) and then placed bare-metal stents distal to proximal in an effort to cover the dissection flap (Figure 45-10). Once patency

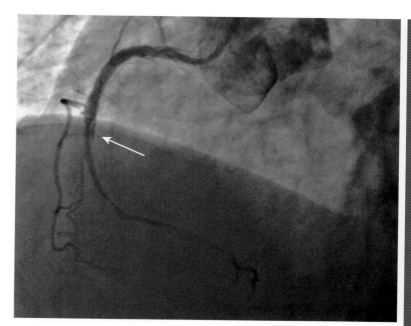

FIGURE 45-6. This right coronary angiogram was obtained shortly after the patient noted the onset of severe chest pain associated with ST-segment elevation. The artery is now closed and there is a dissection flap at the distal end of the stent (*arrow*).

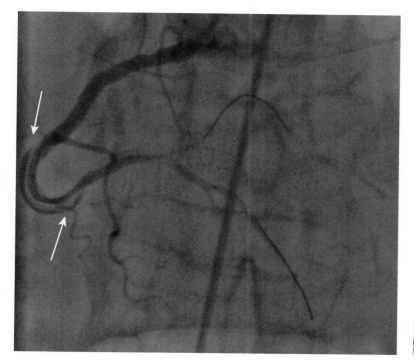

FIGURE 45-7. With great difficulty, wires were successfully placed in the posterior descending and posterolateral branches. Note the extensive spiral dissection (arrow).

was restored, the patient no longer complained of chest discomfort, the bradycardia resolved, and the ST segments returned to normal. The final angiographic result after multiple stents were inserted is shown in Figure 45-11 and Video 45-6.

POSTPROCEDURAL COURSE

Following the procedure, he was admitted to the coronary care unit for close observation and monitoring. Troponin I assays peaked at 58 ng/mL. He had no further chest pain but developed heart failure the night after the procedure that quickly responded to diuretics and

was felt to be due to the excessive contrast load he received from the two procedures, particularly the second, more complex one. He was discharged 3 days later on aspirin, clopidogrel, metoprolol, and atorvastatin. At follow-up 2 months later, he had returned to all activities and remained free of symptoms.

DISCUSSION

The unpredictable nature of balloon angioplasty characterizing the early era of percutaneous coronary intervention mandated the need for surgical backup for all coronary interventional procedures. Without the

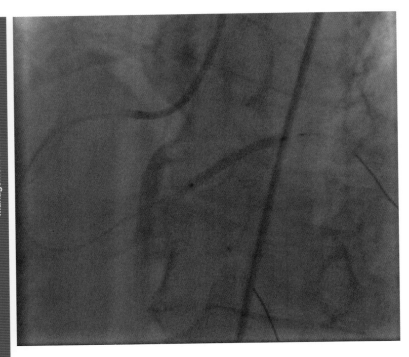

FIGURE 45-8. Stenting of the posterolateral branch.

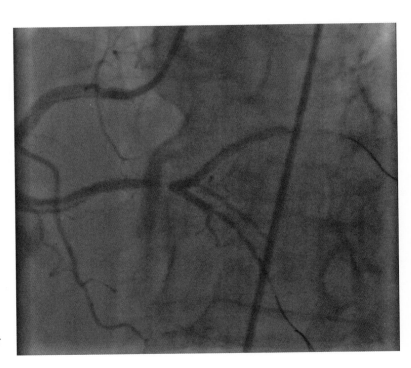

FIGURE 45-9. Angiogram after stenting the posterior descending artery.

coronary stents, technology, and pharmacology we enjoy today, flow-limiting dissections, threatened or abrupt closure, and coronary perforations could only be managed surgically. During this early era, emergency bypass surgery was needed in up to 5% of balloon angioplasties. In the stent era, this has been reduced to less than 0.5%.[1–3]

In the modern era, indications for emergency surgery include the presence of triple vessel disease (40% of cases), dissection or acute closure (43% of cases),

perforation (8% of cases), and failure to cross the lesion (8% of cases).[4] Unfortunately, as evidenced by the case presented here, there do not appear to be clear-cut risk factors that identify which patients are at increased risk for this complication.[5] Clearly, patients requiring PCI of calcified, complex stenoses or chronic total occlusion should not undergo these procedures at institutions without surgical backup. However, the case shown here is an example of a patient with a very straightforward coronary lesion that was initially successfully treated

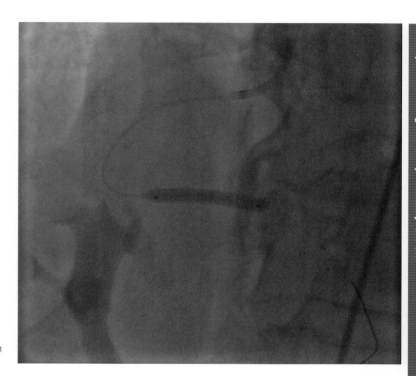

FIGURE 45-10. Stents were placed distal to proximal in an effort to cover the entire dissection.

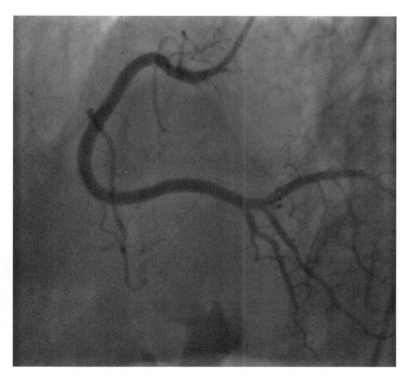

FIGURE 45-11. Final angiographic result after insertion of multiple stents.

percutaneously but would have required emergency bypass for an extensive dissection if the operator had not been fortunate or skilled enough to successfully treat the complication percutaneously.

Despite the low rate of emergency bypass surgery in the modern era, current professional guidelines continue to classify elective coronary interventional procedures without on-site surgical backup as a Class III indication.[6] Emergency angioplasty performed to reperfuse an

ST-segment elevation acute myocardial infarction is classified as a IIb indication, with multiple caveats as follows[6]:

"Primary PCI for patients with STEMI might be considered in hospitals without onsite cardiac surgery provided that appropriate planning for program development has been accomplished, with performance by experienced physician operators (more than 75 total PCIs and, ideally, at least 11 primary PCIs per year for STEMI), an experienced catheterization team on a 24 hours per day, 7 days per week call schedule with a well-equipped catheterization laboratory with digital imaging equipment, a full array of interventional equipment, and intraaortic balloon pump capability, and provided that there is a proven plan for rapid transport to a cardiac surgery operating room in a nearby hospital with appropriate hemodynamic support capability for transfer. The procedure should be limited to patients with STEMI or MI with new or presumably new left bundle-branch block on ECG and should be performed in a timely fashion (goal of balloon inflation within 90 minutes of presentation) by persons skilled in the procedure (at least 75 PCIs per year) and at hospitals performing a minimum of 36 primary PCI procedures per year."

These recommended guidelines remain controversial but have not been modified in the 2007 and 2009 PCI updates. Currently, many community hospitals throughout the nation perform elective PCI without on-site surgical backup and/or perform primary PCI for ST-segment elevation MI without adhering to these numerous stipulations. The number of such centers continues to grow.[7] The most recent data from the National Cardiovascular Data Registry (NCDR) reported that 13% of participating hospitals perform PCI without on-site surgical backup, representing 2.8% of patients undergoing PCI in that registry.[8] Although this data is not randomized and patients may have been carefully selected at the sites without surgical backup, the centers performing PCI without on-site surgical backup had similar rates of emergent CABG and risk-adjusted mortality when compared to centers with on-site surgical backup, despite lower annual PCI procedural volumes. Several other published reports suggest that elective PCI at centers without on-site surgical backup is safe and feasible.[9-11] However, a large report consisting of Medicare enrollees found a higher mortality for patients undergoing non-primary or rescue PCI at centers without on-site surgical backup.[12] Clearly, this issue will not be resolved until a large-scale, randomized trial is performed.

Although the risk is small, in the author's experience, when emergency surgery is needed, it is needed desperately and it is needed immediately. Abrupt vessel closure of an artery supplying a large vascular territory will not be tolerated very long without serious morbidity or death. Similarly, a perforation that cannot be sealed in the cardiac catheterization laboratory is a true emergency requiring immediate attention. Stabilization for transfer to an institution miles away may not be possible in some cases. In addition, the delays involved in arranging for transfer and physically transporting a patient to another institution for emergency surgery will likely be associated with serious and potentially unnecessary morbidity. One study estimates that one in four patients referred for emergency bypass surgery after failed PCI would be placed at increased risk of harm if delays to surgery were present.[13]

This debate will likely continue, but if faced with the prospect of a similar procedure on his or her own heart, at what type of institution would the interventional cardiologist choose to have a coronary intervention performed?

KEY CONCEPTS

1. In the modern era, emergency bypass surgery is required in less than 0.5% of patients undergoing PCI.
2. Even straightforward interventions may suffer unexpected complications requiring emergency surgery.
3. Delays to emergency surgery are associated with increased morbidity and mortality.
4. Professional societies continue to recommend that elective PCI be performed at facilities with on-site surgical backup; however, this may change as data accumulate regarding the safety of PCI at hospitals without on-site surgical backup.

Selected References

1. Detre KM, Holubkov R, Kelsey S, et al: Percutaneous transluminal coronary angioplasty in 1985-1986 and 1977-1981: the National Heart, Lung, and Blood Institute Registry, N Engl J Med 318:265–270, 1988.
2. Seshadri N, Whitlow PL, Acharya N, Houghtaling P, Blackstone EH, Ellis SG: Emergency coronary artery bypass surgery in the contemporary percutaneous coronary intervention era, Circulation 106:2346–2350, 2002.
3. Yang EH, Gumina RJ, Lennon RJ, Holmes DR, Rihal CS, Singh M: Emergency coronary artery bypass surgery for percutaneous coronary interventions. Changes in the incidence, clinical characteristics, and indications from 1979-2003, J Am Coll Cardiol 46:2004–2009, 2005.
4. Roy P, de Labriolle A, Hanna N, Bonello L, Okabe T, Slottow TLP, Steinberg DH, Torguson R, Kaneshige K, Xue Z, Satler LF, Kent KM, Suddath WO, Pichard AD, Lindsay J, Waksman R: Requirement for emergency coronary artery bypass surgery following percutaneous coronary intervention in the stent era, Am J Cardiol 103:950–953, 2009.
5. Shubrooks SJ, Nesto RW, Leeman D, Waxman S, Lewis SM, Fitzpatrick P, Dib N: Urgent coronary bypass surgery for failed percutaneous coronary intervention in the stent era: is backup still necessary? Am Heart J 142:190–196, 2001.
6. Smith SC Jr, Feldman TE, Hirshfeld JW Jr, Jacobs AK, Kern MJ, King SB III, Morrison DA, O'Neill WW, Schaff HV, Whitlow PL, Williams DO: ACC/AHA/SCAI 2005 guideline update for percutaneous coronary intervention: a report of the American College of Cardiology/American Heart Association Task Force on Practice Guidelines (ACC/AHA/SCAI Writing Committee to Update the 2001 Guidelines for Percutaneous Coronary Intervention), J Am Coll Cardiol 47:1–121, 2006.
7. Dehmer GJ, Kutcher MA, Dey SK, Shaw RE, Weintraub WS, Mitchell K, Brindis RG on behalf of the ACC-NCDR: Frequency of percutaneous coronary interventions at facilities without on-site cardiac surgical backup – a report from the American College of Cardiology – National Cardiovascular Data Registry (ACC-NCDR), Am J Cardiol 99:329–332, 2007.
8. Kutcher MA, Klein LW, Ou FS, Wharton TP, Dehmer GJ, Singh M, Anderson HV, Rumsfeld JS, Weintraub WS, Shaw RE, Sacrinty MT, Woodward A, Peterson ED, Brindis RG on behalf of the National Cardiovascular Data Registry (NCDR): Percutaneous coronary interventions in facilities without cardiac surgery on site: a report from the National Cardiovascular Data Registry (NCDR), J Am Coll Cardiol 54:16–24, 2009.
9. Ting HH, Garratt KN, Singh M, Kjelsberg MA, Timimi FK, Cragun KT, Houlihan RJ, Boutchee KL, Crocker CH, Cusma JT, Wood DL, Holmes DR: Low risk percutaneous coronary interventions without on-site cardiac surgery: Two years' observational experience and follow-up, Am Heart J 145:278–284, 2003.
10. Paraschos A, Callwood D, Wightman MB, Tcheng JE, Phillips HR, Stiles GL, Daniel JM, Sketch MH: Outcomes following elective

percutaneous coronary intervention without on-site surgical backup in a community hospital, *Am J Cardiol* 95:1091–1093, 2005.

11. Frutkin AK, Mehta SK, Patel T, Menon P, Safley DM, House J, Barth CW, Grantham JA, Marso SP: Outcomes of 1090 consecutive, elective, nonselected percutaneous coronary interventions at a community hospital without onsite cardiac surgery, *Am J Cardiol* 101:53–57, 2008.

12. Wennberg DE, Lucas FL, Siewers AE, Kellett MA, Malenka DJ: Outcomes of percutaneous coronary interventions performed at centers without and with onsite coronary artery bypass graft surgery, *JAMA* 292:1961–1968, 2004.

13. Lofti M, Mackie K, Dzavik V, Seidelin PH: Impact of delays to cardiac surgery after failed angioplasty and stenting, *J Am Coll Cardiol* 43:3337–3342, 2004.

SECTION FOUR
Peripheral and Noncoronary Interventions

The field of interventional cardiology began when Dr. Andreas Gruentzig performed the first balloon angioplasty of a coronary artery in a human in September, 1977. Since then, decades of intense research along with refinements in techniques and equipment have led to an explosion in the number of percutaneous coronary revascularization procedures worldwide.

The techniques and equipment used to perform coronary interventions became readily applicable to other vascular beds. Thus, advances in percutaneous procedures to treat peripheral arterial disease developed in parallel with coronary interventional procedures. In recent years, interventional cardiologists have become proficient in the percutaneous treatment of atherosclerotic lesions in the arteries of the abdominal aorta and lower extremities, subclavian arteries, and cerebrovascular arteries. In addition, aortic aneurysms, once managed only through vascular surgical procedures, are increasingly treated with percutaneous techniques.

Traditionally, cardiac catheterization of patients with valvular and structural heart disease focused primarily on diagnosis. For most of these conditions, open surgical techniques were the only therapeutic option. Recently, however, novel devices and methods have been developed to percutaneously treat many complex forms of heart disease. Congenital heart defects, such as atrial or ventricular septal defects, patent foramen ovale, coarctation of the aorta, and patent ductus arteriosus are now routinely treated with percutaneous methods. In addition, some structural and valvular defects, such as hypertrophic obstructive cardiomyopathy, aortic valve stenosis, mitral stenosis, and mitral regurgitation are approachable percutaneously using existing devices and methods or by technologies currently in advanced stages of development. The percutaneous procedures designed to manage valvular heart disease are particularly exciting, as they may offer a nonsurgical option to patients who are deemed inoperable or who are at too high a risk for traditional surgery.

This section provides an introduction to some of the peripheral vascular and structural heart disease procedures currently in use or under investigation. While some of these techniques are only available within the confines of a research protocol, it is likely that the next generation of interventional cardiologists will have routine access to these techniques and procedures and that they will become standard treatment for these forms of heart disease.

Balloon Pericardial Window

Michael Ragosta, MD, FACC, FSCAI

CASE PRESENTATION

A 65-year-old woman presents with a recurrent pericardial effusion. Her history began 4 years earlier when she was diagnosed with adenocarcinoma of the breast. She underwent lumpectomy without adjunctive chemotherapy or radiation. Several months earlier, she had complained of shortness of breath and was found to have a large, malignant left pleural effusion treated with thoracentesis. Beginning 3 weeks prior to the present admission, she again developed progressive shortness of breath along with cough, fatigue and a 12-pound weight loss. Evaluation at a local hospital demonstrated an enlarged cardiac silhouette on chest x-ray consistent with a pericardial effusion, and a left-sided pleural effusion with mild pulmonary vascular congestion. A CT scan of the chest suggested neoplastic disease progression. There was left upper lobe atelectasis and consolidation, encasement of the pulmonary artery with a mass, pathological mediastinal lymphadenopathy, and a large pericardial effusion. She was referred for further management of the effusion.

Upon presentation, she was in mild distress from dyspnea, but remained hemodynamically stable with a blood pressure of 150/70 mmHg and, although physical examination confirmed elevation of the jugular venous pressure, there was no pathologic pulsus paradoxus. The electrocardiogram showed sinus tachycardia with low voltage and echocardiography revealed a large circumferential pericardial effusion (Figure 46-1) along with right ventricular collapse and right atrial inversion consistent with tamponade. She underwent pericardiocentesis with removal of 750 mL of serosanguineous fluid. Cytological analysis of the fluid subsequently confirmed adenocarcinoma. A pericardial drain remained in place and she was admitted for continued observation. Over the ensuing 2 days, more than 200 mL of fluid drained from the pericardial space each day. She was referred to the cardiac catheterization laboratory for a balloon pericardial window.

CARDIAC CATHETERIZATION

The patient was positioned on the cardiac catheterization table with the head and torso elevated at roughly 45 degrees. The pigtail catheter drain placed 2 days earlier was removed from the pericardial space. Using sterile technique, and following administration of local anesthesia, a long solid-core needle was positioned into the pericardial space from the subxiphoid approach. An additional 60 mL of fluid was removed from the

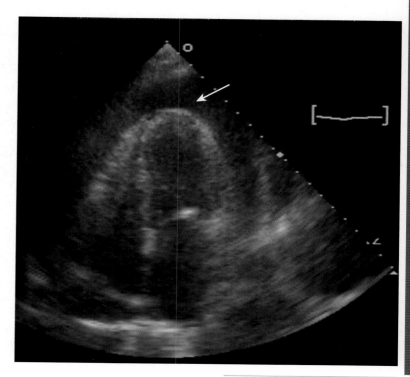

FIGURE 46-1. Transthoracic echocardiogram demonstrating a large, circumferential pericardial effusion (*arrow*).

pericardial space. A 0.038 inch "extra-stiff" Amplatz J-tipped guidewire was advanced through the needle into the pericardial space and the needle was removed. After administration of additional local anesthesia around the entry site, the operator created a tissue tract by passing a 10 French dilator over the guide wire. A valvuloplasty balloon (3 cm long and 20 mm in diameter) was prepared with dilute contrast and advanced along the wire so that the entire balloon was below the skin and the balloon centered across the inferior pericardial border. Prior to this step, the patient was placed in a fully recumbent position to prevent kinking of the catheter and allow easier passage. Using a 60 cc syringe, the balloon was gently inflated under fluoroscopic guidance (Figure 46-2) and a prominent "waist" was noted where the balloon crossed the pericardium. Additional inflation of the balloon led to complete balloon expansion (Figures 46-3, 46-4 and Video 46-1). The balloon was then removed over the guidewire and replaced with a pigtail catheter to remove any residual fluid. The pigtail catheter was then withdrawn and an occlusive dressing was applied to the wound.

POSTPROCEDURAL COURSE

A chest x-ray performed immediately after the procedure did not show any evidence of pneumothorax; a small left pleural effusion was present. The next day,

an echocardiogram was obtained and showed no recurrence of the pericardial effusion. After discharge from the hospital, she received 11 cycles of chemotherapy (paclitaxel) and remained free of recurrent effusion at follow-up 19 months later.

DISCUSSION

Recurrent effusion is an important limitation to pericardiocentesis and is particularly problematic for patients with malignant effusions, in whom life expectancy is limited. Percutaneous balloon pericardiotomy is an effective and less invasive alternative to a surgical pericardial window for palliation of recurrent malignant pericardial effusions.[1] Performed with a valvuloplasty balloon at the time of pericardiocentesis and creating a rent or tear in the pericardium, the procedure allows drainage of pericardial fluid into the pleural and/or peritoneal space, thus preventing reaccumulation of pericardial fluid and its hemodynamic consequences. This procedure is most effective in patients with malignant effusions and should be avoided in patients with uremic pericarditis because of the increased risk of bleeding. In a multicenter registry involving 130 patients with mostly malignant pericardial effusion, balloon pericardial window was successful in 85% of patients, with success defined as no recurrence or need for surgery. The procedure was unsuccessful in 18 patients (15%);

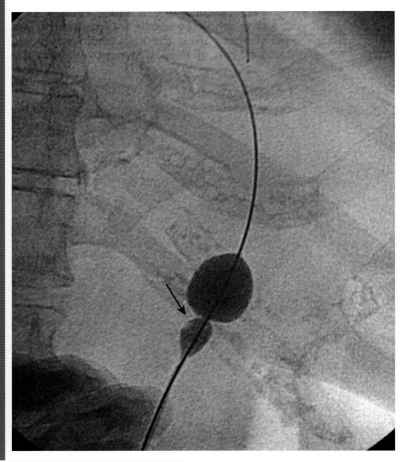

FIGURE 46-2. In this figure, a valvuloplasty balloon is centered on the pericardium and slowly inflated until a "waist" appears (arrow).

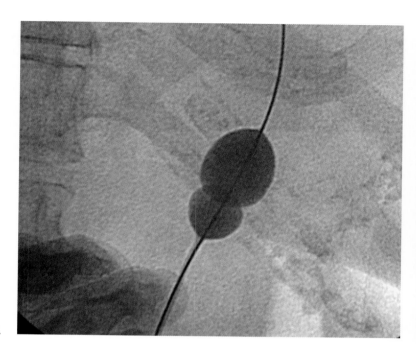

FIGURE 46-3. The valvuloplasty balloon is further inflated.

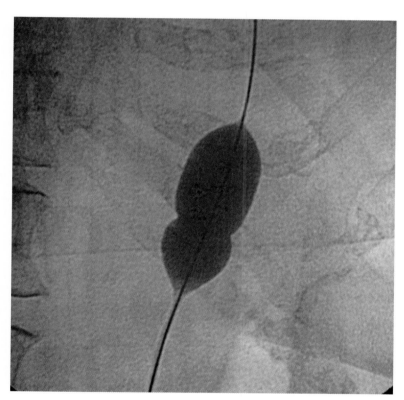

FIGURE 46-4. Full expansion of the valvuloplasty balloon creating a pericardial window.

complications consisted of bleeding requiring surgery in five patients (all of whom had uremic pericardial effusions) and recurrence in 13 patients.[2]

The procedure should be avoided in patients with active infections in the overlying tissues or pericardial space and in those with significant coagulopathy. Balloon pericardial window may not be effective in individuals with large left pleural effusions, as these may prevent adequate drainage to the left pleural space. It also may be ineffective in those who have had extensive chest radiation or surgical scarring, as these conditions may interfere with fluid reabsorption. Complications of percutaneous balloon pericardiotomy include significant pleural effusion, pneumothorax, hemopericardium, hemothorax, infection, and periprocedural pain.

KEY CONCEPTS

1. Balloon pericardial window is an alternative to a surgical window and is effective at reducing recurrence of tamponade in patients with recurrent effusions, particularly those due to malignancy.

Selected References

1. Ziskind AA, Pearce AC, Lemmon CC, Burstein S, Gimple LW, Herrmann HC, McKay R, Block PC, Waldman H, Palacios IF: Percutaneous balloon pericardiotomy for the treatment of cardiac tamponade and large pericardial effusions: description of technique and report of the first 50 cases, *J Am Coll Cardiol* 21:1–5, 1993.
2. Ziskind AA, Lemmon CC, Rodriguez S, Burstein S, Johnson SA, Feldman T, Chow WH, Gimple LW, Palacios IF: Final report of the percutaneous balloon pericardiotomy registry for the treatment of effusive pericardial disease, *Circulation* 90:I–647A, 1994.

Patent Foramen Ovale Closure for Recurrent Stroke

Lawrence W. Gimple, MD, FACC, FSCAI, and D. Scott Lim, MD, FACC, FSCAI

CASE PRESENTATION

A 46-year-old man with a history of recent stroke underwent a head MRI scan and was found to have evidence for both an acute posterior parietal infarct as well as an older frontal infarct. He originally presented with right facial droop and slurred speech; this gradually improved over several months. He underwent several studies to explore the cause of his stroke; a carotid ultrasound with Doppler and hematologic evaluation for a hypercoagulable state found no abnormalities. A transesophageal echocardiogram was performed and demonstrated a long, tunnel-like patent foramen ovale (PFO). Right-to-left shunting on a contrast echo "bubble study" was seen at rest and was apparent even without a Valsalva maneuver. His medications included atorvastatin and aspirin. There was no history of drug or nickel allergy. The medical history was otherwise significant for snoring and he had a family history of premature coronary artery disease. On physical examination, the patient was normotensive and the oxygen saturation was 98% on room air. Jugular venous pressure was normal, the lungs were clear, and there were no pathological murmurs. There was no cyanosis or edema and the pulses were symmetric. The ECG exhibited sinus rhythm and was otherwise normal.

CARDIAC CATHETERIZATION

The patient was referred for percutaneous closure of the patent foramen ovale. The operator attained venous access in the right femoral vein using two vascular sheaths, 11 Fr and 9 Fr respectively. No contrast was used during this procedure, and the PFO closure was done using fluoroscopic and intracardiac echocardiographic guidance. An ACUSON AcuNav intracardiac ultrasound catheter was advanced through the 11 Fr sheath to the right atrium. The ICE catheter was rotated clockwise to attain views of the tricuspid valve and, subsequently, of the aortic valve. The catheter was retroflexed to view the septum (Video 47-1). After the intraatrial septum was well visualized and the absence of a thrombus attached to the PFO was confirmed, the patient was given 75 U/kg of unfractionated heparin. Subsequently, a 6 French multipurpose A2 catheter was passed to the right atrium through the 9 French sheath. The catheter was rotated posteriorly, easily crossing the patent foramen ovale into the left atrium with minimal manipulation. A 0.035 inch J-tip Amplatzer exchange length guidewire was passed into the left atrium and the multipurpose catheter removed. Stable wire position in a left pulmonary vein was confirmed by respiratory, but not cardiac, motion of the wire. A 9 French, 45 degree curved Amplatzer delivery sheath preloaded with a 25 mm Amplatzer Cribiform Septal Occluder was advanced across the interatrial septum and the left atrial disk was delivered under fluoroscopic and intracardiac echocardiographic guidance (Figure 47-1 and Video 47-2). The delivery catheter was pulled back until the left atrial disk was snugly apposed to the septum, and the right atrial disk was delivered out of the sheath but remained attached to the delivery cable while positioning was confirmed

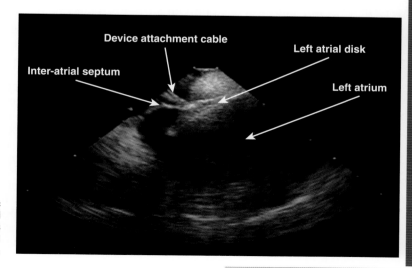

FIGURE 47-1. This image is a still frame from an intracardiac echocardiogram recorded from the right atrium. The left atrial disk has been deployed within the left atrium but remains attached to the device delivery cable. The interatrial septum can be seen in the appropriate position behind the left atrial disk.

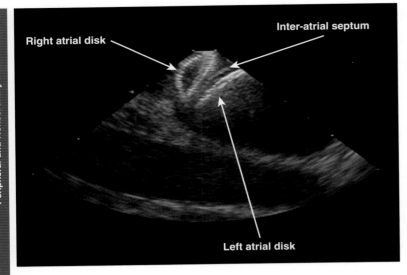

Right atrial disk

Inter-atrial septum

Left atrial disk

FIGURE 47-2. This image is a still frame from an intracardiac echocardiogram recorded from the right atrium. Both disks have been appropriately deployed. The left atrial disk can be seen on the left atrial side of the interatrial septum while the right atrial disk lies on the right atrial side of the septum. Note that gentle traction has been placed on the attachment cable to allow visualization of both disks with the interatrial septum lying between the two disks.

both by fluoroscopy and by intracardiac echocardiography (Figure 47-2 and Video 47-3). Once a stable position was confirmed and each disk was observed by intracardiac echo in appropriate position with the interatrial septum appearing between the left atrial and right atrial disks, the Septal Occluder was released by rotating the delivery cable in a counterclockwise direction until the delivery cable was disconnected from the Occluder. The position was again confirmed by both fluoroscopy and by intracardiac echocardiography, including injection of agitated saline into the femoral vascular sheath to confirm absence of bubble contrast moving from right to left (Video 47-4).

POSTPROCEDURAL COURSE

Following the procedure, the patient was admitted to the hospital for observation. He remained symptom-free during his stay. Device positioning was documented by chest radiography and by transthoracic echocardiography later in the day. The patient was treated with aspirin (325 mg daily) and clopidogrel (75 mg daily) for 1 month and provided instructions regarding antibiotic prophylaxis for endocarditis. At 1 month follow-up, the patient underwent repeat transthoracic echocardiography which confirmed a stable Septal Occluder position and absence of shunting. The clopidogrel was discontinued but aspirin prescribed indefinitely due to the history of prior stroke.

DISCUSSION

In the United States, stroke is the third leading cause of mortality. Because nearly 23% of strokes are recurrent (occur in patients with prior strokes), secondary prevention is an important component of caring for these patients. A patent foramen ovale (PFO) has been reported in approximately 27% of patients evaluated

by autopsy with otherwise structurally normal hearts. When evaluated by contrast echocardiography, nearly 15% of patients over age 39 without a history of stroke are found to have a PFO. Typically, the echocardiographic diagnosis of PFO is made when contrast microbubbles cross the interatrial septum from right to left within 3 to 4 cardiac cycles of right atrial opacification. Although a patent foramen ovale can provide a mechanism by which paradoxical emboli may pass from the right atrium into the left-sided circulation, there are still inadequate data to document the frequency by which this phenomenon results in stroke (or recurrent stroke). Similarly, it has not yet been possible to document with appropriate clinical trials that PFO closure can prevent such strokes. In addition, the optimal patient cohort to potentially treat with PFO closure has not been adequately defined by such randomized clinical trials.

At present, there are no Class I indications for the treatment of stroke and PFO (August/2009). Both the American Heart Association/American Stroke Association (AHA/ASA) and the American College of Chest Physicians (ACCP) guidelines recommend antiplatelet therapy for patients with ischemic stroke or transient ischemic attack and PFO (AHA/ASA Class IIa, ACCP Grade 1A), unless there are other, independent indications for warfarin (atrial fibrillation, hypercoagulable state; AHA/ASA Class IIa, ACCP Grade 1C). With respect to the prevention of stroke, these guidelines argue that there are no adequate randomized clinical data to recommend PFO closure in patients with a first stroke and a PFO. There is a Class IIb indication for PFO closure in patients with recurrent stroke despite optimal medical therapy.

It is important to note that the Food and Drug Administration (FDA) has not specifically approved any device for PFO closure following stroke, and that it strongly endorses the need for randomized clinical trials to address this important issue. Ideally, all patients treated for PFO and stroke would be enrolled in these randomized clinical trials.

KEY CONCEPTS

1. It is difficult to be certain if a neurologic event may be related to a PFO because of the high prevalence of PFO in structurally normal hearts.
2. In patients younger than 55 years, there is an association between PFO and cryptogenic stroke; however, there is considerable uncertainty regarding the risk of recurrent stroke, with estimates ranging from 1.5% to 12.5%.
3. Although device closure of PFO in the setting of cryptogenic stroke has become common practice, there is currently no FDA-approved indication for PFO closure in the setting of stroke.
4. The complication rate associated with device closure varies, with a mean complication rate of 2.3% across multiple studies.
5. Current guidelines from the AHA/ASA and the American College of Chest Physicians recommend antiplatelet therapy following PFO closure. The AHA/ASA guidelines are Class IIa, Level of Evidence B. Current guidelines cite a lack of evidence to make a recommendation about device closure in patients with cryptogenic stroke. Per these guidelines, PFO may be considered in patients with recurrent cryptogenic stroke despite medical therapy (Class IIb, Level of Evidence C).
6. There is widespread agreement that the benefit of PFO closure in patients with cryptogenic stroke is uncertain. For this reason, clinicians should be encouraged to refer patients to ongoing randomized clinical trials.

Selected References

1. Ogara PT, Messe SR, Tuzcu EM, et al: Percutaneous device closure of patent foramen ovale for secondary stroke prevention, *J Am Coll Cardiol* 53:2014–2018, 2009.
2. Meissner I, Khandheria BK, Heit JA, et al: Patent foramen ovale: innocent of guilty? Evidence from a prospective population-based study, *J Am Coll Cardiol* 47:440–445, 2006.

Alcohol Septal Ablation for Hypertrophic Obstructive Cardiomyopathy

Michael Ragosta, MD, FACC, FSCAI

CASE PRESENTATION

A 62-year-old woman with hypertrophic obstructive cardiomyopathy was referred for alcohol septal ablation. Her physician first noted a murmur around age 50 during a routine physical examination performed prior to knee surgery, and echocardiographic evaluation confirmed severe asymmetric septal hypertrophy. The septum measured in excess of 2 cm. There was also systolic anterior motion of the mitral valve and a resting gradient in the left ventricular outflow tract of 50 to 80 mmHg with a provokable gradient of 115 mmHg. She was prescribed beta-blocker therapy and initially was asymptomatic; however, over the past few years she had noted progressive dyspnea with exertion, presyncope, and chest tightness. Her symptoms have progressed to the point where she is unable to perform housework without having to stop because of dyspnea or dizziness. In addition to arthritis, she has a history of paroxysmal atrial fibrillation and becomes severely symptomatic during these episodes. She is currently in sinus rhythm and is maintained on warfarin and metoprolol. There is no family history of sudden cardiac death or hypertrophic cardiomyopathy. On physical examination, she appeared healthy with a blood pressure of 160/80 mmHg in both arms. Jugular venous pressure was normal and lung fields were clear. The cardiac exam was notable for the presence of normal first and second

sounds with a loud systolic crescendo-decrescendo murmur heard over the apex and radiating to the base; this murmur increased dramatically when the patient moved from the supine to upright position. A 12-lead electrocardiogram revealed her to be in sinus rhythm with left ventricular hypertrophy. She was referred for cardiac catheterization and possible alcohol septal ablation.

CARDIAC CATHETERIZATION

Right heart catheterization revealed a mean right atrial pressure of 4 mmHg, a pulmonary artery pressure of 34/14 with a mean of 21 mmHg, and a mean pulmonary capillary wedge pressure of 13 mmHg. The aortic pressure waveform exhibited the characteristic "spike and dome" morphology seen in hypertrophic obstructive cardiomyopathy (Figure 48-1). A multipurpose catheter with an end-hole and two side-holes at the tip was positioned in the left ventricular cavity. Simultaneous recording of left ventricular and femoral arterial pressure revealed a systolic gradient in excess of 100 mmHg at baseline; with provocation using a post-premature ventricular contraction the gradient exceeded 200 mmHg (Figures 48-2, 48-3). A slow pull-back of the catheter recorded no pressure gradient across the aortic valve (Figure 48-4). Left coronary angiography demonstrated several septal perforators appropriate for alcohol septal ablation (Figure 48-5 and Video 48-1).

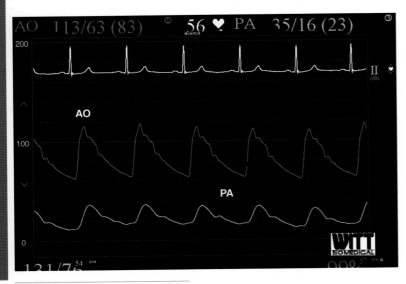

FIGURE 48-1. This is an aortic pressure (AO) tracing demonstrating the characteristic "spike and dome" configuration to the aortic waveform present in hypertrophic obstructive cardiomyopathy (PA = pulmonary artery pressure).

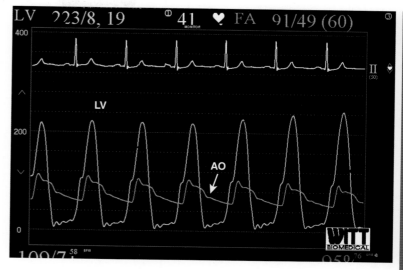

FIGURE 48-2. A large gradient is present at rest in the left ventricular outflow tract.

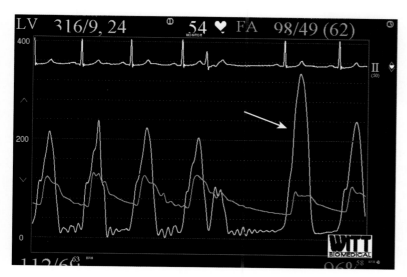

FIGURE 48-3. After provocation with a premature ventricular contraction (*PVC*), there is a marked increase in the degree of obstruction, shown in the post-PVC beat. The aortic pressure has also dropped in the post-PVC beat (*arrow*), known as the "Brockenbrough-Braunwald" sign.

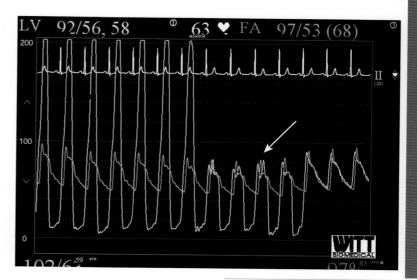

FIGURE 48-4. As the end-hole catheter positioned in the left ventricle is slowly withdrawn, the presence of an intraventricular pressure gradient is appreciated; there is no gradient across the aortic valve (*arrow*).

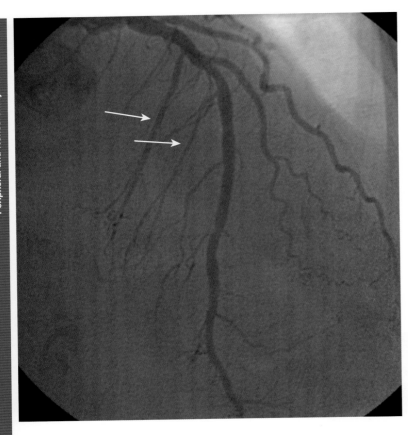

This right anterior oblique left coronary angiogram with cranial angulation demonstrates the presence of several prominent septal perforators (*arrows*) from the left anterior descending artery.

To perform the alcohol septal ablation procedure, the operator first positioned a temporary pacemaker into the right ventricular apex and tested the threshold to ensure capture. An angioplasty guide catheter was engaged into the left coronary ostium and 50 U/kg of unfractionated heparin were administered. A floppy-tipped, 0.014 inch guidewire was advanced into the larger of the first septal branches and a 2.0 mm diameter by 8 mm long over-the-wire balloon catheter was advanced over the wire into the proximal segment of the first septal perforator. The operator inflated the balloon and injected iodinated contrast into the left coronary artery to prove that the balloon was occlusive, thus isolating the septal perforator from the left coronary circulation (Figure 48-6 and Video 48-2). The operator then removed the 0.014 inch wire from the balloon catheter and, with the balloon still inflated, injected iodinated contrast through the lumen of the balloon to show that there was no leakage of contrast from the septal artery to the left anterior descending artery (Figure 48-7 and Video 48-3). With the balloon inflated in this septal perforator, the pressure gradient was observed to decrease by 30 mmHg. Meanwhile, apical long axis views of the left ventricle were obtained by transthoracic echocardiogram and 0.1 cc of an echo contrast agent (Definity) was injected into the lumen of the inflated balloon catheter. This resulted in a contrast effect within the septum localized to the upper septum at the site of contact of the anterior leaflet of the mitral valve. Confident that the instrumented septal perforator represented an appropriate target for alcohol ablation, and rechecking that the balloon remained inflated, the operator slowly injected 3.5 cc of denatured ethanol through the lumen of the inflated balloon catheter over 5 minutes, allowing it to dwell for 5 additional minutes before deflating the balloon. Alcohol injection completely obliterated the left ventricular outflow tract pressure gradient, and restored a normal appearance to the aortic pressure waveform (Figure 48-8). Conduction remained normal during the procedure and the patient reported moderate chest pain. After alcohol injection, angiography confirmed occlusion of the first septal perforator (Figure 48-9 and Video 48-4).

POSTPROCEDURAL COURSE

The temporary pacemaker was left in place and she was admitted to the coronary care unit for observation and recovery. Chest pain continued for several hours and was managed with morphine. The postprocedure electrocardiogram showed a new right bundle branch block. On telemetry, she remained in sinus rhythm with no need for the temporary pacemaker; this was removed after 24 hours. Her blood level of creatine phosphokinase (CPK) rose to 1682 U/L 24 hours after the procedure. Metoprolol 25 mg twice a day was resumed, and a repeat echocardiogram 3 days after the procedure found a small left ventricular outflow tract gradient of no more than 20 mmHg. She was discharged on the fourth day postprocedure. At follow-ups 3 months and 1 year later, she noted marked symptomatic improvement.

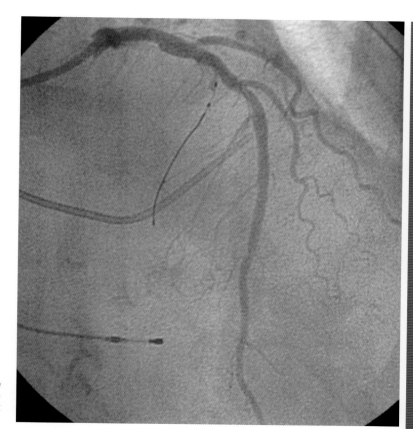

FIGURE 48-6. An angioplasty guidewire is positioned in the first septal perforator and an over-the-wire balloon is inflated in the proximal segment while contrast is injected in the left coronary artery.

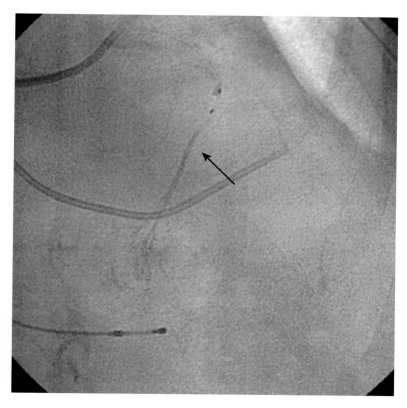

FIGURE 48-7. With the guidewire removed, contrast is injected into the lumen of the inflated balloon to show that there is no leakage of contrast into the left anterior descending artery. Only the first septal perforator fills with contrast (*arrow*).

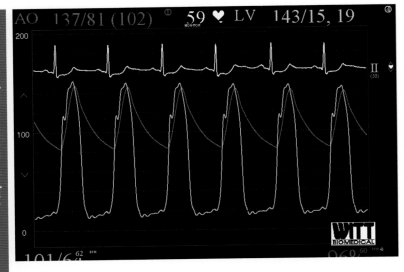

WITT
BIOMEDICAL

FIGURE 48-8. Hemodynamics collected after alcohol septal ablation show resolution of the gradient and normalization of the aortic pressure waveform.

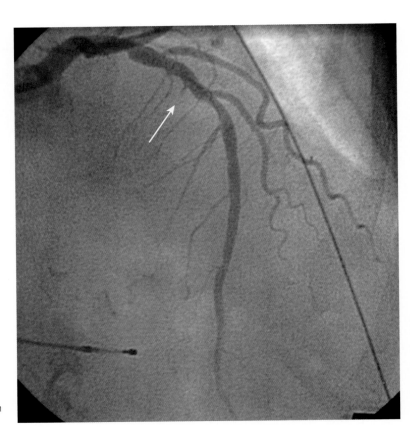

FIGURE 48-9. Following alcohol septal ablation, an angiogram confirms occlusion of the first septal perforator (*arrow*).

DISCUSSION

Hypertrophic cardiomyopathy is an autosomal dominant condition characterized by abnormal left ventricular hypertrophy in the absence of conditions causing compensatory hypertrophy, such as hypertension or valvular aortic stenosis. There are both obstructive and nonobstructive forms. Obstruction, when present, is due to systolic anterior motion of the mitral valve; thus this finding must be present to diagnose the obstructive form of hypertrophic cardiomyopathy.

Many patients with hypertrophic cardiomyopathy are either asymptomatic or minimally symptomatic. Symptoms may be caused by several mechanisms including obstruction (syncope or presyncope, dyspnea, chest pain), diastolic dysfunction (dyspnea), low cardiac output (fatigue), or palpitations (arrhythmia). Sudden cardiac death is a feature of some forms of hypertrophic cardiomyopathy, but is unusual in older patients. The major risk factors for sudden cardiac death in this condition include history of ventricular fibrillation or sustained ventricular tachycardia, family history of premature

TABLE 48-1 Indications for Surgical Myectomy or Alcohol Septal Ablation in Obstructive Hypertrophic Cardiomyopathy

Presence of NYHA Class 3, 4 symptoms on medical therapy or intolerant of medical therapy
Left ventricular outflow tract gradient > 50 mmHg at rest or following physiologic provocation
Significant septal hypertrophy (thickness > 1.8 mm)
Presence of systolic anterior motion of the mitral valve

sudden death, unexplained syncope, marked left ventricular hypertrophy (>30 mm), abnormal exercise blood pressure, and the presence of nonsustained ventricular tachycardia on Holter monitor.[1]

Most patients are effectively treated medically with beta-blockers and calcium channel blockers. Rarely, more aggressive management is warranted. This includes surgical myectomy and alcohol septal ablation. The indications for these procedures are similar and are summarized in Table 48-1. There remains heated controversy regarding the choice of these two procedures in the management of this condition.[2,3] Advantages of surgical myectomy include the fact that it is capable of treating nearly all forms of obstruction with a high degree of success and with low complication rates at experienced centers. Surgical myectomy has been available for more than 40 years and there is excellent long-term outcome data available.[4] Its disadvantages include the fact that it is major surgery and there are few centers and surgeons with significant experience in this procedure. Alcohol septal ablation is an attractive and much less invasive option. It is also highly successful in selected individuals but is highly dependent upon appropriate septal anatomy for optimal results. Although there are no randomized controlled data, alcohol septal ablation generally compares favorably to surgical myectomy with a similar extent of symptomatic improvement and reduction in outflow tract obstruction. The potential long-term effects of the myocardial scar created by the procedure continue to concern many experts in this field and about 8% to 10% of patients require a permanent pacemaker as a consequence of the procedure. The beneficial effects on the left ventricular outflow tract gradient, septal thickness, and symptom status remain stable over time.[5] Recent, nonrandomized data suggest that surgical myectomy in patients less than 65 years of age resulted in better survival (free from death and severe symptoms) compared to alcohol septal ablation.[6] Thus, alcohol septal ablation is usually reserved for patients with severe symptoms due to obstruction who are on medical therapy, who have appropriate septal anatomy, and who either are not candidates for surgical myectomy or are in an older age group.

The success of alcohol septal ablation can be enhanced with the incorporation of myocardial contrast echocardiography.[7] This technique ensures that the selected septal perforator supplies the portion of the septum responsible for the obstruction. On occasion, there may be more than one candidate septal perforator; contrast echo guidance can help localize the best choice for alcohol injection. In most cases, the gradient resolves immediately upon injection of alcohol. As shown in this case, a small gradient may return in the days after the procedure but over time, as the scar heals and with relief of obstruction, the gradient continues to decrease.[8]

The main risk of the procedure is complete heart block, which complicates 8% to 10% of procedures. For this reason, a well-functioning temporary pacemaker is required for all procedures prior to alcohol injection and should remain in place for at least 24 hours with continued, in-hospital rhythm monitoring for at least 3 to 4 days. A right bundle branch block, also observed in this case, complicates 68% of alcohol septal ablation procedures.[9] Thus, in the presence of an underlying left bundle branch block, development of complete heart block can be expected. Rare but potentially serious complications include injury to the left anterior descending artery during instrumentation of the septal perforator and leakage of alcohol into the left anterior descending artery causing an anterior infarction.

KEY POINTS

1. Patients with hypertrophic obstructive cardiomyopathy with severe symptoms on medical therapy may be appropriate for alcohol septal ablation if they have suitable septal anatomy, particularly if they are not candidates for surgical myectomy or are in an older age group.
2. Contrast echocardiography can assist the operator target the correct septal perforator and optimize the result.
3. Heart block complicates 9% of cases; a temporary pacemaker is required to support the procedure. A right bundle branch block can be expected in 68% of cases.
4. In properly selected individuals, alcohol septal ablation improves symptoms and reduces outflow tract obstruction similar to surgical myectomy. Long-term outcome data are not yet available for this procedure and there remain concerns about the long-term effects of the created scar.

Selected References

1. Maron BJ, McKenna WJ, Danielson GK, Kappenberger LJ, Kuhn HJ, Seidman CE, Shah PM, Spencer WH, Spirito P, TenCate FJ, Wigle ED: ACC/ESC clinical expert consensus document on hypertrophic cardiomyopathy: a report of the American College of Cardiology Foundation Task Force on clinical expert consensus documents and the European Society of Cardiology Committee for practice guidelines, *J Am Coll Cardiol* 42: 1687–1713, 2003.
2. Maron BJ, Dearani JA, Ommen SR, Maron MS, Schaff HV, Gersh BJ, Nishimura RA: The case for surgery in obstructive hypertrophic cardiomyopathy, *J Am Coll Cardiol* 44:2044–2053, 2004.
3. Hess OM, Sigwart U: New treatment strategies for hypertrophic obstructive cardiomyopathy. Alcohol ablation of the septum: the new gold standard? *J Am Coll Cardiol* 44:2054–2055, 2004.
4. Ommen SR, Maron BJ, Olivotto I, Maron MS, Cecchi F, Betocchi S, Gersh BJ, Acherman MJ, McCully RB, Dearani JA, Schaff HV, Danielson GK, Tajik AJ, Nishimura RA: Long-term effects of

surgical septal myectomy on survival in patients with obstructive hypertrophic cardiomyopathy, *J Am Coll Cardiol* 46:470–476, 2005.

5. Fernandes VL, Nielsen C, Nagueh SF, Herrin AE, Slifka C, Franklin J, Spencer WH: Follow-up of alcohol septal ablation for symptomatic hypertrophic obstructive cardiomyopathy. The Baylor and Medical University of South Carolina experience 1996–2007, *J Am Coll Cardiol Interv* 1:561–570, 2008.

6. Sorajja P, Valeti U, Nishimura RA, Ommen SR, Rihal CS, Gersh BJ, Hodge DO, Schaff H, Holmes DR: Outcome of alcohol septal ablation for obstructive hypertrophic cardiomyopathy, *Circulation* 118:131–139, 2008.

7. Holmes DR, Valeti US, Nishimura RA: Alcohol septal ablation for hypertrophic cardiomyopathy: Indications and technique, *Catheter Cardiovasc Interv* 66:375–389, 2005.

8. Yoerger DM, Picard MH, Palacios IF, Vlahakes GJ, Lowry PA, Fifer MA: Time course of pressure gradient response after first alcohol septal ablation for obstructive hypertrophic cardiomyopathy, *Am J Cardiol* 97:1511–1514, 2006.

9. Runquist LH, Nielsen CD, Killip D, Gazes P, Spencer WH: Electrocardiographic findings after alcohol septal ablation therapy for obstructive hypertrophic cardiomyopathy, *Am J Cardiol* 90:1020–1022, 2002.

Aortic Balloon Valvuloplasty

Michael Ragosta, MD, FACC, FSCAI

CASE PRESENTATION

A 61-year-old woman with severe aortic stenosis was referred for aortic balloon valvuloplasty. She has a complex past medical history including a renal transplant 7 years ago with a baseline creatinine of 2.0 mg/dL, prior coronary bypass graft surgery 10 years earlier, peripheral vascular disease, diabetes, hypertension, ongoing tobacco abuse with chronic obstructive pulmonary disease, and known aortic stenosis. She presented with increasing dyspnea and two- to three-pillow orthopnea punctuated by an episode of paroxysmal nocturnal dyspnea. On examination, her blood pressure was 110/64 with a heart rate of 119 beats/minute. She was in marked respiratory distress with prominent rales, a murmur of severe aortic stenosis, and elevated jugular venous pressure. Her laboratory values were notable for a rise in creatinine from her baseline of 2.0 mg/dL to 3.4 mg/dL. An echocardiogram confirmed severe aortic stenosis with a peak instantaneous gradient of more than 100 mmHg and reduced left ventricular function with an estimated ejection fraction of 35% to 40%. She was placed on 100% non-rebreather face mask, which resulted in adequate oxygenation, and was sent urgently to the cardiac catheterization laboratory.

CARDIAC CATHETERIZATION

Cardiac catheterization consisted only of a hemodynamic study in order to avoid worsening renal function from exposure to iodinated contrast agents. Her baseline hemodynamics revealed severe heart failure with a mean right atrial pressure of 11 mmHg, a pulmonary artery pressure of 53/27 mmHg and a mean pulmonary capillary wedge pressure of 33 mmHg. The cardiac output was 4.8 L/minute. Using a straight wire to cross the aortic valve, the operator placed a dual-lumen pigtail catheter into the left ventricle and measured a baseline peak-to-peak systolic gradient across the aortic valve of 94 mmHg, yielding a calculated valve area of 0.7 cm² (Figure 49-1). An extra-stiff, 0.038 inch Amplatz guidewire was advanced through the pigtail catheter into the left ventricle and the pigtail catheter removed. The originally inserted 6 French arterial sheath was replaced with a 12 French sheath, and a 5 cm long by 18 mm diameter valvuloplasty balloon was advanced and centered across the aortic valve. Using a 30-cc syringe filled with dilute contrast, the balloon was inflated by hand (Figure 49-2 and Video 49-1). The balloon was deflated and removed over the guidewire and replaced with the dual lumen pigtail catheter. The operator noted that the transaortic peak-to-peak systolic pressure gradient only diminished by 20 mmHg. Thus, a 5 cm long by 22 mm diameter balloon was advanced, centered across the aortic valve, and inflated. The transaortic pressure gradient after the second balloon inflation is shown in Figure 49-3, with the peak-to-peak systolic gradient noted to fall to 44 mmHg, yielding a valve area of 1.1 cm².

POSTPROCEDURAL COURSE

Following the valvuloplasty, she felt symptomatically improved with less respiratory distress and was rapidly weaned to 4 liters of oxygen by nasal cannula. Her renal function returned to baseline over the subsequent days

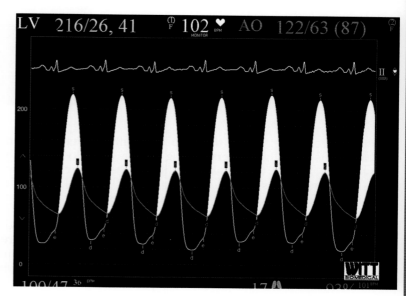

FIGURE 49-1. These waveforms represent simultaneous left ventricular and central aortic pressure and demonstrate a peak-to-peak systolic pressure gradient of 94 mmHg. Note also the marked elevation of left ventricular end diastolic pressure at 40 mmHg.

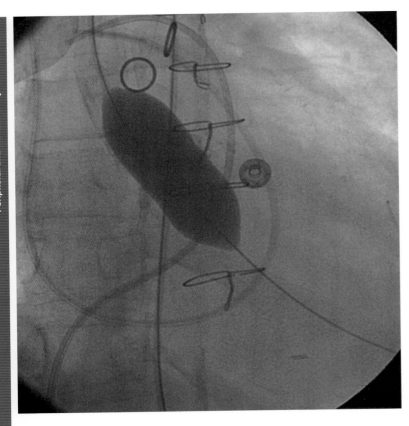

FIGURE 49-2. Balloon valvuloplasty was performed with a 20 mm diameter by 5 cm balloon.

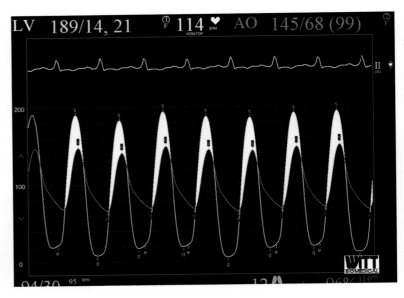

FIGURE 49-3. The pressure waveforms were collected after balloon valvuloplasty. The pressure gradient had decreased to 44 mmHg and left ventricular end diastolic pressure had dropped to 20 mmHg.

after the procedure. With the improvement in her clinical status and the understanding that a valvuloplasty represented a temporary solution to her aortic stenosis, attention was turned to her potential surgical candidacy. Six days after the valvuloplasty, with her creatinine at baseline, she underwent coronary angiography that demonstrated total occlusion of the circumflex and right coronary arteries and severe stenosis of the proximal left anterior descending artery, with patent vein grafts to the right coronary and circumflex arteries but an occluded left subclavian artery supplying the left internal mammary to the left anterior descending artery. Heavy calcification of the aorta was also noted. Clinically improved, she decided to wait until after the holidays to consider surgery on her aortic valve and was discharged 9 days after the valvuloplasty; however, she was readmitted the next day with severe dypnea and found to be in congestive heart failure with acute renal failure. This time, she required mechanical ventilation and an intraaortic balloon pump was inserted to improve her heart failure. An echocardiogram showed reduced left ventricular function and a peak instantaneous gradient of 80 mmHg. Unfortunately, she was not able to be weaned from the ventilator and dialysis was initiated because of continued deterioration in renal function. Consultation with cardiothoracic surgery was obtained. A reoperation consisting of an aortic valve replacement with correction of the subclavian occlusion supplying the left internal mammary artery in a patient in Class IV heart failure with serious comorbid conditions including excessive aortic calcification and advanced lung and kidney disease was deemed to be of unacceptable risk. After extensive discussions with the patient and her family, her level of care was changed to comfort measures and she expired several days later.

DISCUSSION

Aortic balloon valvuloplasty is an effective method to treat congenital aortic stenosis, but its efficacy in calcific aortic stenosis is limited. Original reports from the 1980s confirmed its role primarily as a palliative procedure. In one series of 170 patients with severe aortic stenosis undergoing balloon valvuloplasty, the peak transaortic gradient fell from about 70 mmHg to 36 mmHg with the valve area increasing from an average of 0.6 to 0.9 cm^2.[1] Thus, patients are still left with significant aortic stenosis and, although symptoms typically improve, the restenosis rate is very high, with at least 50% of patients experiencing restenosis within 6 to 12 months. Importantly, aortic balloon valvuloplasty does not improve long-term survival, which remains very poor and not different from the expected survival for untreated severe aortic stenosis.[2,3] For these reasons, aortic balloon valvuloplasty is recommended as a Class IIb indication only as a bridge to aortic valve surgery in hemodynamically unstable patients (i.e., severe heart failure or shock) with severe aortic stenosis at high risk for emergency aortic valve surgery or as a palliative procedure in a patient with severe symptomatic aortic stenosis who is not an operative candidate.[4] The procedure was chosen for the patient presented in this case because she was felt to be unsuitable for an emergent heart operation due to progressive renal failure and refractory pulmonary edema. The goal of the procedure was to improve her hemodynamic status such that her renal failure and heart failure would improve to a point that valve replacement surgery could proceed at a much lower risk. The procedure resulted in the usual and expected degree of hemodynamic improvement and initially, clearly improved her clinical status. Unfortunately, her comorbid illnesses, particularly her renal failure, exacerbated her condition, precluding her candidacy for aortic valve surgery and she succumbed to the disease.

The usual procedural technique is described in this case. The retrograde approach is fairly simple, but requires up to a 12 French sheath; this may be an issue in patients with peripheral vascular disease. An alternative is to position the balloon anterograde across the aortic valve via a transseptal puncture, using an Inoue balloon.[5] This approach requires a great deal of skill but can reduce the risk of vascular complication. When the retrograde approach is used, it may prove difficult to position the balloon during inflations because of the tendency to "spit" or "watermelon seed." Brief bursts of rapid ventricular pacing at ventricular rates of 180 to 200 beats per minute can be employed to transiently lower the cardiac output and allow the balloon to inflate without movement.

In the current era, balloon valvuloplasty is being commonly used as an adjunct to percutaneous aortic valve replacement, facilitating passage and positioning of the prosthesis. The safety, efficacy, and role of percutaneous aortic valves are currently under study. Initial reports are promising. Had it been available, this might have been an effective therapy in the patient presented here.

KEY POINTS

1. Aortic balloon valvuloplasty results in only modest improvements in hemodynamics with an average change in pressure gradient of about 30 to 40 mmHg and a valve area increase of about 0.3 cm^2.
2. The procedure is limited by a very high restenosis rate and does not improve survival.
3. The procedure is indicated as a bridge to valve surgery in a clinically unstable patient with severe aortic stenosis and as a palliative procedure in severely symptomatic patients with severe aortic stenosis who are not candidates for surgery. In the current era, this procedure will likely be needed to facilitate the performance of percutaneous aortic valves.

Selected References

1. Safian RD, Berman AD, Diver DJ, McKay LL, Come PC, Riley MF, Warren SE, Cunningham MJ, Wyman M, Weinstein JS, Grossman W, McKay RG: Balloon aortic valvuloplasty in 170 consecutive patients, *N Engl J Med* 319:125–130, 1988.
2. Otto CM, Mickel MC, Kennedy JW, Alderman EL, Bashore TM, Block PC, Brinker JA, Diver D, Ferguson J, Holmet DR: Three-year outcome after balloon aortic valvuloplasty. Insights into prognosis of valvular aortic stenosis, *Circulation* 89:642–650, 1994.
3. Lieberman EB, Bashore TM, Hermiller JB, Wilson JS, Pieper KS, Keeler GP, Pierce CH, Kisslo KB, Harrison JK, Davidson CJ: Balloon aortic valvuloplasty in adults: failure of procedure to improve long-term survival, *J Am Coll Cardiol* 26:1522–1528, 1995.
4. Bonow RO, Carabello BA, Chatterjee K, de Leon AC Jr, Faxon DP, Freed MD, Gaasch WH, Lytle BW, Nishimura RA, O'Gara PT, O'Rourke RA, Otto CM, Shah PM, Shanewise JS: 2008 focused update incorporated into the ACC/AHA 2006 guidelines for the management of patients with valvular heart disease: a report of the American College of Cardiology/American Heart Association Task Force on Practice Guidelines (Writing committee to develop guidelines for the management of patients with valvular heart disease), *J Am Coll Cardiol* 52:e1–e142, 2008.
5. Sakata Y, Syed Z, Salinger MH, Feldman T: Percutaneous balloon aortic valvuloplasty: antegrade transseptal vs. conventional retrograde transarterial approach, *Catheter Cardiovasc Interv* 64(3):314–321, 2005.

Renal Artery Stenosis Resulting From Fibromuscular Dysplasia

Michael Ragosta, MD, FACC, FSCAI

CASE PRESENTATION

An 81-year-old retired pediatric nurse with longstanding hypertension was referred for further evaluation of uncontrolled hypertension and dyspnea. She was diagnosed with hypertension at least 40 years earlier and is currently on adequate doses of amlodipine, olmesartan, and furosemide with blood pressures remaining in the 140 to 170 mmHg systolic and 85 to 95 mmHg diastolic range. Her only symptom is exertional dyspnea; there is no chest pain, orthopnea, or paroxysmal nocturnal dyspnea. Additional medical history includes prior stroke with no residua 12 years ago, diabetes mellitus, chronic obstructive pulmonary disease, dyslipidemia, and hypothyroidism. Her baseline renal function was normal with a creatinine of 0.9 mg/dL. Her primary care physician ordered an MRI of the renal arteries; this suggested right renal artery stenosis. Because of her exertional dyspnea and atherosclerotic risk factors, she was referred for coronary and renal angiography.

CARDIAC CATHETERIZATION

A diagnostic cardiac catheterization was performed first and revealed mild coronary atherosclerosis with no significant obstruction and preserved left ventricular function. Selective right renal angiography demonstrated the characteristic findings of fibromuscular dysplasia with a "beaded" appearance of the renal artery and the presence of linear "webs" (Figure 50-1 and Video 50-1). This abnormality was also present to a lesser degree in the left renal artery (Figure 50-2 and Video 50-2). After administering 70 U/kg of unfractionated heparin, balloon dilatation was performed at these sites using a 5.5 mm diameter by 20 mm long balloon, which improved the angiographic appearance (Figures 50-3, 50-4 and Videos 50-3, 50-4).

POSTPROCEDURAL COURSE

She was observed overnight with no complications. Follow-ups 1 month and 1 year later confirmed excellent control of her blood pressure on olmesartan and furosemide alone.

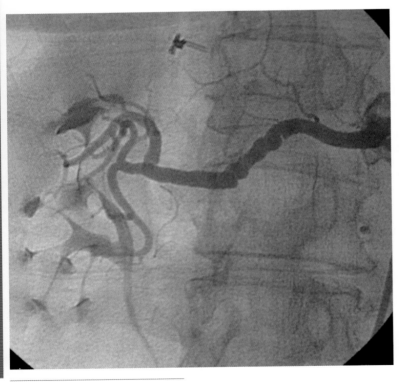

FIGURE 50-1. This is a selective right renal arteriogram demonstrating the classic "string of beads" appearance to the renal artery.

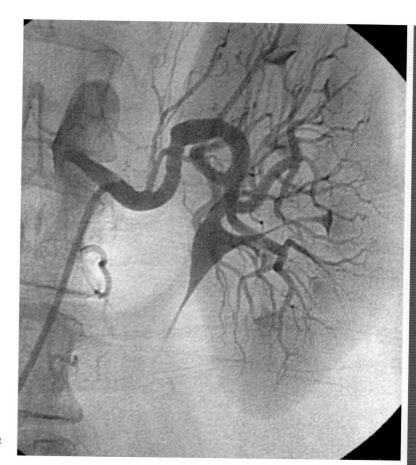

FIGURE 50-2. There are also more subtle findings consistent with fibromuscular dysplasia present in the left renal artery.

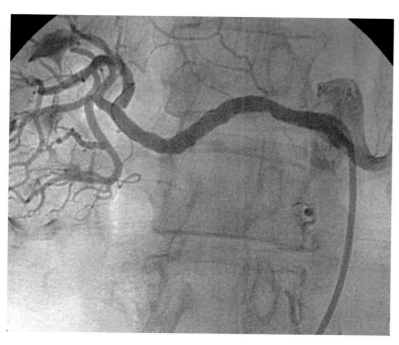

FIGURE 50-3. This is the result after balloon angioplasty of the right renal artery.

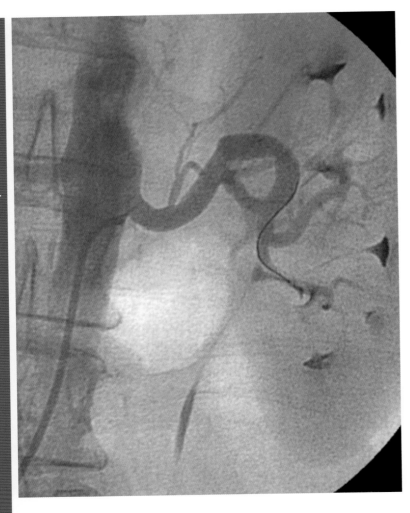

FIGURE 50-4. This is the result after balloon angioplasty of the left renal artery.

DISCUSSION

Renal artery stenosis is most commonly caused by atherosclerosis, typically affecting the ostium and proximal segment of the renal artery. In roughly 10% of cases, fibromuscular dysplasia is the cause.[1] This condition is more common in young females (less than 50 years old) and involves the distal portion of the renal artery or its branches. Although usually attributed to young women, it has also been recognized as a cause of secondary hypertension in elderly individuals, as shown in this case.[2]

The diagnosis of fibromuscular dysplasia is made based on the classic angiographic appearance, often referred to as a "string of beads" (Figure 50-5). This finding is due to luminal occupation with webs and ridges of dysplastic media. It is sometimes difficult to decide if these webs and ridges obstruct the lumen to a significant degree. When the angiogram is ambiguous, additional information regarding the hemodynamic significance of an abnormal segment can be determined by measurement of a pressure gradient.[3]

In general, fibromuscular dysplasia is treated with balloon angioplasty alone. Disruption of the abnormal webs and ridges with a balloon alone is often adequate and stenting is reserved for treatment of flow-limiting dissections caused by the balloon. The clinical response to balloon angioplasty is excellent, with more than 90% cured or improved after the procedure and restenosis occurring in about 20%.[4]

KEY CONCEPTS

1. Fibromuscular dysplasia accounts for 10% of cases of renal artery stenosis and, although it usually affects young or middle-aged women, it may be seen in the elderly.
2. Diagnosis is based upon the classic angiographic finding of a "string of beads" due to numerous dysplastic webs and ridges.
3. Balloon angioplasty is an excellent treatment, with stenting reserved for treatment of dissection.

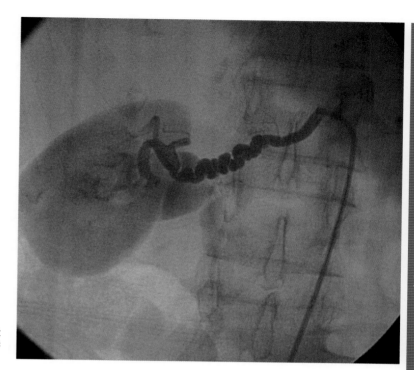

FIGURE 50-5. This angiogram was obtained in a different patient and is an impressive demonstration of the classic angiographic appearance of this condition.

Selected References

1. Safian RD, Textor SC: Renal artery stenosis, *N Engl J Med* 344:431–442, 2001.
2. Pascual A, Bush HS, Copley JB: Renal fibromuscular dysplasia in elderly persons, *Am J Kidney Dis* 45:E63–E66.
3. Birrer M, Do DD, Mahler F, et al: Treatment of renal artery fibromuscular dysplasia with balloon angioplasty: A prospective follow-up study, *Eur J Vasc Endovasc Surg* 23:146–152, 2002.
4. Mahmud E, Brocato M, Palakodeti V, et al: Fibromuscular dysplasia of renal arteries: Percutaneous revascularization based on hemodynamic assessment with a pressure measurement guidewire, *Catheter Cardiovasc Interv* 67:434–437, 2006.

Percutaneous Aortic Valve Replacement

Michael Ragosta, MD, FACC, FSCAI

CASE PRESENTATION

An 86-year-old man with previously known, asymptomatic aortic stenosis presented for an outpatient follow-up after a recent hospital admission for congestive heart failure and progressive angina. Before his admission with heart failure, he had noted several months of increasing shortness of breath with exertion and associated with chest tightness. During the office visit, his cardiologist obtained an echocardiogram that revealed severe, calcific aortic stenosis with a peak velocity of 4 m/sec, a peak instantaneous gradient of 66 mmHg, and a calculated valve area of 0.7 cm^2, with preserved left ventricular function and an estimated pulmonary artery pressure of 70 mmHg (Figures 51-1, 51-2 and Video 51-1). In addition to the known aortic stenosis, his past medical history is extensive and includes chronic obstructive pulmonary disease, persistent atrial fibrillation, non–insulin-dependent diabetes mellitus, hypertension, dyslipidemia, obstructive sleep apnea, and coronary artery disease, with coronary bypass surgery performed 13 years earlier consisting of a left internal mammary artery to the left anterior descending artery, and saphenous vein grafts to the first and second obtuse marginals, to a large first diagonal, and to the right coronary arteries. He also has mild dementia, manifested primarily by short-term memory loss, but he remains functional and interactive with his family. Medications included metformin, ramipril, aspirin, furosemide, atorvastatin, and warfarin. He was referred for cardiac catheterization for further evaluation.

CARDIAC CATHETERIZATION

A hemodynamic evaluation found elevated right-sided heart pressures with a mean right atrial pressure of 19 mmHg and prominent V waves consistent with severe tricuspid regurgitation, pulmonary artery pressure of 63/18 mmHg (mean of 37 mmHg), and mean pulmonary capillary wedge pressure of 26 mmHg, with a cardiac output of 4.8 L/min and a valve area of 0.8 cm^2. The native coronary arteries were all occluded but the left internal mammary and saphenous vein grafts remained patent and free of disease. Abdominal

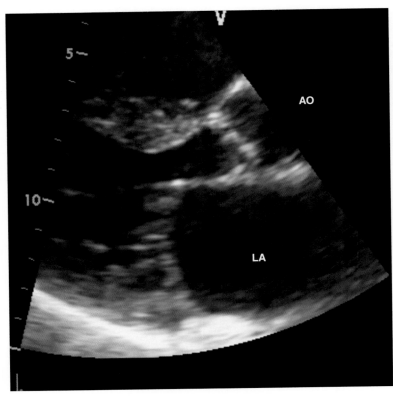

FIGURE 51-1. A parasternal long-axis view of the patient's aortic valve is shown here demonstrating calcific aortic stenosis.

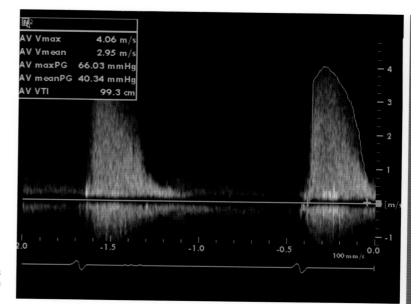

FIGURE 51-2. The Doppler velocity across the aortic valve is shown here and measured 4 m/sec, consistent with severe aortic stenosis.

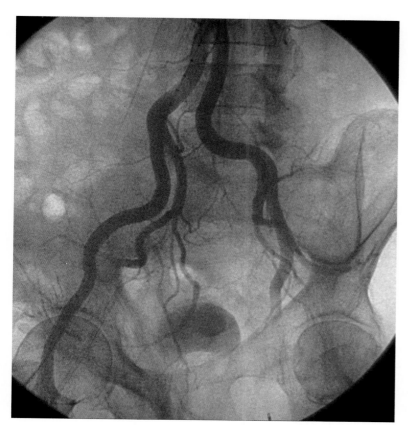

FIGURE 51-3. Abdominal aortography found healthy, large caliber iliac and femoral vessels; there is moderate tortuosity of the left iliac artery, but this straightened with the use of a stiff guidewire.

aortography found normal, large-caliber iliac arteries with moderate left-sided tortuosity (Figure 51-3).

Based on his advanced age, comorbid conditions, and reoperation status, he was deemed a high surgical risk with an estimated surgical mortality with conventional aortic valve replacement of 10.7% (based on the Society of Thoracic Surgeons scoring system). After consultation with cardiac surgery, he was enrolled in a randomized controlled trial comparing the outcome of a percutaneous aortic valve replacement using the Edwards SAPIEN valve to conventional aortic valve replacement (the PARTNER trial) and was randomized to the percutaneous transfemoral approach.

He returned to the cardiac catheterization laboratory for percutaneous aortic valve replacement. With an annulus size of 20 mm, the operator planned to insert a 26 mm valve. After the administration of general anesthesia, a 24 French sheath was inserted into the left common

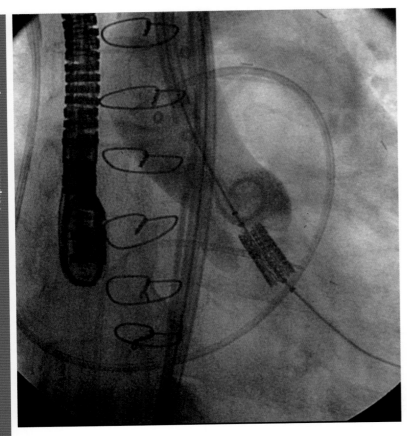

FIGURE 51-4. Optimal position of the aortic valve prosthesis is shown in this AP caudal aortogram; note that two thirds of the valve lies on the left ventricular side and one third on the aortic side.

femoral artery under direct surgical exposure. A temporary transvenous pacemaker was positioned in the right ventricular apex via a 6 French venous sheath in the right femoral vein and a Swan-Ganz catheter was positioned in the pulmonary artery from the right internal jugular vein, allowing measurement of baseline pressures and cardiac output. Heparin was administered intravenously. The operator crossed the aortic valve with a straight wire and advanced a dual-lumen pigtail catheter to measure simultaneous left ventricular and aortic pressures. A 0.035 inch extra-stiff Amplatz wire was inserted and the dual-lumen pigtail catheter was exchanged for a valvuloplasty balloon. Using first a 20 mm diameter by 6 cm long, followed by a 22 mm diameter by 3 cm long balloon, each balloon was centered on the aortic valve and, during balloon inflation, rapid ventricular pacing at 170 beats/min was performed to decrease the cardiac output and prevent the balloon from sliding into the aorta or ventricle. The balloon catheter was removed over an extra-stiff Amplatz wire and exchanged for a 26 mm Edwards SAPIEN valve using the Retroflex I delivery catheter. The valve prosthesis was advanced over the wire and centered on the calcified valve using aortography to guide positioning. Optimal position was present when two thirds of the prosthesis lay in the ventricular side and one third on the aortic side (Figure 51-4 and Video 51-2). Rapid ventricular pacing was performed and the balloon was inflated, deploying the valve (Video 51-3). After valve insertion, hemodynamic assessment found no pressure gradient and aortography confirmed excellent position without aortic regurgitation (Video 51-4).

POSTPROCEDURAL COURSE

Following valve deployment, the 24 French sheath was removed and the arteriotomy repaired surgically. He was transferred to a surgical intensive care unit and extubated shortly after. He recovered uneventfully and was discharged on the second postoperative day with the addition of clopidogrel to his medical regimen. He remained free of heart failure and angina at a follow-up visit 6 months later with an echocardiogram showing normal ventricular function and a well-functioning prosthesis.

DISCUSSION

Surgical replacement of the aortic valve is an effective method of relieving symptoms and reducing mortality in patients with symptomatic, severe calcific aortic stenosis.[1] Unfortunately, many patients with severe, calcific aortic stenosis are usually very elderly and have accrued other comorbid conditions during their long lives that may result in an unacceptable surgical risk. In addition to advanced age, these include pulmonary disease, renal insufficiency, prior stroke, prior cardiac surgery, and a general frail status from coexisting arthritis, degenerative neurological conditions, and diminished functional status. These patients are often deemed poor surgical candidates and have few other options. Medical therapy is ineffective and balloon aortic valvuloplasty offers no more than a temporary palliative effect.[2]

Percutaneous aortic valve replacement offers the potential for a lower-risk alternative to conventional surgery. First described by Cribier in 2000 using an anterograde transseptal approach,[3] current devices are inserted either by a transfemoral retrograde approach as shown in this case, or, alternatively, by a minimally-invasive transapical approach if the iliofemoral vessels are diseased, too small, or too tortuous to allow passage of the large devices.

To date, there are two devices in advanced stages of development, the Edwards SAPIEN valve and the CoreValve. The Edwards device consists of a valve constructed of equine pericardium mounted within a balloon expandable stent and is available in a 23 mm (for annulus sizes of 18 to 20 mm) and 26 mm size (for annulus sizes of 20 to 24 mm). The first generation devices are mounted on 22 French and 24 French catheters for 23 mm and 26 mm valves, respectively. The CoreValve consists of a bovine pericardial valve within a self-expanding nitinol frame and is available in 24 and 28 mm sizes; both valves are mounted on an 18 French catheter. Both valves have been shown to be safe and effective in registry reports of patients with severe, symptomatic aortic stenosis at high risk for aortic valve replacement.[4,5] The results of randomized controlled trials comparing these devices to conventional surgery in high-risk patients are currently in progress and their role in low-risk patients is unknown at present.

KEY CONCEPTS

1. Surgical replacement of the aortic valve remains the optimal therapy for symptomatic calcific aortic stenosis; however, many patients are elderly and have significant comorbid conditions, thereby increasing the risk of surgery. This has led to the development of lower-risk alternatives to traditional surgery.

2. Percutaneous aortic valve replacement offers an alternative to surgery but remains under investigation in the United States at the present time. Two approaches, transfemoral and transapical, are under development. The transfemoral approach uses large-bore sheaths and thus requires healthy, large-caliber iliac and femoral vessels without significant tortuosity or calcification.

3. Ongoing randomized controlled trials will ultimately establish the role for these exciting devices.

Selected References

1. Schwarz F, Baumann P, Manthey J, Hoffmann M, Schuler G, Mehmel HC, Schmitz W, Kubler W: The effect of aortic valve replacement on survival, *Circulation* 66:1105–1110, 1982.
2. Lieberman EB, Bashore TM, Hermiller JB, Wilson JS, Pieper KS, Keeler GP, Pierce CH, Kisslo KB, Harrison JK, Davidson CJ: Balloon aortic valvuloplasty in adults: Failure of procedure to improve long-term survival, *J Am Coll Cardiol* 26:1522–1528, 1995.
3. Cribier A, Eltchaninoff H, Tron C, Bauer F, Agatiello C, Sebagh L, Bash A, Nusimovici D, Litzler PY, Bessou JP, Leon MB: Early experience with percutaneous transcatheter implantation of heart valve prosthesis for the treatment of end-stage inoperable patients with calcific aortic stenosis, *J Am Coll Cardiol* 43:698–703, 2004.
4. Webb JG, Pasupati S, Humphries K, Thompson C, Altwegg L, Moss R, Sinhal A, Carere RG, Munt B, Ricci D, Ye J, Cheung A, Lichtenstein SV: Percutaneous transarterial aortic valve replacement in selected high-risk patients with aortic stenosis, *Circulation* 116:755–763, 2007.
5. Piazza N, Grube E, Gerckens U, den Heijer P, Linke A, Luha O, Ramondo A, Ussia G, Wenaweser P, Windecker S, Laborde J-C, de Jaegere P, Serruys PW: Procedural and 30-day outcomes following transcatheter aortic valve implantation using the third generation (18 Fr) CoreValve ReValving System: results from the multicentre, expanded evaluation registry 1-year following CE mark approval, *EuroIntervention* 4:242–249, 2008.

Percutaneous Repair of Atrial Septal Defect

D. Scott Lim, MD, FACC, FSCAI

CASE PRESENTATION

A 53-year-old woman was referred for evaluation for lung transplant due to severe pulmonary hypertension in the setting of an atrial septal defect. She noted exertional dyspnea and peripheral edema of 3 years duration, with frequent nonsustained palpitations.

Physical examination revealed mild tachycardia and a resting oxygen saturation of 92% on room air. Jugular veins were distended while sitting, and there was an increased precordial activity with a right ventricular heave. A harsh systolic ejection murmur was present along the left sternal border, but diastole was clear. The abdominal exam was notable for a liver distended 3 centimeters below the right costal margin. Her lower extremities had edema to the ankles but intact peripheral pulses.

A 12-lead surface electrocardiogram demonstrated sinus rhythm with right axis deviation and a narrow RSR' in V1, consistent with right ventricular enlargement. Transthoracic echocardiography demonstrated a markedly dilated right ventricle (Figure 52-1 and Video 52-1) and a tricuspid regurgitant Doppler signal consistent with severe pulmonary hypertension (Figure 52-2). Subcostal imaging demonstrated an atrial septal defect with significant left-to-right shunt across the atrial septum (Figure 52-3 and Video 52-2). There was normal left ventricular size and systolic function. She was referred for percutaneous closure of the atrial septal defect.

CARDIAC CATHETERIZATION

The procedure was performed using conscious sedation. Vascular access initially consisted of a 6 French sheath in the right femoral artery and both 8 and 11 French sheaths in the right femoral vein. The patient received 4000 U of unfractionated heparin intravenously along with 1 g of cefazolin. A 10.5 French intracardiac echocardiography catheter was then inserted through the 11 French sheath and advanced to the right atrium, allowing imaging and sizing of the atrial septal defect as well as confirming normal pulmonary venous return to the left atrium (Figure 52-4 and Video 52-3). A right and retrograde left-heart catheterization was performed for measurement of hemodynamics and shunt calculation. The pulmonary artery pressure was 95/27 mmHg with a mean of 50 mmHg, and oximetry determined a pulmonary to systemic flow ratio (or Qp:Qs) of 1.5:1 on room air. Pulmonary vascular resistance calculated to 9 Wood units. Repeating the hemodynamic measurements on inhaled epoprostenol at 50 ng/kg/min reduced the pulmonary pressure to 70/25 mmHg with a mean of 38 mmHg, with stable systemic pressures and a Qp:Qs ratio of 2.5:1. With pulmonary vasodilator administration, her pulmonary vascular resistance calculated to 3 Wood units-indexed. Selective coronary angiography demonstrated normal coronaries. The decision was made to occlude her atrial septal defect and maintain her on pulmonary vasodilator therapy.

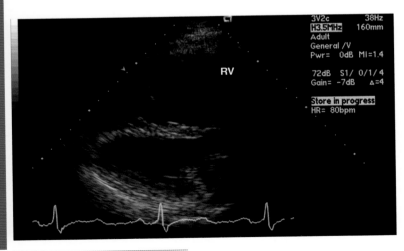

FIGURE 52-1. Parasternal long-axis view showing enlargement of the right ventricle.

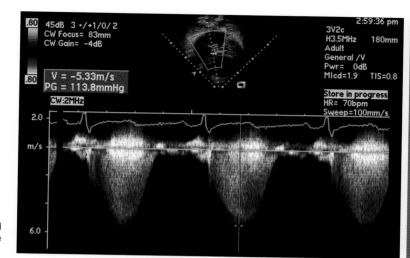

FIGURE 52-2. Doppler evaluation found significant tricuspid regurgitation with increased velocities consistent with severe pulmonary hypertension.

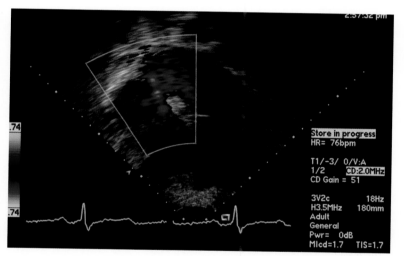

FIGURE 52-3. Subcostal image showing flow across the atrial septal defect.

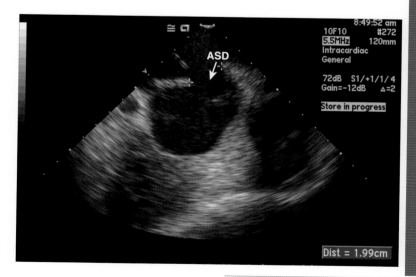

FIGURE 52-4. This is an intracardiac echocardiogram showing the atrial septal defect (measuring 1.99 cm) *(arrow)*.

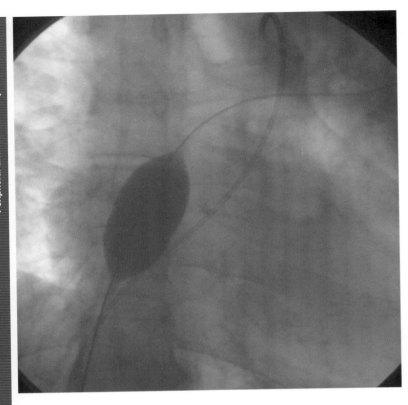

FIGURE 52-5. A compliant sizing balloon was used to determine the size of the defect.

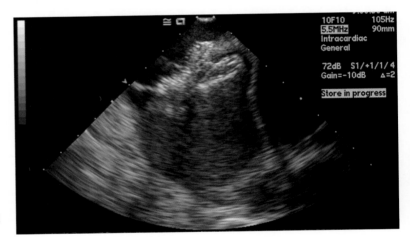

FIGURE 52-6. Closure device positioned across the atrial septal defect.

The atrial septal defect was first sized with a 34 mm sizing balloon, and the stretch diameter was 24 mm (Figure 52-5). A 24 mm Amplatzer septal occluder was then delivered and its position confirmed satisfactorily by intracardiac echocardiography (Figures 52-6, 52-7 and Video 52-4). Repeat hemodynamics confirmed stable pulmonary and wedge pressures. The patient was then monitored in the intensive care unit before being discharged 24 hours later on oral bosentan and sildenafil therapy.

POSTPROCEDURAL COURSE

At 6-month follow-up, she reported no further dyspnea or other symptoms, and a repeat right-heart catheterization found a pulmonary pressure of 35/17 mmHg with a mean of 21 mmHg. She was then weaned off the oral pulmonary vasodilators and has remained symptom-free for a follow-up period of 5 years.

DISCUSSION

A significant atrial septal defect creates a left-to-right shunt due to the higher compliance of the right ventricle and lower right atrial pressures, with a resultant volume overload of the right heart and pulmonary circulation. The natural history of significant atrial septal defects results in a reduced life expectancy (approximately 57% mortality by age 40) and severe pulmonary hypertension in 22%.[1,2] Previously, correction of such atrial septal defects required a surgical approach with cardiopulmonary bypass. In attempting surgery in patients with

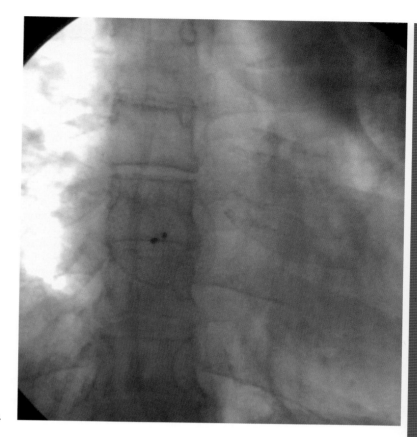

FIGURE 52-7. Fluoroscopic appearance of the closure device.

elevated pulmonary vascular resistance (≥ 7 U/m^2), significant mortality and morbidity may result, and extremely elevated resistance (≤ 15 U/m^2) has been associated with death.[3]

The development of percutaneous devices to close atrial septal defects changes this concept as the defect may be closed without the deleterious effects of cardiopulmonary bypass and with the possibility of simultaneously determining the hemodynamic consequences of defect closure. Prior to final deployment, if it is observed that the hemodynamics worsen when there is occlusion of the defect resulting in volume loading of the left ventricle, then the septal occlusion device may be percutaneously removed.

Frequently, percutaneous closure of atrial septal defects is performed with transesophageal guidance under general anesthesia. However, it has been shown that the effects of general anesthesia can raise the mixed venous oxygen saturation and therefore mask the severity of the shunt.[4]

Therefore, when approaching the diagnostic catheterization of a patient with any cardiovascular shunt, use a baseline hemodynamic evaluation to determine Qp:Qs ratio, pulmonary blood flow, and pulmonary vascular resistance under light procedural sedation. If the findings warrant an intervention, guide the intervention by intracardiac echocardiography or, at that point, provide general anesthesia for airway protection during a transesophageal echocardiogram.

Finally, careful decisions must be made when facing the patient with a cardiac shunt and pulmonary hypertension.

The utility of newer pulmonary hypertension agents allows the possibility of both a safe shunt occlusion and improved patient outcomes. However, in the patient with persistent right-to-left shunting, occluding the atrial septal defect will only worsen the patient's outcome and therefore, in these cases, medical therapy alone is warranted.

KEY CONCEPTS

1. Many atrial septal defects can be repaired by one of several available closure devices.
2. Careful assessment of the pulmonary pressures and shunt ratios is necessary before deciding to close an atrial septal defect.

Selected References

1. Campbell M: Natural history of atrial septal defect, *Br Heart J* 32 (6):820–826, 1970.
2. Craig RJ, Selzer A: Natural history and prognosis of atrial septal defect, *Circulation* 27(4):805–815, 1968.
3. Steele PM, Fuster V, Cohen M, Ritter DG, McGoon DC: Isolated atrial septal defect with pulmonary vascular obstructive disease—long-term follow-up and prediction of outcome after surgical correction, *Circulation* 76(5):1037–1042, 1987.
4. Colonna-Romano P, Horrow JC: Dissociation of mixed venous oxygen saturation and cardiac index during opioid induction, *J Clin Anesth* 6:95–98, 1994.

Renal Artery Stenosis

Michael Ragosta, MD, FACC, FSCAI

CASE PRESENTATION

A 71-year-old woman with a history of hypertension, dyslipidemia, and remote tobacco abuse presents with difficult to control blood pressure despite four medications. Diagnosed with essential hypertension many years earlier, her blood pressure had been well-controlled on an angiotensin-receptor blocker (valsartan) and a diuretic (hydrochlorothiazide). Over the past 6 to 8 months, her blood pressure progressively increased with systolic pressures in the 180 mmHg range and diastolic pressures exceeding 90 mmHg despite the addition of adequate doses of beta-blocker (atenolol) and a calcium channel blocker (amlodipine). Her physical examination was notable only for a blood pressure of 160/90 mmHg. Routine laboratory studies, including renal function, were normal, with a creatinine of 1.1 mg/dL. Suspicious of renal artery stenosis, her physician ordered a magnetic resonance angiogram (MRA) of her renal arteries. This revealed a severe stenosis of the left renal artery and she was referred for renal angiography and intervention.

CATHETERIZATION

Selective right and left renal angiography was performed using a 6 French, 55 cm long internal mammary guide catheter. Selective right renal angiography uncovered a nonsignificant stenosis of the ostium (Figure 53-1 and Video 53-1). Left renal angiography confirmed the findings on MRA with a very severe eccentric stenosis of the proximal segment of the left renal artery apparent (Figure 53-2 and Video 53-2).

The decision was made to perform left renal artery stenting and, after administration of a bolus followed by an infusion of bivalirudin, the operator positioned a 0.014 inch floppy-tipped guidewire in the left renal artery and performed predilatation with a 4.5 mm diameter by 15 mm long rapid exchange balloon (Figures 53-3, 53-4). After balloon predilatation, a 6.0 mm diameter by 15 mm long bare-metal stent on a rapid exchange, a 0.014 inch platform was positioned in the proximal segment of the left renal artery (Figure 53-5). The stent was deployed by inflating the balloon to 10 atmospheres of pressure. An excellent angiographic result was obtained (Figure 53-6 and Video 53-3).

POSTPROCEDURAL COURSE

She was observed overnight and hydrated with normal saline. Blood pressures remained well-controlled after the procedure and she was discharged the next morning on aspirin, clopidogrel, simvastatin, atenolol, amlodipine, furosemide, and losartan. At follow-up 1 month later, her blood pressure measured 100/60 mmHg in both arms and the amlodipine and clopidogrel were discontinued. She returned 6 months later feeling well and brought along her own record of well-controlled blood pressures. On exam, her blood pressure was 130/60 mmHg on atenolol, furosemide, and losartan. A renal ultrasound showed normal kidney size bilaterally and normal Doppler velocities in both the right and left renal arteries.

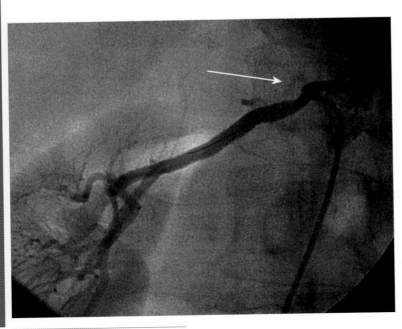

FIGURE 53-1. Selective right renal angiogram demonstrating a mild stenosis of the proximal segment of the right renal artery (*arrow*).

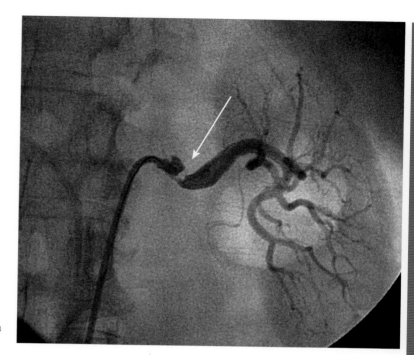

FIGURE 53-2. Selective left renal angiogram revealing a severe stenosis in the left renal artery (*arrow*).

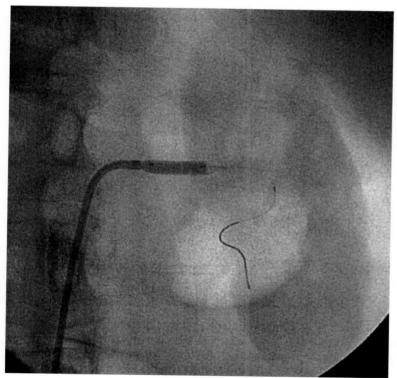

FIGURE 53-3. Balloon inflation in the left renal artery.

DISCUSSION

Renal artery stenosis is the most common cause of secondary hypertension. The underlying pathophysiology of renal artery stenosis is atherosclerosis in 90% of cases and fibromuscular dysplasia in the remaining 10%.[1,2] As demonstrated in this case, most atherosclerotic renal artery lesions affect the ostium and proximal segment of the renal artery while fibromuscular dysplasia, a condition primarily seen in young females, affects the middle third of the artery.[2]

Diagnosis of renal artery stenosis is based on a clinical suspicion of the entity, as symptoms and physical findings are usually absent. Guidelines suggest screening for renal artery stenosis in patients with: 1) onset of hypertension either before age 30 or after age 55; 2) accelerated, malignant, or resistant hypertension; 3) new or worsening renal insufficiency after initiation of angiotensin-converting enzyme inhibitor or angiotensin receptor blocker therapy; 4) unexplained renal atrophy; or 5) unexpected pulmonary edema.[2] Several imaging

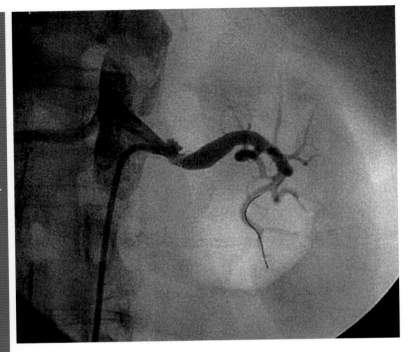

FIGURE 53-4. Result after balloon inflation in the left renal artery.

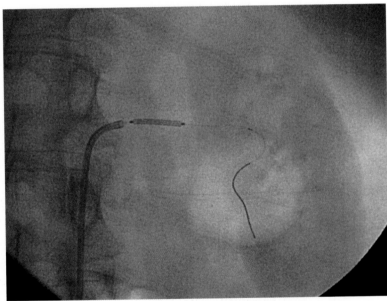

FIGURE 53-5. Position of the stent in the left renal artery.

methods are useful for diagnostic screening including duplex ultrasound, CTA, or MRA, with angiography reserved for patients with abnormal screening tests.

Treatment of renal artery stenosis includes medical therapy, stenting, and surgical revascularization. At present, the data supporting renal artery stenting over optimal medical therapy are limited.[3] Trials comparing medical therapy to renal artery revascularization are difficult to design and implement. First, the hemodynamic significance of renal artery lesions is often unclear, particularly in the presence of moderate stenoses,[4,5] and this may create a heterogenous group of patients in any given study depending on their inclusion criteria. Second, there has not been clear consensus on the need for adjunctive pharmacology or embolic protection.[6] Third,

there is a large selection bias involved in these trials, as many physicians believe they "know the answer" already and are reluctant to enroll patients in a trial in which their patient may be randomized to medical therapy instead of receiving a stent; thus the studies may consist mostly of moderate lesions, as the most severe lesions may not be enrolled. Finally, a variety of endpoints may be used, including blood pressure control, renal function, quality of life and cardiovascular mortality.

Initially, the only available randomized controlled studies consisted of a small number of patients treated with balloon angioplasty rather than stenting, and relied on study endpoints of unclear relevance.[3] These studies showed no difference in blood pressure control between patients treated with balloon angioplasty and those

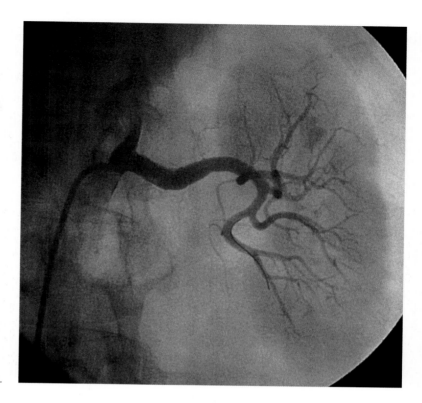

FIGURE 53-6. Post-stent result in the left renal artery.

treated with medical therapy; however, these studies did find that the balloon angioplasty group required less antihypertensive drugs to achieve that control. Given the fact that renal artery stenting, with high procedural success rates and low rates of restenosis, is clearly superior to balloon angioplasty, it was believed that the results of these trials would be different with stenting.

A recently published randomized controlled trial of medical therapy versus stenting for renal artery stenosis in over 800 patients found no clinical benefit from revascularization in terms of renal function, blood pressure, and cardiovascular events but several procedural complications in the revascularization group.[7] Additional, large-scale randomized controlled trials designed to compare renal artery stenting to optimal medical therapy are underway and their results are highly anticipated. The study design, primary endpoints, and results of these trials will likely be exhaustively debated over the years.

Until we have the evidence from these trials, current guidelines recommend renal artery stenting for significant renal artery stenosis in the following clinical settings[2]:

1. Malignant, accelerated, or resistant hypertension (defined as three-drug resistance)
2. Presence of hypertension with a unilateral small kidney
3. Intolerance to antihypertensive agents
4. Bilateral renal artery stenosis or renal artery stenosis supplying a solitary functioning kidney
5. Renal artery stenosis in the presence of unexplained heart failure, pulmonary edema, or refractory unstable angina

There are several important technical issues in the performance of renal artery stenting. Most operators currently use 0.014 or 0.018 inch guidewire-compatible balloons and stents. Guide catheter placement is often straightforward but may be challenging in the presence of iliac or aortic tortuosity or if the renal artery originates at a steep angle from the aorta. One of the most challenging aspects for the operator relates to the ostial involvement of the disease. It is sometimes difficult for the operator to accurately image the ostium and be highly confident that the stent covers this segment adequately. Most operators like to have the end of the stent protrude slightly into the aorta to ensure the ostium is covered.

Complications of renal artery stenting include spasm, renal artery occlusion and loss of the kidney, renal parenchymal hemorrhage from guidewire perforation, dissection, renal artery perforation, distal embolization, and renal failure. Fortunately, these are rare in skilled hands and the procedural success rates exceed 95%. Restenosis after stenting is low (5% to 15%) and primarily relates to the diameter of the stent.

KEY CONCEPTS

1. Renal artery stenosis is an important cause of secondary hypertension and is caused by atherosclerosis in 90% of cases.
2. Renal artery stenosis should be suspected when there is new onset of hypertension, development of uncontrolled hypertension, unexplained renal insufficiency or renal atrophy, or unexpected pulmonary edema.
3. At present, the data supporting renal artery stenting over optimal medical therapy are limited with important ongoing trials expected to shed light on this clinical problem in the future.

Selected References

1. Safian RD, Textor SC: Renal artery stenosis, *N Engl J Med* 344:431–442, 2001.
2. Shetty R, Amin MS, Jovin IS: Atherosclerotic renal artery stenosis: Current therapy and future developments, *Am Heart J* 158:154–162, 2009.
3. Schwarzwalder U, Zeller T: Critical review of indications for renal artery stenting: Do randomized trials give the answer? *Catheter Cardiovasc Interv* 74:251–256, 2009.
4. DeBruyne B, Manoharan G, Pijls NHJ, Verhamme K, Madaric J, Bartunek J, Vanderheyden M, Heyndrickx GR: Assessment of renal artery stenosis severity by pressure gradient measurements, *J Am Coll Cardiol* 48:1851–1855, 2006.
5. Leesar MA, Varma J, Shapira A, Fahsah I, Raza ST, Elghoul Z, Leonard AC, Meganathan K, Ikram S: Prediction of hypertension improvement after stenting of renal artery stenosis. Comparative accuracy of translesional pressure gradients, intravascular ultrasound and angiography, *J Am Coll Cardiol* 53:2363–2371, 2009.
6. Cooper CJ, Haller ST, Coyler W, et al: Embolic protection and platelet inhibition during renal artery stenting, *Circulation* 117: 2752–2760, 2008.
7. The ASTRAL Investigators: Revascularization versus medical therapy for renal artery stenosis, *N Engl J Med* 361:1953–1962, 2009.

Left Subclavian Stenosis

Michael Ragosta, MD, FACC, FSCAI

CASE PRESENTATION

A 61-year-old man with prior inferior infarction and history of recent percutaneous coronary intervention presented with a several month history of left arm weakness and discomfort. He noted that his primary care physician first told him that he has "trouble" measuring a blood pressure from his left arm many years earlier, but the patient reported no symptoms until 4 to 6 months ago. He first noted diminished strength in his left arm during activity and this progressed to pain in his left arm whenever he used it. He denies paresthesias or sensory loss, obvious muscle atrophy, or skin changes. He also denied any neurologic symptoms including dizziness, vertigo, or syncope during arm exertion.

In addition to coronary disease, he has hypertension and dyslipidemia, and he underwent treatment with radiation therapy for prostate cancer. Medications include aspirin, clopidogrel, atorvastatin, metoprolol, and ramipril. He does not smoke and remains employed as a truck driver. On examination, his blood pressure was 146/80 mmHg in the right arm and 90/60 mmHg in the left arm with a noticeably diminished brachial and radial pulse by palpation in the left arm compared to the right arm. On auscultation, there were no appreciable bruits in the carotid or subclavian regions. He was referred for subclavian angiography.

CARDIAC CATHETERIZATION

Angiography of the left subclavian artery revealed a severe stenosis of the subclavian artery proximal to any branches and with clear evidence of left vertebral steal evidenced by absence of anterograde flow in the left vertebral artery (Figure 54-1 and Video 54-1). The operator planned to stent this lesion and positioned a 7 French, 90 cm long sheath in the proximal subclavian artery. Procedural anticoagulation was accomplished with a bolus and infusion of bivalirudin. The lesion was first crossed with a 0.035 inch angled glide wire and a 4 French catheter was placed across the lesion; simultaneous pressure measurements proximal and distal to the stenosis recorded a 30 mmHg systolic pressure gradient across the lesion. The glide wire was exchanged for a 0.035 inch, 300 cm long angled Storq wire and a 7 mm diameter by

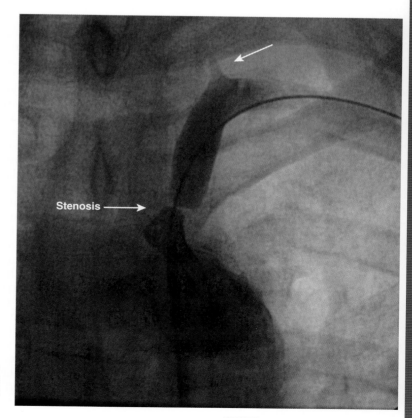

FIGURE 54-1. Angiography of the left subclavian artery showed a severe stenosis proximal to the left vertebral. No anterograde flow was present in the vertebral artery, consistent with vertebral steal (*arrow*).

Stenosis →

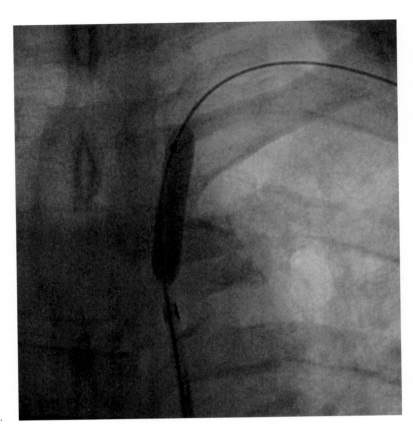

FIGURE 54-2. Balloon angioplasty of the subclavian stenosis.

3 cm long, 0.035 inch, compatible, over-the-wire balloon was advanced to the stenosis and inflated (Figure 54-2). Balloon dilatation restored anterograde flow to the left vertebral artery, but a significant residual stenosis remained (Video 54-2). The operator exchanged the balloon catheter for a 8 mm diameter by 24 mm long balloon-expandable biliary stent and achieved an excellent angiographic result with no residual pressure gradient noted (Figure 54-3 and Video 54-3). There was prompt restoration of the radial pulse noted, with no evidence of distal embolization.

POSTPROCEDURAL COURSE

After an overnight period of observation, he was discharged the next morning. While still in the hospital, he noted immediate improvement in arm strength and no longer noted arm claudication. At 3 month and 1 year follow-up, he remained completely asymptomatic with equal blood pressures in both arms. Eighteen months after the subclavian stent was placed, he developed atypical chest pain and underwent cardiac catheterization. This showed no significant coronary lesions, and arch aortography confirmed wide patency of the subclavian stent (Figure 54-4).

DISCUSSION

Subclavian stenosis is an uncommon manifestation of peripheral vascular disease. Left subclavian disease is more common than disease in the innominate artery or right subclavian artery. Although the overall prevalence of this condition is not entirely clear, significant left subclavian stenosis is present in 2% of the general population, in about 7% of patients referred to a noninvasive vascular laboratory, and in about 5% of patients with coronary disease requiring coronary bypass surgery.[1,2] A blood pressure differential of greater than 15 mmHg is a strong predictor for the presence of significant subclavian stenosis.[2,3]

Many cases of subclavian stenosis are asymptomatic and are clinically evident solely as a difference in blood pressure between the two arms. When symptoms are present, they may be either from limb ischemia (upper extremity claudication, digital embolization) or from subclavian steal. Subclavian steal occurs when a severe stenosis is located proximal to the vertebral artery and causes reversal of blood flow down the vertebral artery, leading to symptoms of dizziness, vertigo, visual disturbances, ataxia, and syncope. In patients who have undergone coronary bypass surgery with a left internal mammary graft, a significant left subclavian stenosis proximal to the left internal mammary artery may cause angina, particularly during exertion involving the left arm (coronary subclavian steal). For this reason, it is important to carefully screen for the presence of subclavian stenosis in patients undergoing cardiac catheterization who are found to have disease requiring coronary bypass surgery. Some physicians routinely perform left subclavian angiography after catheterization in patients found to need coronary bypass surgery; others are more selective and screen for subclavian stenosis only in

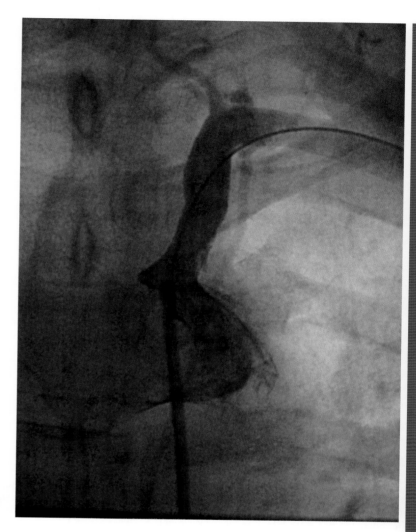

FIGURE 54-3. An excellent angiographic result was obtained after stent placement in the left subclavian artery.

patients with known vascular disease, a subclavian bruit, or a blood pressure differential greater than 15 mmHg on examination.

Treatment options for symptomatic patients include endovascular therapy with balloon-expandable stents or surgical treatment.[1,4] Endovascular therapy is the preferred method for patients with patent but stenotic subclavian arteries; the procedural success rate approaches 100%, and the long-term patency rate is greater than 90%.[4] Balloon-expandable stents are most commonly used. Technically, these are often approached from femoral access but brachial approaches may also be employed, particularly if there is significant tortuosity of the proximal subclavian or aorta. Complications include stroke (1%), distal embolization, and access site hematoma. It is important to delineate the origin and status of the left vertebral artery when considering endovascular therapy. Stenting of lesions adjacent to the left vertebral artery may result in closure or compromise of this important vessel and may result in devastating consequences if the right vertebral is diminutive or closed. Chronically occluded vessels have a much lower procedural success rate (approximately 50%), a higher

acute complication rate and, if successful, a higher restenosis rate than for nonoccluded arteries. A variety of surgical methods may be employed including carotid-subclavian bypass using a synthetic graft or transposition of the sublavian to the common carotid.[1,4] These techniques are also highly effective and are usually performed for symptomatic, chronically occluded subclavian arteries and for lesions at high risk for endovascular repair.

KEY CONCEPTS

1. Severe subclavian stenosis results in a blood pressure differential between arms of greater than 15 mmHg and may cause upper extremity claudication or a variety of neurological symptoms from subclavian steal.
2. Endovascular therapy is the preferred approach for arteries that are stenotic but not occluded; surgical therapy is indicated for chronically occluded arteries or high-risk lesions.

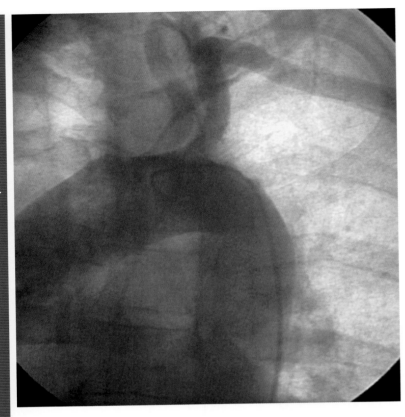

FIGURE 54-4. Aortogram performed 18 months later showed wide patency of the subclavian stent.

Selected References

1. Mahmud E, Cavendish JJ, Salami A: Current treatment of peripheral arterial disease. Role of percutaneous interventional therapies, *J Am Coll Cardiol* 50:473–490, 2007.
2. Shadman R, Criqui MH, Bundens WP, Fronek A, Denenberg JO, Gamst AC, McDermott MM: Subclavian artery stenosis: prevalence, risk factors, and association with cardiovascular disease, *J Am Coll Cardiol* 44:618–623, 2004.
3. Osborn LA, Vernon SM, Reynolds B, Timm TC, Allen K: Screening for subclavian artery stenosis in patients who are candidates for coronary bypass surgery, *Catheter Cardiovasc Interv* 56:162–165, 2002.
4. Brountzos EN, Malagari K, Kelekis DA: Endovascular treatment of occlusive lesions of the subclavian and innominate arteries, *Cardiovasc Interv Radiol* 29:503–510, 2006.

Foreign Body Retrieval

Michael Ragosta, MD, FACC, FSCAI

CASE PRESENTATION

A 50-year-old man with history of a prior non-ST segment elevation myocardial infarction several years earlier presented with worsening angina and was referred for cardiac catheterization. Angina occured while walking less than 2 blocks and has increased in severity over the past year. Pain was promptly relieved by rest and occasionally required one or two sublingual nitroglycerin tablets for relief. Risk factors include ongoing, heavy tobacco abuse (three packs per day), hypertension, and dyslipidemia. His medications, with which he is admittedly poorly compliant, included lisinopril, metoprolol, simvastatin, isosorbide dinitrate, and aspirin. The physical examination was notable only for systolic hypertension, and a 12-lead electrocardiogram and routine blood studies were normal.

CARDIAC CATHETERIZATION

Left ventricular function was normal. Coronary angiography demonstrated complex and multivessel coronary disease. The right coronary artery was essentially totally occluded in the midportion with some anterograde flow

(Figures 55-1, 55-2 and Videos 55-1, 55-2). Although the distal right coronary artery appeared small, the distal right coronary was believed to be larger, based on review of the prior angiogram and from the collateral visible from the left coronary artery (Figure 55-3). A long, moderate lesion was noted in the left anterior descending artery (LAD) (Figure 55-4) and the circumflex system appeared to be without significant stenosis (Figure 55-5). To determine the significance of the lesion, the operator further evaluated the LAD by assessing fractional flow reserve. Using a pressure wire and an intracoronary injection of adenosine to achieve maximum hyperemia, fractional flow reserve of the LAD was 0.69 and thus represented a significant lesion.

The femoral artery sheath was removed and the patient brought to the recovery area. After discussing the options of surgical versus percutaneous revascularization, the patient chose a percutaneous approach and an elective procedure was scheduled for the following week.

He received 300 mg of clopidogrel the night before the procedure. The operator used bivalirudin as the procedural anticoagulant and began with the occluded right coronary artery. A floppy-tipped guidewire easily

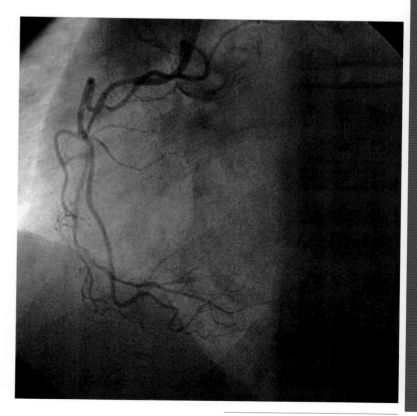

FIGURE 55-1. This is a left anterior oblique projection of the right coronary artery.

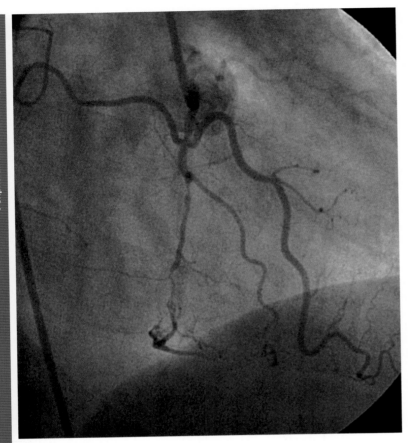

FIGURE 55-2. This is a right anterior oblique projection of the right coronary artery.

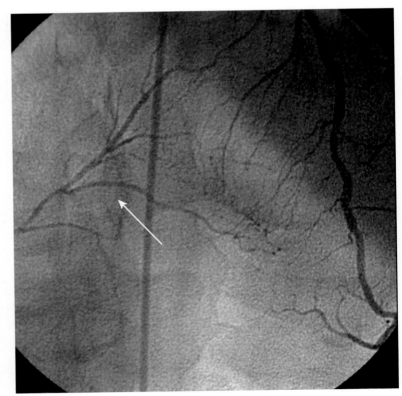

FIGURE 55-3. This angiogram shows the collateral to the right coronary artery (*arrow*).

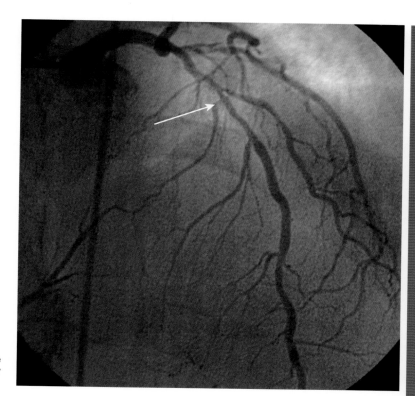

FIGURE 55-4. A long, moderate stenosis was present in the left anterior descending artery (*arrow*) with a fractional flow reserve of 0.69, consistent with a significant stenosis.

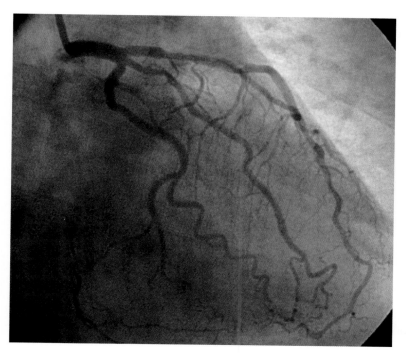

FIGURE 55-5. This is a right anterior oblique projection with caudal angulation of the left coronary artery demonstrating no significant left circumflex disease.

crossed the occluded segment and a 2.0 mm diameter compliant balloon was used to restore patency of the artery. The operator positioned and deployed two 2.5 mm diameter by 28 mm long sirolimus-eluting stents across the lesion. A residual stenosis remained in the proximal segment (Figure 55-6 and Video 55-3) and the operator attempted to position a third sirolimus-eluting stent at this location. Despite the relative ease of passing the

first two stents, the operator could not advance the stent across the lesion and thus decided to remove the stent and dilate the proximal end of the deployed stent as well as the unstented segment with a noncompliant balloon. During the attempt to remove the stent catheter from the coronary artery, the operator encountered significant resistance when the back end of the stent balloon entered the guide catheter. Despite gentle

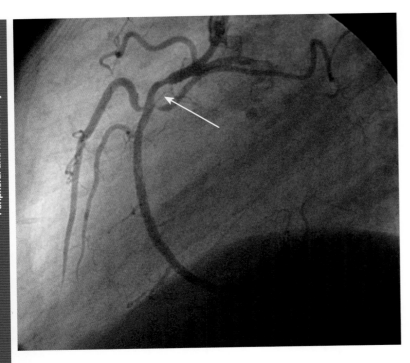

FIGURE 55-6. This is a lateral projection of the right coronary artery obtained after stenting; a residual stenosis is proximal to the stented site (*arrow*).

manipulations, the stent would not enter the guide catheter. Fearing that struts from the back end of the stent edge were raised from the surface of the balloon, and concerned about the possibility of stent embolization, the operator decided to remove the stent catheter and guide together as one unit into the descending aorta. The operator successfully removed the stent from the coronary artery and the stent remained in position on the balloon catheter with the 0.014 inch guidewire in place. The entire apparatus (guide, stent catheter, and guidewire) was withdrawn to the femoral artery sheath. Again, the operator noted resistance when he attempted to withdraw the stent into the femoral artery sheath (Figure 55-7) and decided to snare the end of the stent to prevent stent embolization during removal of the stent catheter. The guide catheter was removed from the femoral sheath by cutting the back end of the balloon catheter. A stiff 0.014 inch floppy-tipped guidewire (Mailman, Boston Scientific) was passed through the sheath to allow continued femoral access during sheath removal. The operator then passed a 4 French, 10 mm Amplatz GooseNeck snare through the femoral sheath alongside the stent catheter. The 0.014 inch guidewire was carefully withdrawn with about 10 cm of wire tip extending beyond the stent catheter. The open loop of the snare was manipulated to capture the 0.014 inch guidewire (Figure 55-8) and then carefully withdrawn to capture the wire near the end of the stent catheter (Figure 55-9 and Video 55-4). The operator removed the sheath, stent catheter, and snare together while maintaining femoral access with the other 0.014 inch stiff guidewire. The stent was successfully removed and a new sheath positioned in the femoral artery over the 0.014 inch wire. The operator decided to accept the angiographic result obtained and did not place any additional stents in the right coronary artery.

POSTPROCEDURAL COURSE

The patient recovered uneventfully without vascular complication and was discharged the next day. His physician planned to bring him back for an intervention on the LAD; however, the patient felt well, with resolution of his angina, and decided not to undergo any further procedures.

DISCUSSION

Stent embolization occurs in about 0.3% of coronary interventions[1,2] and is more common when stents are manually crimped onto the balloon catheter.[1] Risk factors for stent embolization include severe proximal angulation and heavy coronary calcification. Stent embolization in the coronary artery typically occurs when a stent cannot be advanced and the operator tries to withdraw the stent catheter back into the guide. The stent may become caught in the lesion and shear off the balloon or, as demonstrated by this case, struts at the back end of the stent may become raised when the stent catheter is pulled back and is not entirely coaxial to the guide. In either case, if the operator does not detect the resistance or carelessly withdraws the stent catheter despite the resistance, then the stent may come off the balloon. In the case shown here, the operator sensed the resistance at the guide and decided to withdraw the entire apparatus, thereby at least preventing stent embolization into the coronary circulation.

When a stent embolizes into the coronary circulation, potentially serious consequences may arise if the stent cannot be successfully retrieved, including myocardial infarction, emergency surgery, and death.[2-4] An undeployed stent sitting in a coronary artery can be managed in one of several ways. If the stent remains on the 0.014 inch guidewire, a low-profile 1.5 mm

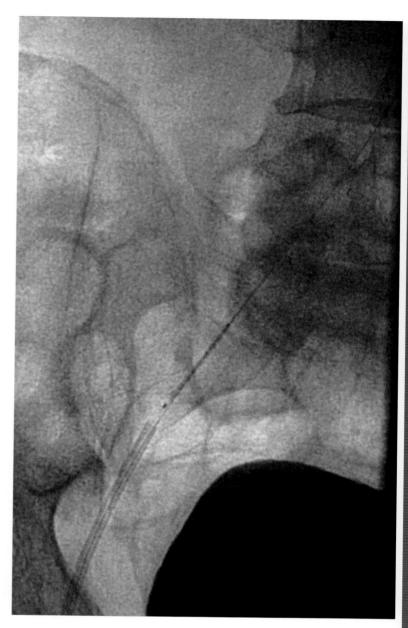

FIGURE 55-7. After the operator experienced resistance during the attempt to withdraw the stent into the guide, the stent catheter was withdrawn to the sheath.

compliant balloon can be advanced within or just distal to the stent, inflated, and pulled into the guide catheter. Another method involves placing a second 0.014 inch guidewire alongside the original guidewire and the undeployed stent and twirling the two wires around each other in an attempt to ensnare the stent. In the author's experience, this technique is often not possible because the undeployed stent is wedged within a lesion and a guidewire cannot be advanced around it. If the stent is not on a 0.014 inch guide wire, the operator may try to snare the stent within the coronary artery or capture it with a set of biopsy forceps; however, the latter method may result in significant arterial injury. Another popular method is to simply crush the undeployed stent against the wall of the coronary artery with a balloon and then another stent. However, this implies the operator will be successful at delivering a new stent to a location within an artery to which the operator could not initially successfully deliver a stent. By whatever method works, the

operator should make an effort to retrieve or deploy the embolized stent to minimize the risk of an adverse event.

Embolization of a stent into the peripheral circulation appears to be a benign event.[3,4] Usually, the stent embolizes into the lower extremity circulation. Often, it cannot be found. The outcome of these peripheral embolization events appears benign, although there are reports of claudication occurring due to stent embolization.

Prevention of embolization is desirable and operators should be sure the coronary is well-prepared before attempting to deliver a stent in a calcified, angulated lesion. Nevertheless, all interventionalists should be familiar with methods of retrieving embolized stents and foreign bodies. As shown in this case, the goose neck snares are easy to use and highly effective at capturing embolized devices. Care should be taken to carefully manage the vascular access site, since removal of the embolized and frequently distorted stent may enlarge the arteriotomy and result in increased access site bleeding.[2]

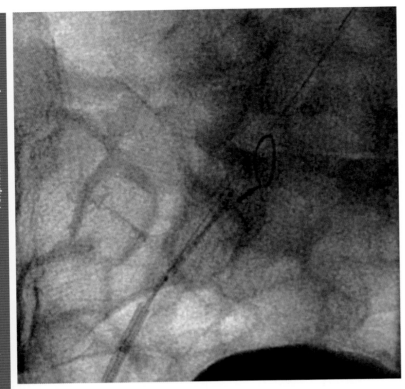

FIGURE 55-8. The snare was used to capture the 0.014 inch guidewire.

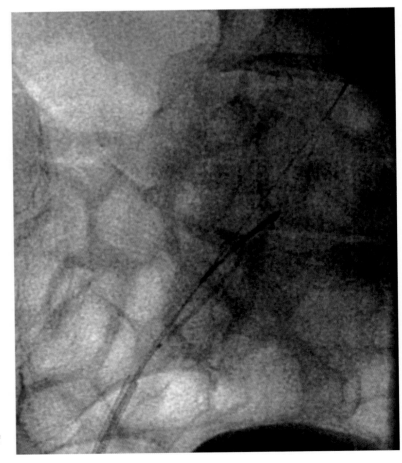

FIGURE 55-9. The wire was firmly captured near the end of the stent catheter.

Key Concepts

1. Stent embolization is rare. Embolization into the coronary circulation is a serious event. In contrast, embolization of a stent into the peripheral circulation is a relatively benign event.
2. Management of stent embolization includes stent retrieval by use of a low-profile balloon, loop snares, or forceps, or by crushing the stent against the arterial wall with another stent.

Selected References

1. Eggebrecht H, Haude M, von Birgelen C, Oldenburg O, Baumgart D, Herrmann J, Welge D, Bartel T, Dagres N, Erbel R: Nonsurgical retrieval of embolized coronary stents, *Catheter Cardiovasc Interv* 51:432–440, 2000.
2. Brilakis ES, Best PJM, Elesber AA, Barsness GW, Lennon RJ, Holmes DR, Rihal CS, Garratt KN: Incidence, retrieval methods, and outcomes of stent loss during percutaneous coronary intervention: a large single center experience, *Catheter Cardiovasc Interv* 65:333–340, 2005.
3. Kozman H, Wiseman AH, Cook JR: Long term outcome following coronary stent embolization or misdeployment, *Am J Cardiol* 88:630–634, 2001.
4. Kammler J, Leisch F, Kerschner K, Kypta A, Steinwender C, Kratochwill H, Lukas T, Hofmann R: Long term follow-up in patients with lost coronary stents during interventional procedures, *Am J Cardiol* 98:367–369, 2006.

Foreign Body Retrieval

Mitral Balloon Valvuloplasty

Michael Ragosta, MD, FACC, FSCAI

CASE PRESENTATION

Several members of the Cardiovascular Division of the University of Virginia visit a medical clinic in Santo Domingo, Dominican Republic each year to provide tertiary care services for indigent patients with rheumatic heart disease. During one of these excursions, a 33-year-old Dominican woman presented with a 1-year history of worsening dyspnea on exertion. She reported fatigue and severe dyspnea with mild exertion but denied orthopnea or paroxysmal nocturnal dyspnea. She had been treated with a diuretic and aspirin with minimal improvement. On physical examination, she appeared healthy with a blood pressure of 110/80 mmHg and a regular pulse at 72 bpm. Her jugular veins were normal and lung fields clear. Cardiac exam revealed a loud first sound, an opening snap, and a diastolic rumble consistent with mitral stenosis without evidence of regurgitation. Her chest x-ray revealed left atrial enlargement, and a 12-lead electrocardiogram showed sinus rhythm with a right axis, evidence of right ventricular hypertrophy, and atrial enlargement (Figure 56-1). Her echocardiogram (Figure 56-2) confirmed the presence of rheumatic mitral stenosis with left atrial enlargement and a mean gradient by Doppler of 5 to 8 mmHg with only trace mitral regurgitation. The Wilkins score calculated to 8, based on the following characteristics: leaflets were severely restricted at the tips with the base showing normal mobility (score of 2); leaflet thickening appeared primarily at the margins (score of 2); there was only minimal leaflet calcification (score of 2); and there appeared to be modest thickening of the subvalvular apparatus (score of 2).

A transesophageal echocardiogram showed no evidence of a left atrial thrombus. She was referred for cardiac catheterization and consideration for mitral balloon valvuloplasty.

CARDIAC CATHETERIZATION

The pulmonary artery pressure measured 50/22 mmHg (Figure 56-3) and the baseline cardiac output measured 5.3 L/min. Simultaneous left ventricular and pulmonary capillary wedge pressures are shown in Figure 56-4. This confirmed a mean transmitral gradient of about 5 mmHg, and the valve area calculated to 1.4 cm². Her symptoms appeared to be out of proportion to these findings and

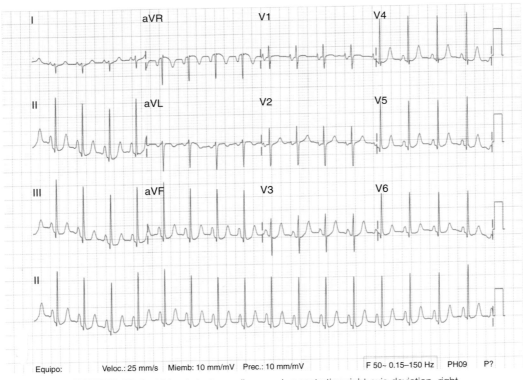

FIGURE 56-1. 12-lead electrocardiogram demonstrating right axis deviation, right ventricular hypertrophy, and left atrial enlargement, consistent with a diagnosis of mitral stenosis.

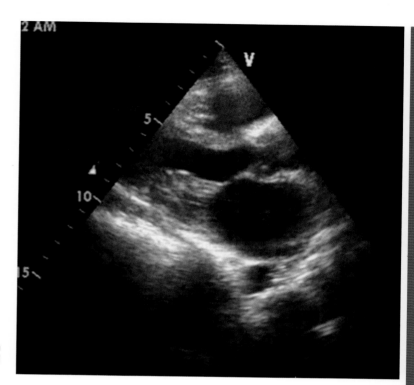

FIGURE 56-2. Long-axis transthoracic echocardiogram showing the classic rheumatic mitral deformity and left atrial enlargement.

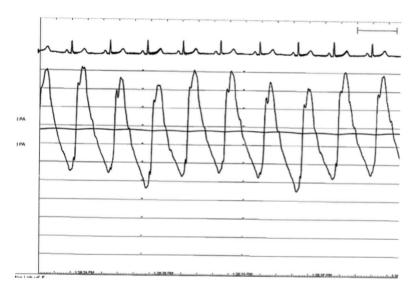

FIGURE 56-3. This is the patient's pulmonary artery pressure (50/23 mmHg).

therefore, while on the cardiac catheterization laboratory table, exercise was performed by having the patient repetitively raise and lower a one liter bag of saline in each arm. The hemodynamic measurements were repeated after just a few minutes of exercise and showed a marked increase in pulmonary artery pressure (systolic pressure >65 mmHg) and an increase in the transmitral gradient to more than 10 mmHg (Figure 56-5). Based on the hemodynamic data, the patient's symptoms, and the favorable echocardiographic findings, the operator proceeded with mitral balloon valvuloplasty.

A transseptal puncture was accomplished and a transseptal sheath placed in the left atrium. Based on the patient's height (142 cm), a 26 mm Inoue balloon was prepared and calibrated to inflate first to 24 mm. The Inoue guidewire was advanced into the left atrium and the atrial septum dilated with a 14 French dilator to accommodate the Inoue balloon. The balloon catheter was then advanced over the wire into the left atrium and the guidewire replaced with a steering wire and advanced to the tip of the balloon. The tip of the balloon was steered across the mitral valve and into the left ventricle. The operator began balloon inflation, first inflating the left ventricular side. The balloon catheter was then pulled back snugly against the valve (Figure 56-6). With continued inflation, the left atrial side inflated (Figure 56-7) and then the central portion of the balloon expanded, resulting in dilatation of the mitral annulus and valve (Figure 56-8 and Video 56-1). The steering wire was removed and simultaneous left ventricular and left

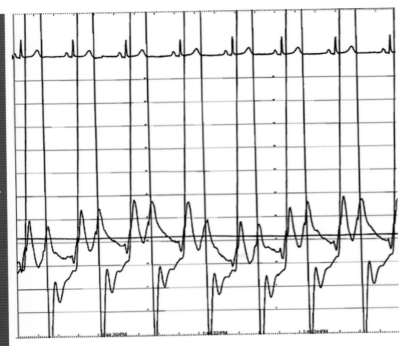

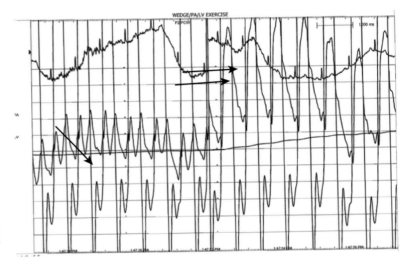

FIGURE 56-4. The simultaneous left ventricular and pulmonary capillary wedge pressures are shown here with the patient at rest. There is a mean transmitral gradient of 5 mmHg.

FIGURE 56-5. With exercise, the transmitral gradient increased to about 10 mmHg (*arrow*); pulmonary artery pressure also increased (*double arrow*).

atrial pressures were measured, with no significant residual transmitral gradient found (Figure 56-9). An echocardiogram found no mitral regurgitation; this was confirmed by ventriculography (Video 56-2).

POSTPROCEDURAL COURSE

Her postprocedural course was uncomplicated. Echocardiography performed the following day found no mitral regurgitation and a 4 mmHg gradient. At follow-up evaluation, she felt well with resolution of her dyspnea and fatigue.

DISCUSSION

With the near elimination of rheumatic fever, rheumatic mitral stenosis has become very rare and is seen in the United States primarily among immigrants from

developing countries where the condition still remains prevalent. In developing countries, individuals afflicted with severe mitral stenosis may suffer severely, both in terms of their symptoms as well as socioeconomically, as they are often unable to work or care for their families.

Medical therapy of rheumatic mitral stenosis includes antibiotic prophylaxis, beta-blockers to allow increased diastolic filling time, diuretics, and warfarin for thromboembolic protection in patients with atrial fibrillation.[1] These agents are useful during the long asymptomatic or minimally symptomatic phase of the disease. Exertional symptoms are often present in patients with valve areas less than 1.6 cm^2 and in patients that develop pulmonary hypertension. Patients with severe mitral stenosis (valve areas less than 1.2 cm^2) usually are significantly impaired by the condition and typically require relief of valve obstruction either surgically or by balloon valvuloplasty. Both open commissurotomy

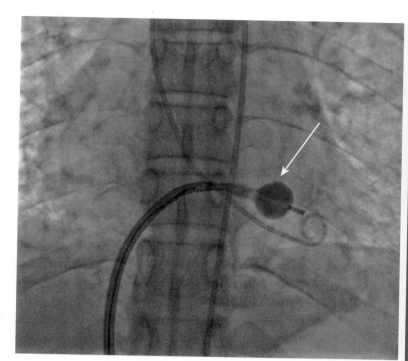

FIGURE 56-6. The Inoue balloon is positioned from a transseptal approach across the mitral valve and is inflated; the left ventricular side inflates first, as shown here (*arrow*). A pigtail catheter is in the left ventricle.

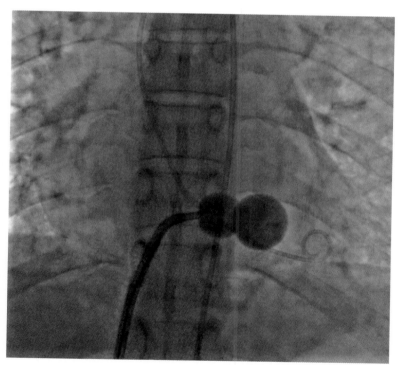

FIGURE 56-7. The balloon is pulled against the mitral annulus, and further inflation results in inflation of the left atrial side of the balloon.

and mitral valve replacement are effective surgical options and percutaneous mitral balloon valvuloplasty appears as effective as open commissurotomy in patients with appropriate valvular anatomy.[2]

The early generation techniques for mitral balloon valvuloplasty relying on a single or double balloon were less effective and associated with a higher complication rate, including acute mitral regurgitation or cardiac perforation from balloon slippage. The Inoue balloon, used in this case, is characterized by differential expansion and allows the balloon to inflate in a more stable and predictable manner.[2] This device has improved the efficacy and safety of this procedure and is currently the most commonly used device for percutaneous mitral valvuloplasty.

Indications for mitral balloon valvuloplasty are listed in Table 56-1.[3] The pathology of the mitral valve as seen by echocardiography is an important predictor of

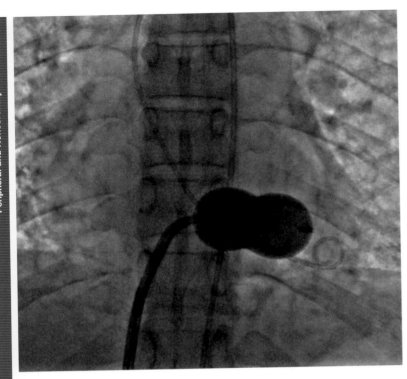

FIGURE 56-8. The balloon is now fully inflated and dilating the mitral valve orifice.

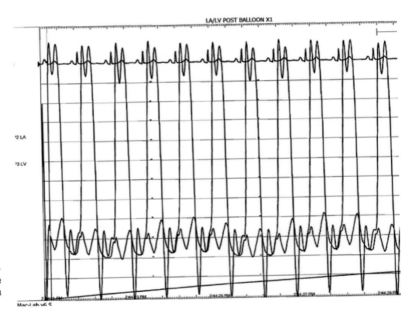

FIGURE 56-9. Following balloon valvuloplasty, the simultaneous left ventricular and pulmonary capillary wedge pressures were measured and the gradient was reduced to a negligible amount.

success.[4,5] The Wilkins score takes into consideration the important pathologic features predicting success (Table 56-2). A score of 1 to 4, ranging from mild to severe abnormalities, is used to describe four variables: leaflet mobility, leaflet thickening, leaflet calcification, and subvalvular thickening. A Wilkins score less than 8 is favorable for mitral balloon valvuloplasty.[4,5] Although a score over 8 is associated with inadequate hemodynamic results and a higher complication rate, patients with significant symptoms who are poor operative candidates may still derive benefit from mitral valvuloplasty.

The procedure is contraindicated in the presence of significant (more than 2+) mitral regurgitation and in the presence of a left atrial thrombus. For these reasons, patients require transesophageal echocardiography prior to the procedure to exclude left atrial thrombus. Complications of the procedure include tamponade during performance of the transseptal puncture, stroke, peripheral embolization, arrhythmia, residual left-to-right shunt from the atrial septal puncture, and development of severe mitral regurgitation.

The long-term efficacy of mitral balloon valvuloplasty is excellent. Young patients with favorable anatomy do

TABLE 56-1 Indications for Mitral Balloon Valvuloplasty[3]

Grading of Mitral Stenosis (MS)

	Mean Gradient (mmHg)	PA Systolic Pressure (mmHg)	Valve Area (cm²)
Mild	<5	<30	>1.5
Moderate	5-10	30-50	1.0-1.5
Severe	>10	>50	<1.0

Class I Indications

- Symptomatic (NYHA Class II, III or IV) with moderate or severe MS and suitable valve anatomy
- Asymptomatic patients with moderate or severe MS and suitable valve anatomy with pulmonary hypertension (PA systolic >50 mmHg at rest or >60 mmHg with exercise).

Class IIa Indications

- Patients who are poor surgical candidates with severe symptoms (Class III-IV) with moderate or severe MS and nonpliable, calcified valves

Class IIb Indications

- Asymptomatic patients with moderate or severe MS and favorable anatomy with new-onset atrial fibrillation
- Symptomatic patients with valve area >1.5 cm² and pulmonary pressure >60 mmHg, wedge pressure >25 mmHg or mean transmitral gradient >15 with exercise
- As an alternative to surgery in patients with Class III-IV severe MS and nonpliable, calcified valves

Class III Indications

- Mild MS
- Left atrial thrombus
- Moderate or severe mitral regurgitation

TABLE 56-2 Echocardiographic Scoring System Used to Predict Success of Mitral Valvuloplasty[4]

Score	Leaflet Mobility	Leaflet Thickening	Leaflet Calcification	Subvalvular Thickening
1	Highly mobile, only tips restricted	Normal (4-5 mm)	Single area of echo brightness	Minimal thickening below mitral leaflets
2	Midleaflet and base have normal mobility	Midleaflet normal, thick at margins (5-8 mm)	Scattered areas of brightness confined to leaflet margins	Thickened chordal structures up to 1/3 chordal length
3	Valve moves forward in diastole only from base	Entire leaflet thickened (5-8 mm)	Brightness extends to midportion of leaflets	Thickening extending to distal 2/3 of chords
4	No movement of leaflets in diastole	Marked thickening (>8-10 mm)	Extensive brightness throughout	Extensive thickening and shortening of chordal structures to papillary muscles

KEY CONCEPTS

1. Rheumatic mitral stenosis is uncommon in the U.S. but remains a significant problem in developing nations.
2. Patients with severe mitral stenosis, symptoms, and appropriate valve anatomy without mitral regurgitation or left atrial thrombus are excellent candidates for mitral balloon valvuloplasty.
3. Long-term results for mitral valvuloplasty are excellent and similar to open commissurotomy.

better than older patients with more calcified valves. Overall, between 60% and 90% of patients are alive and free of symptoms with no further intervention on the mitral valve 5 to 10 years after the procedure.[2] In a large cohort of patients treated in the U.S. between 1986 and 2000, 82% of patients with a Wilkins score of less than 8 were alive at 12-year follow-up.[5] Balloon valvuloplasty can be repeated in patients who have had prior balloon valvuloplasty (i.e., mitral valve restenosis) and in patients who have had prior open commisurotomy, although the results are less favorable as compared to an initial procedure.[2]

Mitral balloon valvuloplasty is a technically demanding procedure. It requires skill in transseptal puncture and a thorough understanding of the nuances of the hemodynamics of mitral stenosis. Perhaps the greatest challenge to the operator is determining when to stop. This decision requires a great deal of judgment and experience. In the present case, a single inflation resulted in an excellent hemodynamic result. However, if after balloon inflation, a residual gradient greater than 5 mmHg or valve area less than 1.5 cm² remains and there is no more than 1+ mitral regurgitation, additional balloon inflations using progressive increases in balloon size by increments of 1 mm can be performed, with hemodynamic measurements and assessment for degree of mitral regurgitation performed after each inflation until a satisfactory result is obtained.

Selected References

1. Carabello BA: Modern management of mitral stenosis, *Circulation* 112:432–437, 2005.
2. Nobuyoshi M, Arita T, Shirai S, Hamasaki N, Yokoi H, Iwabuchi M, Yasumoto H, Nosaka H: Percutaneous balloon mitral valvuloplasty. A review, *Circulation* 119:e211–e219, 2009.
3. Bonow RO, Carabello BA, Chatterjee K, et al: ACC/AHA 2006 practice guidelines for the management of patients with valvular heart disease: Executive summary. A report of the American College of Cardiology/American Heart Association task force on practice guidelines (Writing committee to revise the 1998 guidelines for the management of patients with valvular heart disease), *J Am Coll Cardiol* 48:598–675, 2006.
4. Wilkins GT, Weyman AE, Abascal VM, Block PC, Palacios IF: Percutaneous balloon dilatation of the mitral valve: an analysis of echocardiographic variables related to outcome and the mechanism of dilatation, *Br Heart J* 60:299–308, 1988.
5. Palacios IF, Sanchez PL, Harrell LC, Weyman AE, Block PC: Which patients benefit from percutaneous mitral balloon valvuloplasty? Prevalvuloplasty and postvalvuloplasty variables that predict long-term outcome, *Circulation* 105:1465–1471, 2002.

Percutaneous Mitral Valve Repair

D. Scott Lim, MD, FACC, FSCAI

CASE PRESENTATION

An 84-year-old woman, with a history of a heart murmur for more than 15 years, presented with congestive heart failure and severe mitral regurgitation. She had undergone a diagnostic catheterization 5 years earlier for dyspnea, which found moderate (2+) mitral regurgitation and a mild global reduction in left ventricular function (ejection fraction 50%), with normal coronary arteries. Diagnosed with a nonischemic cardiomyopathy, she was treated medically and did well until 1 year prior to this presentation.

She now reports progressive and severe shortness of breath with exertion, limiting her ability to perform all her usual activities. An echocardiogram found severe mitral regurgitation and deterioration in left ventricular function (ejection fraction 35% to 40%). The mechanism of her mitral regurgitation appeared to be from tethered leaflets. She was referred to a cardiac surgeon for consideration of mitral valve replacement. After her consultation, she initially declined surgery, but then developed overt congestive heart failure requiring hospital admission. At this point, she agreed to participate in a randomized controlled trial comparing mitral valve surgery to percutaneous repair of the mitral valve using a MitraClip (EVEREST II trial) and was randomized to the MitraClip arm of the trial.

Her past medical history is notable for diabetes, asthma, paroxysmal atrial fibrillation, and hypertension, and she was treated with lisinopril, furosemide, amiodarone, and warfarin. On physical examination, she appeared markedly younger than her stated age. Blood pressure measured 124/58 mmHg, heart rate was 80 and regular, and jugular venous pressure was normal. On cardiac exam, the first sound was inaudible and the second sound was loud, consistent with pulmonary hypertension. A long, 3/6 holosystolic murmur was present at the apex. A 12-lead electrocardiogram demonstrated sinus rhythm with left anterior fascicular block, an intraventricular conduction delay, and left ventricular hypertrophy. Routine blood analysis revealed mild renal insufficiency with a creatinine of 1.7 mg/dL.

CARDIAC CATHETERIZATION

The procedure was performed under general anesthesia and was guided by transesophageal echocardiography. Vascular access initially consisted of an 8 French sheath in the right femoral vein, and a 6 French sheath in the left femoral artery. Baseline hemodynamics were assessed and found a pulmonary artery pressure of 56/40 mmHg,

a mean pulmonary capillary wedge pressure of 40 mmHg, and a cardiac output of 4.0 L/minute. A transseptal catheterization was performed and mean left atrial pressure measured 35 mmHg.

Following transseptal puncture, she received 4000 U of unfractionated heparin and maintained an activated clotting time (ACT) over 250 seconds. The transseptal sheath was exchanged for a 24 French MitraClip steerable guide. Through this guide, the MitraClip was advanced through the left atrium and oriented to the mitral valve using transesophageal echo guidance. Once the device was in the left ventricle, the clip was opened (Figure 57-1 and Video 57-1). Careful adjustments were made using echo guidance in order to position the clip at the site of maximum regurgitation. The device was gently pulled back and the leaflets were grabbed (Videos 57-2, 57-3). After the leaflets were grabbed and the clip closed (Figures 57-2, 57-3), the degree of mitral regurgitation was assessed and found to be satisfactorily reduced (Video 57-4). At this point, the clip was released. There was only minimal, 1+ residual regurgitation. Hemodynamics were reassessed. There was no diastolic pressure gradient between the left atrium and left ventricle (Figure 57-4). The guide was withdrawn to the right atrium and exchanged for a 16 French short sheath. Right heart pressures were repeated and showed an increase in cardiac output to 8.0 L/minute with a significant decrease in left atrial pressure. The sheaths were removed with manual pressure. No contrast was used, and fluoroscopy time was 18.6 minutes.

POSTPROCEDURAL COURSE

She recovered uneventfully from general anesthesia and was observed overnight. She was discharged 48 hours later without complication; clopidogrel was added to her medication regimen. During 2 years of follow-up, she remained free of symptoms with no significant mitral regurgitation on transthoracic echocardiograms.

DISCUSSION

Mitral valve surgery is effective but carries significant morbidity. Many patients are not operative candidates or are at high risk from surgery. Quite recently, a novel percutaneous approach was has been developed for treatment of patients with nonrheumatic mitral regurgitation that involves the placement of a metal clip (MitraClip, Evalve, Menlo Park, CA) on the regurgitant portions of the mitral valve.[1,2] This approach was derived from a known surgical approach of edge-to-edge leaflet repair

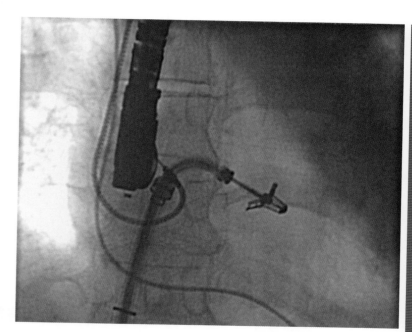

FIGURE 57-1. Via a transseptal approach, the MitraClip is positioned across the mitral valve and the clip opened.

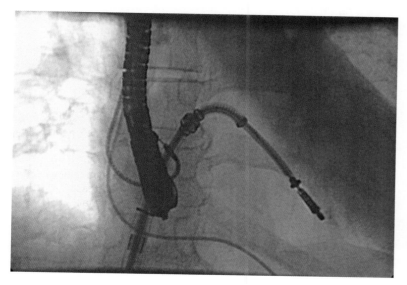

FIGURE 57-2. After the mitral leaflets have been successfully grabbed, the clip is closed and the degree of mitral regurgitation assessed. If the improvement in mitral regurgitation is judged inadequate, then the clip can be opened and the leaflets released, and the device can be repositioned and the leaflets grabbed at a different location.

as described by Alfieri.[3,4] The MitraClip is introduced from a percutaneous, transvenous, transseptal approach to the mitral valve. The traditional imaging modality in the catheterization laboratory of fluoroscopy is of limited utility in this procedure, as it cannot visualize the mitral leaflets. Therefore, the procedure is guided by simultaneous transesophageal imaging, using both two- and three-dimensional echocardiography (see Figure 57-3). Therefore, it is important that the interventionalist be skilled in transesophageal imaging to complement his or her catheterization skills.

By placing the MitraClip on the central portions of the anterior and posterior leaflets, it acts to anchor prolapsing or flail segments, as well as to coapt tethered leaflets, so that it reduces the time and force required to close the valve. By decreasing mitral regurgitation, the left ventricular volumes are reduced, leading to beneficial effects on left ventricular remodeling.[5] Anatomically, the MitraClip creates a tissue bridge between the two leaflets, which limits dilation of the mitral annulus in the septal-lateral dimension, and supports the durability of this repair.[2]

This novel approach to percutaneous mitral valve repair was evaluated in the EVEREST trials. EVEREST I was the safety and feasibility registry, which enrolled 55 patients in a nonrandomized clinical trial.[6] EVEREST II was the pivotal clinical trial in which 279 patients with 3+ or 4+ mitral regurgitation were randomized to either the MitraClip therapy or standard surgical therapy (either mitral valve repair or replacement). It is important to note that this involved low- and moderate-risk patients, in comparison to the EVEREST High-Risk Registry, which enrolled 79 patients who were not operative candidates to the MitraClip therapy. In the initial

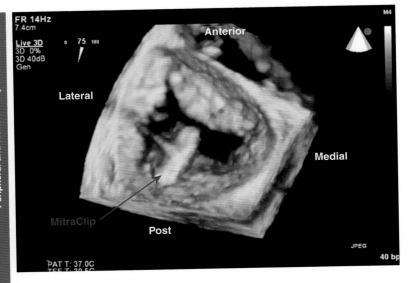

FR 14Hz
7.4cm

Live 3D
3D 0%
3D 40dB
Gen

Anterior

Lateral

Medial

MitraClip

Post

JPEG

40 bp

PAT T: 37.0C

FIGURE 57-3. Three-dimensional transesophageal echocardiographic image of the MitraClip and its orientation to the mitral valve is shown here.

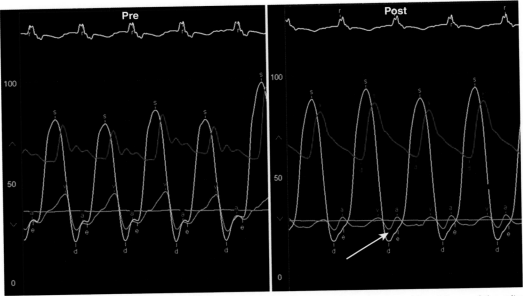

Pre

Post

FIGURE 57-4. Hemodynamics obtained pretreatment show marked elevation of the left atrial pressure. After delivery of the mitral clip, the left atrial pressure has fallen and there is an insignificant pressure gradient between the left atrium and left ventricle (*arrow*).

nonrandomized experience with the MitraClip, procedural success (reduction of mitral regurgitation to 2+ or less) was achieved in 74%, and 66% were alive and without having mitral valve surgery or MR >2+ at 12 months. It is also important to note that this represents the initial experience with this novel technology, which has a steep learning curve. Ongoing follow-up from the randomized trial continues, but the initial data appear promising.

A separate registry was created for patients with severe mitral regurgitation from either degenerative (prolapse or flail) or functional etiologies (mitral regurgitation secondary to ischemic or nonischemic cardiomyopathy) who were not operative candidates – the EVEREST High-Risk Registry. This registry rapidly enrolled 79 patients, as there was significant support for it from surgical colleagues. Data presented showed that while at 30 days the predicted mortality for the

group was 18.2%, the actual mortality was 7.7%, with 76% survival at 1 year and 79% of the survivors being in the New York Heart Association symptom class I or II.[7] These data give support to the concept that particularly for these nonoperative patients, novel percutaneous options are attractive.

KEY CONCEPTS

1. Novel devices to treat mitral regurgitation by a percutaneous approach are under intense investigation.
2. The MitraClip is a percutaneously delivered device that coapts the mitral leaflets in a similar manner to an Alfieri stitch. Preliminary data suggest it is an effective method of treating some forms of mitral regurgitation.

Selected References

1. Fann JI, St Goar FG, Komtebedde J, Oz MC, Block PC, Foster E, Butany J, Feldman T, Burdon TA: Beating heart catheter-based edge-to-edge mitral valve procedure in a porcine model: efficacy and healing response, *Circulation* 110(8):988–993, 2004.
2. St Goar FG, Fann JI, Komtebedde J, Foster E, Oz MC, Fogarty TJ, Feldman T, Block PC: Endovascular edge-to-edge mitral valve repair: short-term results in a porcine model, *Circulation* 108 (16):1990–1993, 2003.
3. Alfieri O, Maisano F, De Bonis M, Stefano PL, Torracca L, Oppizzi M, La Canna G: The double-orifice technique in mitral valve repair: a simple solution for complex problems, *J Thorac Cardiovasc Surg* 122(4):674–681, 2001.
4. Maisano F, Torracca L, Oppizzi M, Stefano PL, D'Addario G, La Canna G, Zogno M, Alfieri O: The edge-to-edge technique: a simplified method to correct mitral insufficiency, *Eur J Cardiothorac Surg* 13(3):240–245, 1998; discussion 245–246.
5. Herrmann HC, Kar S, Siegel R, Fail P, Loghin C, Lim S, Hahn R, Rogers JH, Bommer WJ, Wang A, et al. Effect of percutaneous mitral repair with the MitraClip device on mitral valve area and gradient, *EuroIntervention* 4(4):437–442, 2009.
6. Feldman T, Kar S, Rinaldi M, Fail P, Hermiller J, Smalling R, Whitlow PL, Gray W, Low R, Herrmann HC, et al. Percutaneous mitral repair with the MitraClip system: safety and midterm durability in the initial EVEREST (Endovascular Valve Edge-to-Edge Repair Study) cohort, *J Am Coll Cardiol* 54(8): 686–694, 2009.
7. Whitlow PL, Kar S, Pederson W, Lim S, Foster E, Glower D, Feldman T: MitraClip therapy in the EVEREST High Risk Registry: One Year Results, *EuroIntervention* 4:437–442, 2008.

Iliac Artery Disease

Jason T. Call, MD

CASE PRESENTATION

A 64-year-old woman with a history of hypertension, hyperlipidemia, and tobacco use noted progressive bilateral calf discomfort during activity. These symptoms slowly progressed, and ultimately they became so severe that she stopped participating in tennis, her favorite activity. She discussed these symptoms with her primary care physician. Her physician interpreted these symptoms as claudication and ordered non-invasive vascular testing. Her resting ankle brachial index (ABI) was 0.75 on the right and 0.58 on the left (Figure 58-1). After exercise, her right ABI dropped to 0.60 and her left ABI dropped to 0.21. In addition, exercise caused significant bilateral calf pain, with the left side hurting more than the right. She was subsequently referred for angiography.

ANGIOGRAPHY

Abdominal angiography found normal renal arteries and distal aorta. Angiography of the pelvic vessels demonstrated a severe stenosis of the left external iliac artery (Figures 58-2, 58-3). Initially, there did not appear to be appreciable disease in the right iliac system to account for the findings on the noninvasive study; however, there was significant vessel overlap. The femoral and runoff vessels appeared normal bilaterally.

The left external iliac lesion was felt to be consistent with her noninvasive studies and likely accounted for her symptoms. The etiology of her right leg findings was not apparent on the initial angiograms. The operator decided to proceed with intervention of the left external iliac. Arterial access had initially been obtained in the right common femoral artery for the diagnostic angiograms. A long, 6 French Ansel 2 sheath was taken up and over the aortoiliac bifurcation and positioned proximal to the left external iliac lesion. A bolus of unfractionated heparin was administered intravenously to achieve a therapeutic activated clotting time of greater than 250 seconds. The operator positioned an 0.018 inch guidewire distally (Figure 58-4) and dilated the stenosis with a 5 mm diameter by 40 mm long balloon (Figure 58-5). Following balloon angioplasty, substantial residual narrowing remained due to elastic recoil. The operator then deployed a 7 mm diameter by 40 mm long self-expanding

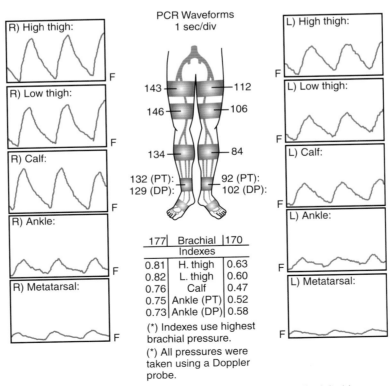

FIGURE 58-1. Baseline, resting, noninvasive studies showing bilateral inflow disease worse on the left side.

PCR Waveforms
1 sec/div

R) High thigh:

R) Low thigh:

R) Calf:

R) Ankle:

R) Metatarsal:

L) High thigh:

L) Low thigh:

L) Calf:

L) Ankle:

L) Metatarsal:

143   112
146   106
134   84
132 (PT):   92 (PT):
129 (DP):   102 (DP):

177	Brachial	170
	Indexes	
0.81	H. thigh	0.63
0.82	L. thigh	0.60
0.76	Calf	0.47
0.75	Ankle (PT)	0.52
0.73	Ankle (DP)	0.58

(*) Indexes use highest brachial pressure.
(*) All pressures were taken using a Doppler probe.

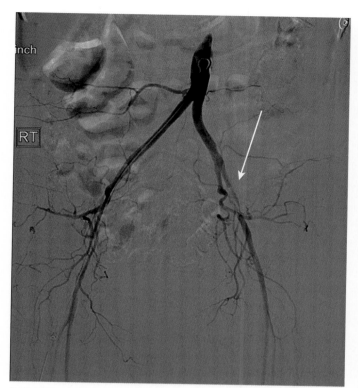

FIGURE 58-2. Pelvic arteriogram showing a high-grade left external iliac stenosis (*arrow*).

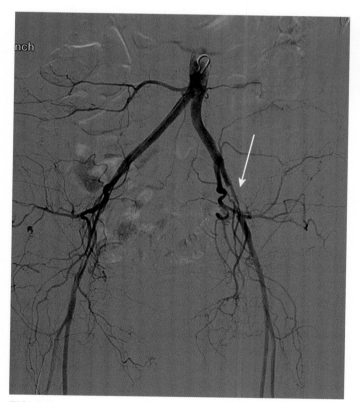

FIGURE 58-3. Pelvic angiogram obtained with additional filling of contrast showing a high grade, left external iliac stenosis.

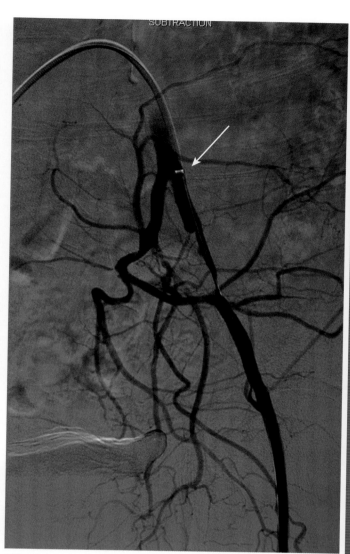

FIGURE 58-4. A long sheath was placed selectively into the left common iliac from the right side (*arrow*) and the external iliac stenosis was crossed with a 0.018 inch guidewire.

nitinol stent and postdilated the stent with the 5 mm diameter by 40 mm long balloon. The post-stent angiogram revealed an excellent result (Figure 58-6) and angiography of the distal runoff showed no distal emboli.

Following the procedure on the left external iliac artery, the operator withdrew the long sheath over a 0.035 inch wire. Pressure monitoring during the pullback uncovered a 60 mmHg pressure gradient between the distal aorta and the distal right external iliac. Another angiogram was performed, which found a stenosis just proximal to the inguinal ligament (Figure 58-7). The lesion did not resolve with intraarterial nitroglycerin. Although it did not appear severe angiographically, this stenosis was associated with a significant pressure gradient and likely accounted for the patient's right leg symptoms and the findings on the noninvasive studies. The distal right external iliac stenosis was then treated with

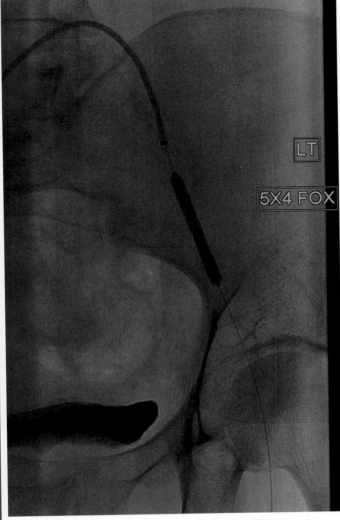

FIGURE 58-5. Balloon dilatation of the left external iliac stenosis.

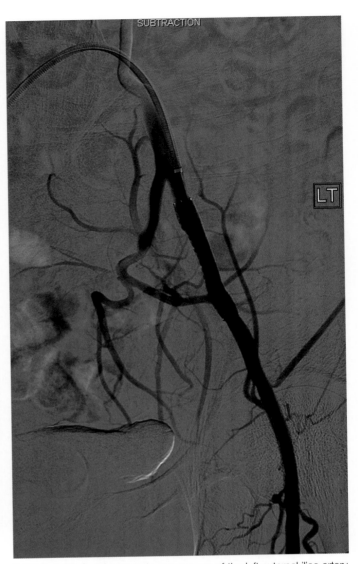

FIGURE 58-6. Angiographic appearance of the left external iliac artery following angioplasty and stenting.

a 5 mm diameter by 40 mm long balloon for a prolonged inflation (Figures 58-8, 58-9). The operator was not entirely satisfied with the angiographic result and placed a 7 mm diameter by 40 mm long self-expanding nitinol stent, post dilated with the 5 mm diameter by 40 mm long balloon. The final angiograms demonstrated an excellent result with no evidence of distal embolization (Figure 58-10).

POSTPROCEDURAL COURSE

The arterial sheath was removed by manual pressure when the activated clotting time fell below 180 seconds and the patient was prescribed bed rest for 4 hours. She was discharged later that same day. At follow-up 1 month later, noninvasive testing was repeated and found a right ABI of 1.02 and a left ABI of 0.99 at rest (Figure 58-11). With exercise, the right ABI was 1.00 and the left ABI was 1.01. Her symptoms had completely resolved and she was able to return to her tennis game.

DISCUSSION

Over 8 million individuals in the United States have peripheral arterial disease. Many are asymptomatic; however, at least a third experience claudication, and up to 5% develop limb-threatening ischemia.[1] Noninvasive physiologic testing helps determine the degree of arterial insufficiency and provides information regarding the location of the stenoses. Conventional angiography remains the gold standard to define the arterial anatomy and diagnose luminal obstruction. Adjunctive techniques performed during angiography are also helpful to assess the disease severity and include measurement of translesional pressure gradients and intravascular ultrasound. In fact, in this case, based solely on the angiogram, the disease in the right external iliac artery might have been disregarded; the measurement of a translesional pressure gradient determined that this disease was, in fact, significant.

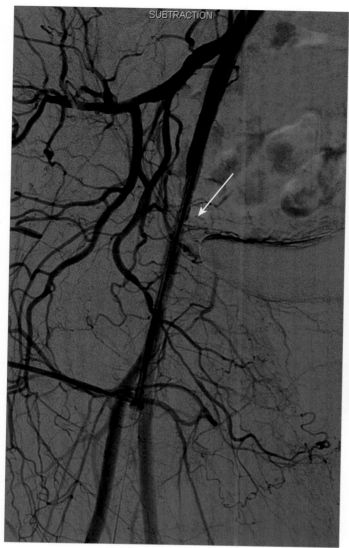

FIGURE 58-7. Although the right external iliac stenosis did not appear severe on angiography (*arrow*), a 60 mmHg translesional pressure gradient was measured.

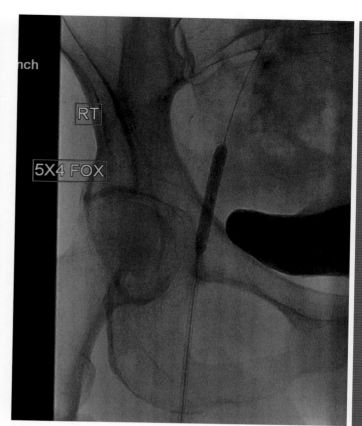

FIGURE 58-8. Balloon dilatation of the right external iliac.

Endovascular therapy has emerged as the leading method to relieve lifestyle-limiting symptoms. The decision between endovascular therapy and surgical therapy often depends on the severity and location of the lesions, as well as patient comorbidities and the overall functional status of the patient.

Inflow disease, defined as a stenosis located above the inguinal ligament, is present in approximately 30% of patients with claudication. Patients with isolated inflow disease may complain of typical calf claudication, but may also have thigh and/or buttock claudication; men will often complain of impotence.

The management of inflow disease is outlined in the TransAtlantic Inter-Society Consensus Document on Management of Peripheral Arterial Disease (TASC), which was last revised in 2007.[2] In this document, a classification system has been devised to help guide in the management of inflow disease (Table 58-1). Based on the excellent long-term patency rates with endovascular therapy, aortoiliac disease classified as TASC A or B is

considered best treated initially by endovascular techniques. Lesions classified as TASC D are managed surgically. Lesions characterized as TASC C have a lower likelihood of long-term success with an endovascular approach. In this category, patient variables such as comorbidities and overall functional status become extremely important in the decision process. Surgical management is usually recommended in patients with TASC C lesions and low surgical risk due to better long-term outcomes with regards to patency. However, in these categories, it may be reasonable to proceed with an initial endovascular approach as long as surgical targets are not compromised. As the field of endovascular therapy evolves, new devices and novel techniques may improve the long-term patency and new data originating from larger series and randomized controlled trials may change these recommendations to a primary endovascular strategy.

While the TASC criteria are helpful in decision-making, it should be emphasized that patency rates do not always equate with clinical outcomes; the ultimate goal is to improve the patient's quality of life. In addition, the TASC criteria are based on an interpretation of the angiogram and subtle changes in the description of a lesion can significantly change the classification. For instance in the case presented here, the disease would be classified as TASC A based on the presence of bilateral external iliac stenosis <3 cm; the classification changes to TASC C if these lesions are interpreted as 3 to 10 cm in length.

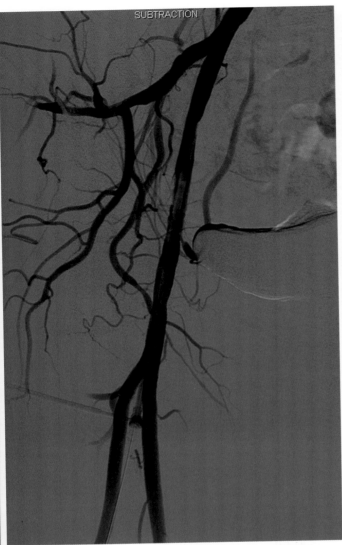

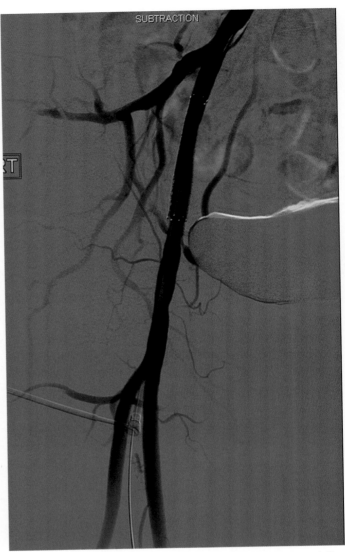

FIGURE 58-9. Disrupted plaque in the right external iliac after balloon angioplasty.

FIGURE 58-10. Angiographic appearance of the right external iliac following angioplasty and stenting.

TABLE 58-1 TASC Classification of Aortoiliac Disease[2]

Classification	Characteristics
Type A	• Unilateral or bilateral stenosis of the common iliac artery • Short (<3cm) unilateral or bilateral stenosis of the external iliac artery
Type B	• Short (<3 cm) stenosis of the infrarenal aorta • Unilateral occlusion of the common iliac artery • Single or multiple stenoses of the external iliac artery totaling 3-10 cm without involving the common femoral artery • Unilateral external iliac stenosis not involving the origin of the internal iliac or common femoral artery
Type C	• Bilateral common iliac occlusions • Bilateral external iliac stenoses 3-10 cm, not extending into the common femoral arteries • Unilateral external iliac stenosis extending into the common femoral artery • Unilateral external iliac artery occlusion involving the origin of the internal iliac and/or common femoral arteries • Heavily calcified unilateral external iliac artery occlusion with or without involvement of the origins of the internal iliac and/or common femoral arteries
Type D	• Infrarenal aortoiliac occlusion • Diffuse disease involving the aorta and both iliac arteries requiring treatment • Diffuse multiple stenoses involving the unilateral common iliac, external iliac, and common femoral arteries • Unilateral occlusions of both common and external iliac arteries • Bilateral occlusions of the external iliac arteries • Iliac stenoses in patients with abdominal aortic aneurysm requiring treatment and not amenable to endograft placement or other lesions requiring open aortic or iliac surgery

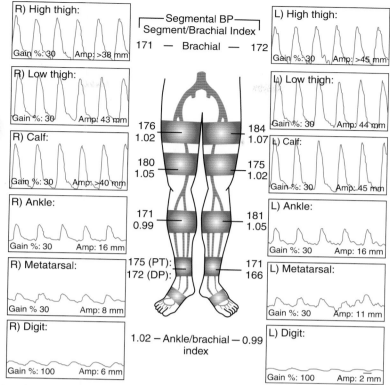

FIGURE 58-11. Follow-up noninvasive studies 1 month after the procedure showing normalization of resting values.

KEY CONCEPTS

1. Noninvasive testing and the patient's symptoms provide information on the location of the disease and are helpful in planning the angiogram.
2. Intraprocedural testing such as the assessment of translesional pressure gradients may be necessary to fully evaluate the circulation.
3. The TASC document helps guide treatment decisions for inflow disease.
4. Endovascular therapy for inflow disease has a high rate of technical success, with long-term durability dependent on lesion characteristics and patient variables.

Selected References

1. Creager MA, Loscalzo J: Vascular Diseases of the Extremities. In Fauci AS, Braunwald E, Kasper DL, Hauser SL, Longo DL, Jameson JL, Loscalzo J, editors: *Harrison's Principles of Internal Medicine,* ed 17, New York, NY, 2008, McGraw-Hill, pp 1568–1570.
2. Norgren L, Hiatt WR, Dormandy JA, Nehler MR, Harris KA, Fowkes FGR on behalf of the TASC II Working Group: Intersociety consensus for the management of peripheral arterial disease (TASC II), *Eur J Vasc Endovasc Surg* 33:S1–S70, 2007.

Stenosis in a Superficial Femoral Artery

Jason T. Call, MD

CASE PRESENTATION

A 74-year-old diabetic man with hypertension and prior tobacco use, whose medications included aspirin, a statin, and an ACE inhibitor, developed bilateral calf claudication. Eventually, his leg symptoms progressed and he was unable to exercise, greatly limiting his lifestyle. His physician detected diminished pulses distally and assessed these symptoms with noninvasive studies (Figure 59-1). These demonstrated moderate bilateral arterial insufficiency at the level of the superficial femoral artery (SFA). He was referred for angiography.

ANGIOGRAPHY

The patient's symptoms were worse in the left leg; thus angiography of the left leg was performed first from an arterial sheath placed in the right femoral artery. It showed high-grade, sequential lesions in the mid-SFA (not shown). These were successfully treated with a self-expanding stent. Following that procedure, diagnostic angiography of the right leg was performed and demonstrated two high-grade lesions in the SFA with an ulcerated stenosis of the proximal segment of the right SFA (Figures 59-2, 59-3) and a longer, severe stenosis in the mid- to distal segment (Figure 59-4). The patient was discharged after this procedure on the left leg and experienced resolution of his left leg claudication with normalization of his left leg noninvasive studies. However, he continued to be limited by right leg claudication. Therefore, approximately 3 months after his left leg intervention, he presented for endovascular treatment of the right leg.

Access was obtained from the left common femoral artery. An Omniflush catheter was used to lay out the iliac vessels, and a 6 French long sheath was placed "up and over" from the left femoral to the right external iliac artery. An intravenous bolus of unfractionated heparin was administered to achieve a therapeutic activated clotting time of more than 250 seconds. The proximal and distal lesions were crossed with a hydrophilic glide

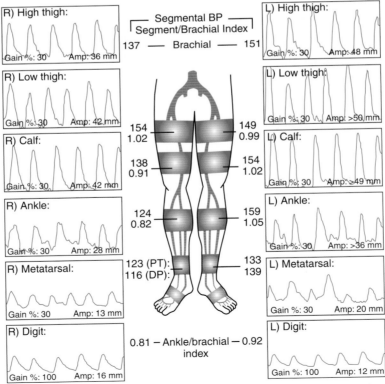

FIGURE 59-1. Preprocedure noninvasive studies demonstrating bilateral disease at the level of the superficial femoral arteries.

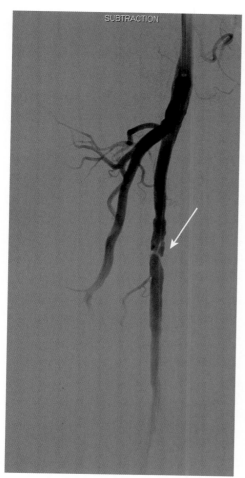

FIGURE 59-2. Angiography found a severe, eccentric stenosis in the proximal segment of the superficial femoral artery (*arrow*).

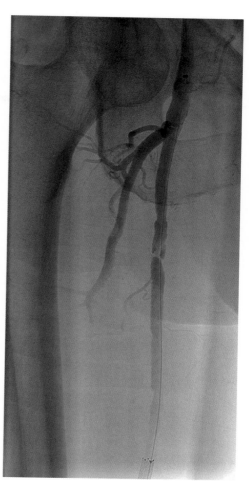

FIGURE 59-3. This is a nonsubtracted image of the proximal stenosis in the SFA.

wire. A catheter was then used to exchange the glide wire for a 0.018 inch guidewire. The distal SFA was treated first using a 5 mm diameter by 60 mm long balloon in two overlapping locations. The distal lesion was found to be difficult to expand (Figure 59-5); ultimately, the balloon appeared fully expanded at 12 atmospheres of pressure. A post balloon angiogram showed residual stenosis and elastic recoil; thus the operator deployed a 7 mm diameter by 150 mm long self-expanding nitinol stent across the extent of the distal lesions. The stent was postdilated with the 5 mm diameter by 60 mm long balloon (Figure 59-6) and the post-stent angiogram demonstrated an excellent result (Figure 59-7).

The proximal stenosis was then dilated with the 5 mm diameter by 60 mm long balloon (Figure 59-8). This disrupted the plaque, but a significant stenosis remained; therefore the operator placed a 7 mm diameter by 60 mm long self-expanding nitinol stent, postdilating it with the 5 mm diameter balloon used earlier. The final angiogram found no residual stenosis or angiographic complication (Figure 59-9).

POSTPROCEDURAL COURSE

Following this procedure, the 6 French sheath was left in place until the activated clotting time fell below 180 seconds. Hemostasis was achieved with manual pressure

followed by 4 hours of bed rest. He was discharged later that same day on aspirin and clopidogrel. At follow-up 1 month later, he had resolution of his symptoms and normalization of his noninvasive tests both at rest and after exercise (Figures 59-10, 59-11).

DISCUSSION

Disease of the superficial femoral artery is present in 80% to 90% of patients with claudication.[1] At the time of angiography, this vessel is often found to be completely occluded, with collateralization and reconstitution of the distal vessel from the profunda femoris. In fact, the profunda femoris is considered to be the "lifeline" to the lower leg, as the collaterals it provides are usually adequate to avoid limb-threatening ischemia. They are usually not adequate, however, to prevent claudication.

The high incidence of SFA disease may relate to the unusual forces that it undergoes, especially in the distal portion of the vessel, including flexion, torsion, compression, and extension. These forces lead to nonlaminar flow and endothelial injury, both of which can promote atherosclerosis. These forces also make endovascular therapy challenging. Traditional balloon-expandable stents cannot be used in the SFA, as they would be

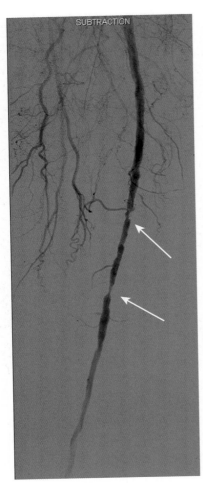

FIGURE 59-4. Complex disease in the mid- and distal segments of the right SFA (*arrows*).

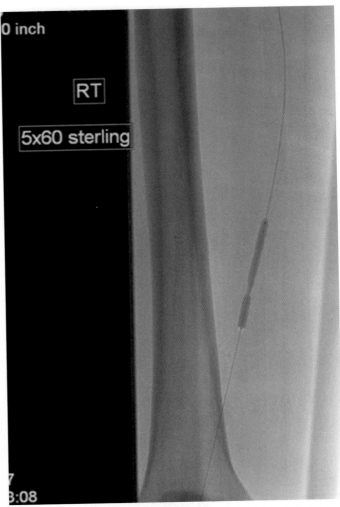

FIGURE 59-5. Balloon dilatation of the mid- to distal right SFA showing persistence of the waist in the balloon, which resolved at higher atmospheres.

deformed and compressed by these same forces. Instead, self-expanding stents are employed. These are most commonly made of nitinol, which has a unique property of "memory" that allows the stent to be expanded to the size it was created, providing continual outward forces against the artery and thus resisting external compression. Typically, a stent is chosen one millimeter in diameter larger than the reference vessel diameter to allow uniform apposition and to accommodate for the dynamic forces that the stent undergoes.

There are a variety of other techniques used to treat SFA disease. These include balloon dilatation alone, scoring balloons, freezing balloons, atherectomy devices (including shaving devices, lasers, and drills), and covered stents, all of which have advantages and disadvantages and specific niche applications. However, despite all of this technology, restenosis rates of SFA lesions are typically 20% to 30% at 1 year.

As with aortoiliac disease, the TASC working group has created a classification system for femoral/popliteal disease (Table 59-1).[2] Again, similar to aortoiliac disease, endovascular treatment is preferred for TASC A and B lesions and surgery is preferred for TASC D lesions. TASC C lesions are usually treated surgically unless the patient is a poor surgical candidate, although endovascular approaches are reasonable in some patients as

long as the intervention does not "burn any bridges" regarding future surgical options. The lesions presented in this case would be considered TASC B as there were multiple SFA lesions which individually were less than 5 cm each (the distal SFA lesion was actually two lesions that were treated as one).

Above-the-knee surgical bypass with autologous vein or prosthetic material has acceptable 5-year patency rates, typically approaching 75%. The outcome after surgery also depends on the status of the inflow and outflow vessels as well as the presence of a healthy section of distal artery to receive the anastomosis. Restenosis remains a significant issue for femoropopliteal lesions and there are a variety of options available if restenosis occurs, including balloon angioplasty, debulking techniques (laser, shavers, drills), restenting, and restenting with a covered stent. There are few data available comparing the outcomes of these various strategies. Patients with recurrent restenosis and significant symptoms should be considered for surgical bypass. It is important for the interventionalist to keep this in mind so as to not limit future surgical options by placing stents in locations where a distal surgical anastomosis may be necessary.

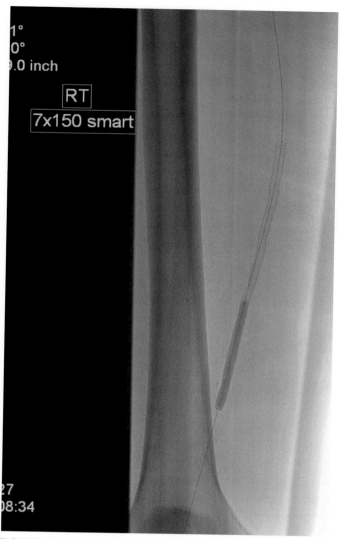

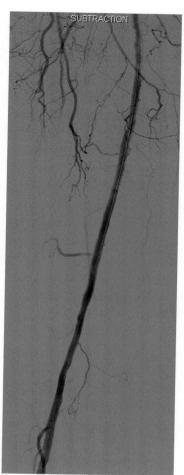

SUBTRACTION

FIGURE 59-7. Angiographic result of the mid- to distal right SFA lesions after angioplasty and stenting.

FIGURE 59-6. Postdilatation of nitinol stents in the right mid- to distal SFA.

TABLE 59-1 TASC Classification of Femoropopliteal Disease[2]

Classification	Characteristics
Type A	• Single stenosis ≤10 cm in length • Single occlusion ≤5 cm in length
Type B lesions	• Multiple lesions (stenoses or occlusions) each ≤5 cm • Single stenosis or occlusion ≤15 cm not involving the infrageniculate popliteal artery • Single or multiple lesions in the absence of continuous tibial vessels to improve inflow for a distal bypass • Heavily calcified occlusion ≤5 cm in length • Single popliteal stenosis
Type C lesions	• Multiple stenoses or occlusions totaling >15 cm with or without heavy calcification • Recurrent stenoses or occlusions that need treatment after two endovascular interventions
Type D lesions	• Chronic total occlusions of common femoral or superficial femoral arteries (>20 cm, involving the popliteal artery) • Chronic total occlusion of popliteal artery and proximal trifurcation vessels

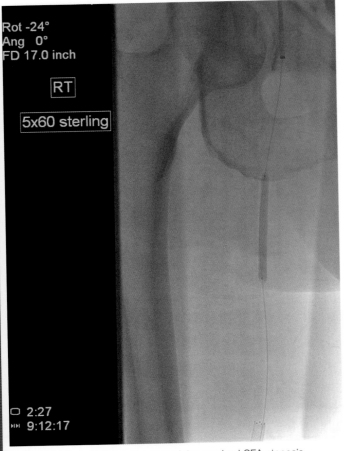

FIGURE 59-8. Balloon dilatation of the proximal SFA stenosis.

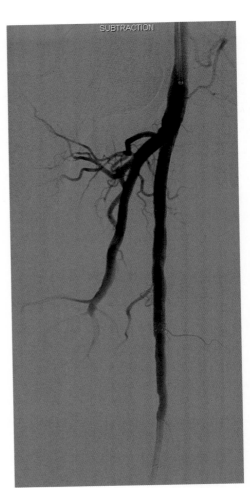

FIGURE 59-9. Final angiographic result of proximal SFA lesion after balloon angioplasty and stenting.

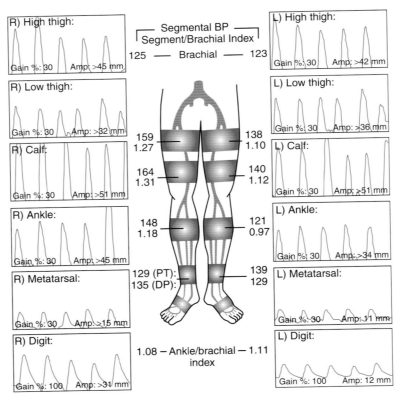

FIGURE 59-10. Noninvasive studies at rest 1 month postprocedure.

EXERCISE PRESSURE MEASUREMENT

	Rest	1	2	3	4	5	6	7	8	9	10
R Ankle (DP):	135	161									
L Ankle (PT):	139	151									
R Brachial:	125	145									
R ABI	1.08	1.11									
L ABI	1.11	1.04									

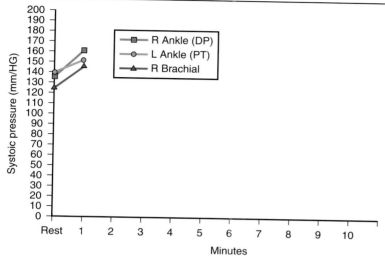

PT exercised 3 1/2 mins at 2.0 mph and 10% grade with no leg symptoms test stopped due to fatigue

FIGURE 59-11. Exercise ABIs 1 month postprocedure.

KEY CONCEPTS

1. Lesions of the superficial femoral artery (SFA) are common in patients with peripheral vascular disease. Extrinsic forces on the SFA contribute to its susceptibility to atherosclerosis and restenosis.
2. Numerous devices are effective for the treatment of SFA disease including balloon angioplasty, atherectomy devices, and self-expanding stents.
3. TASC A and B lesions in the femoral-popliteal segments are routinely managed by an endovascular approach.
4. Given the high rate of restenosis, the interventionalist should attempt to preserve future surgical options during endovascular procedures. This includes leaving reasonable anastomotic sites free of stents.

Selected References

1. Creager MA, Loscalzo J: Vascular Diseases of the Extremities. In Fauci AS, Braunwald E, Kasper DL, Hauser SL, Longo DL, Jameson JL, Loscalzo J, editors: *Harrison's Principles of Internal Medicine*, ed 17, New York, NY, 2008, McGraw-Hill, pp 1568–1570.
2. Norgren L, Hiatt WR, Dormandy JA, Nehler MR, Harris KA, Fowkes FGR: on behalf of the TASC II Working Group: Inter-Society consensus for the management of peripheral arterial disease (TASC II), *Eur J Vasc Endovasc Surg* 33:S1–S70, 2007.

Chronic Occlusion of a Superficial Femoral Artery

Jason T. Call, MD

CASE PRESENTATION

A 76-year-old woman developed worsening leg claudication, progressing nearly to rest pain. She had numerous atherosclerotic risk factors including diabetes, hypertension, hyperlipidemia, and prior tobacco abuse, and had an extensive atherosclerosis history including coronary artery disease, renal artery stenosis, cerebrovascular disease, and peripheral arterial disease. Six months prior to her current presentation, she underwent lower extremity angiography and was found to have bilateral iliac artery lesions along with disease in the superficial femoral arteries. At that point, her physician decided to first treat the inflow disease with stents and then reevaluate the patient's symptoms. Following the bilateral iliac stenting procedure, she continued to have lifestyle-limiting claudication and her right leg symptoms progressed to occasional nocturnal rest pain. The noninvasive studies obtained after iliac stenting showed severe arterial insufficiency in both legs at the level of the thigh (Figure 60-1) consistent with the disease in the superficial femoral artery (SFA). Her physician recommended repeat angiography and possible SFA intervention.

ANGIOGRAPHY

Arterial access was obtained in the left common femoral artery and a 4 French Omniflush catheter was used to perform angiography. Aortography confirmed wide patency of the common iliac stents (Figure 60-2). Selective right femoral angiography and runoff was performed by passing a hydrophilic glide wire over the bifurcation using the Omniflush catheter and then exchanging for a 4 French RIM catheter. Angiography found a mild stenosis in the common femoral artery, followed by a diffusely diseased segment of the proximal SFA of moderate stenosis and then a long segment of total occlusion (Figure 60-3). There was reconstitution of the distal SFA above the adductor canal via collaterals from the profunda femoris (Figures 60-4 through 60-6). Below the knee, the anterior tibial was occluded; however,

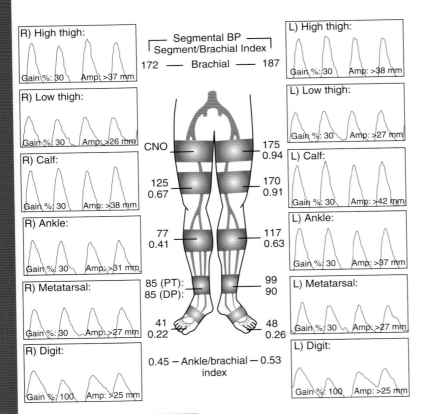

FIGURE 60-1. Baseline noninvasive studies obtained after treatment of the iliac lesions with stents, showing bilateral arterial insufficiency with pressures and waveforms suggesting superficial femoral artery disease.

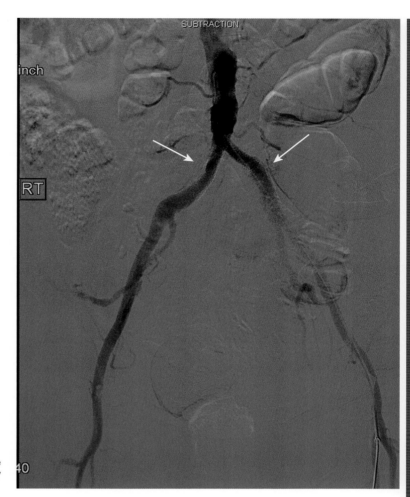

FIGURE 60-2. Angiogram obtained for assessment of the superficial femoral disease shows patency of the previously placed stents in the common iliacs (*arrows*).

two-vessel runoff was present to the foot via the posterior tibial and peroneal arteries. Based on the patient's profound symptoms, her anatomy, and her comorbid conditions, it was decided to proceed with an intervention to the right SFA.

An Amplatz wire was placed through the RIM catheter in the right external iliac. Attempts were made to get a 6 French long Ansel sheath to pass over the bifurcation from the left femoral artery over the Amplatz wire; however, the sheath would not advance past the previously placed iliac stents. A longer dilator and a 0.018 inch system were tried without success. In order to avoid damage to the prior iliac stents, the operator decided to access the right femoral artery in an antegrade fashion. Access to the right common femoral artery was obtained with a micropuncture kit and a 6 French Ansel sheath was inserted. Following the administration of unfractionated heparin, the occluded segment of the right SFA was probed with a glide wire backloaded on a hydrophilic catheter (VERT catheter). With gentle manipulations, the catheter and wire successfully crossed the SFA occlusion and the distal tip of the guidewire appeared to move freely within the popliteal artery. The glide wire was removed; contrast injected through the catheter confirmed intraluminal placement (Figure 60-7). Systemic heparin was administered to achieve

a therapeutic activated clotting time of more than 250 seconds. A 0.018 inch interventional guidewire was inserted and the hydrophilic catheter exchanged for a balloon catheter. The entire SFA was then dilated with a 4 mm diameter by 80 mm long balloon (Figure 60-8). Substantial residual stenosis and recoil remained after balloon dilatation, and thus the operator decided to place multiple stents. Beginning in the distal SFA, a 6 mm diameter by 150 mm long, self-expanding nitinol stent was deployed, followed by a 6 mm diameter by 120 mm long self-expanding nitinol stent. A 1 to 2 cm gap was initially left at the ostium of the SFA. The stented segment and ostial SFA were further dilated with the 4 mm by 80 mm balloon to high atmospheres (Figure 60-9). Subsequent angiography confirmed an excellent result in the stented segment (Figure 60-10); however, the ostium of the SFA had greater than 30% residual stenosis and an ulcerated dissection (Figure 60-11). The operator placed another stent (6 mm diameter by 20 mm long self-expanding nitinol), taking great care to avoid impingement on the profunda femoris and postdilated with a 4 mm diameter by 80 mm long balloon (Figure 60-12). The final angiogram demonstrated sealing of the dissection with no residual stenosis, no impingement on the profunda femoris, and no signs of distal embolization (Figure 60-13).

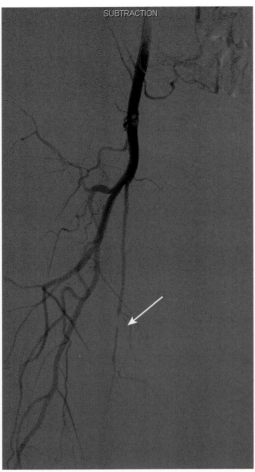

FIGURE 60-3. Angiogram of the right common femoral and proximal superficial femoral artery demonstrating occlusion of the SFA (*arrow*) and patency of the profunda femoris.

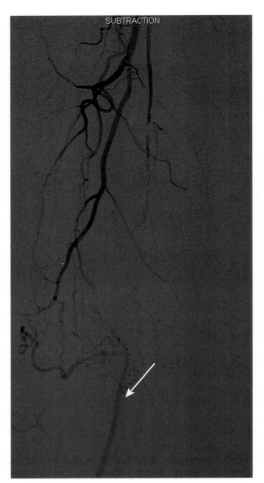

FIGURE 60-4. A long occlusion of the mid-SFA is present and reconstitutes at the popliteal artery (*arrow*).

POSTPROCEDURAL COURSE

Both sheaths were left in place and removed by manual compression when the activated clotting time fell below 180 seconds. The patient remained on bed rest for 4 hours following sheath removal and was hydrated with normal saline. After she was able to ambulate without difficulty, she was discharged the same day. At follow-up 1 month later, she had experienced resolution of her right leg symptoms. Noninvasive testing found near-normalization of her right lower extremity ankle-brachial index (ABI) (Figure 60-14). Her left leg symptoms were only moderate and she decided to continue with medical therapy and exercise. At 6 months, she noted stable symptoms. Noninvasive testing found a slight drop in her ABIs, likely due to moderate restenosis of her right SFA stents.

DISCUSSION

Disease of the SFA is found in 80% to 90% of patients with claudication.[1] Guidelines were created to help manage patients with peripheral arterial disease involving the femoral-popliteal arteries.[2] The TASC criteria classifies femoropopliteal lesions from A to D, with TASC A and B lesions typically being treated percutaneously and TASC D lesions being treated surgically, due to the poor long-term patency of endovascular therapy for this subset. Surgery is preferred for TASC C lesions unless the patient has substantial comorbid conditions resulting in excessive surgical risk. The lesions in the case presented here would be classified TASC C or D and the long term patency would likely have been greater with surgical rather than endovascular revascularization. However, the decision regarding the method of revascularization is complex and must consider other medical conditions, patient preference, and technical feasibility. For example, in this case, the presence of multiple comorbid conditions including advanced age, diabetes, and both prior myocardial infarction and stroke increased her risk of surgery. Endovascular therapy was thought to be lower-risk and appeared technically feasible. Importantly, this mode of revascularization would be unlikely to interfere with surgical options if

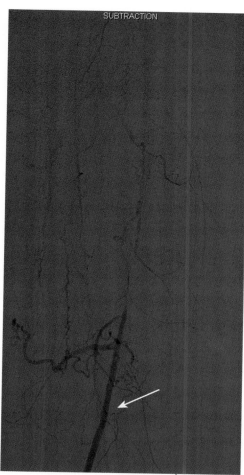

FIGURE 60-5. Another view of the long occlusion of the mid-SFA with reconstitution of the popliteal from collaterals (*arrow*).

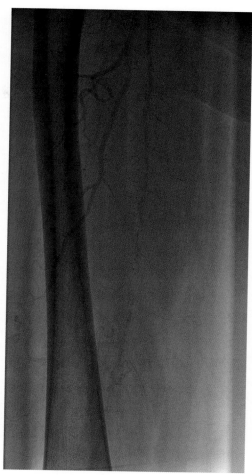

FIGURE 60-6. This is the nonsubtracted image showing the location of SFA occlusion as well as the degree of calcification.

needed at a later date, leading to the decision to pursue endovascular therapy.

With the recent advances in technique and device technology, many chronic SFA occlusions are currently approachable with a high rate of success, offering hope to patients who may have not had other options. One such method is the SAFARI technique (subintimal arterial flossing with antegrade-retrograde intervention) where the operator approaches the occlusion from both above and below with a second access site in the pedal vessels or popliteal artery. The traditional technique approaches the occlusion from above with a guidewire and catheter. Using this technique, the operator may pass the wire and catheter into a dissection plane just distal to the exit site of the occlusion and find it difficult to reenter the true lumen. Several devices have been created to facilitate reentry into the true lumen (the Outback and Pioneer catheters). Armed with these devices, the interventionalist may attempt to cross a chronically occluded SFA using the traditional wire technique and, if the wire fails to reenter the true lumen distally, then employ one of these devices to redirect the wire into the true lumen. With this approach, procedural success rates greater than 80% to 90% are common.

Once a wire has been positioned distally, a variety of techniques have been proposed to treat the occluded segment. These include balloon angioplasty, directional or orbital atherectomy, self-expanding stents, and covered self-expanding stents. There are little data available comparing these techniques and most information is generated from registries and self-reported case series. With this in mind, at the present time, there does not appear to be a clearly superior mode of therapy for the treatment of a chronically occluded SFA. The relatively high rate of restenosis, on the order of 20% to 50%, remains a major limitation for all of these devices.[3] There are also limited data available addressing the issue of restenosis. Nevertheless, with current endovascular techniques, aggressive medical therapy, and close follow-up, the majority of these patients have an improvement in their quality of life.

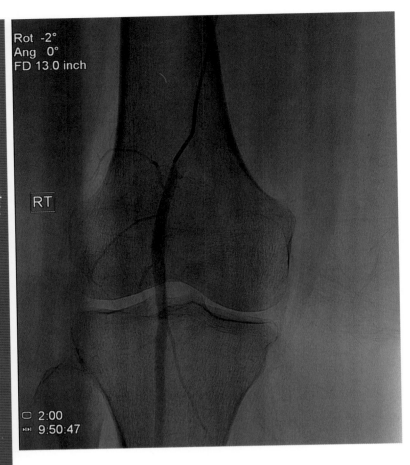

FIGURE 60-7. Injection through the VERT catheter after the SFA has been crossed, demonstrating intraluminal positioning of the catheter.

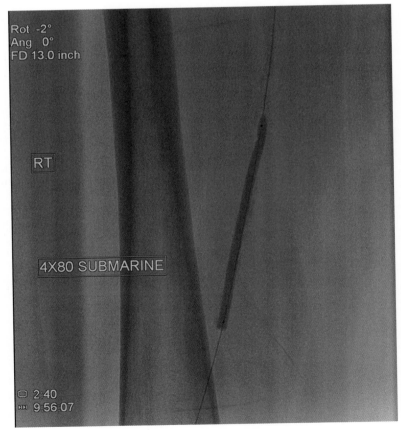

FIGURE 60-8. Balloon dilatation of the SFA.

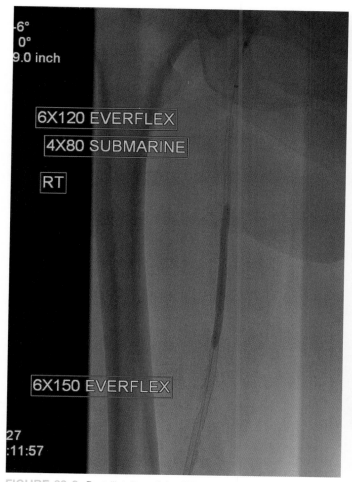

FIGURE 60-9. Postdilatation of the SFA self-expanding stents.

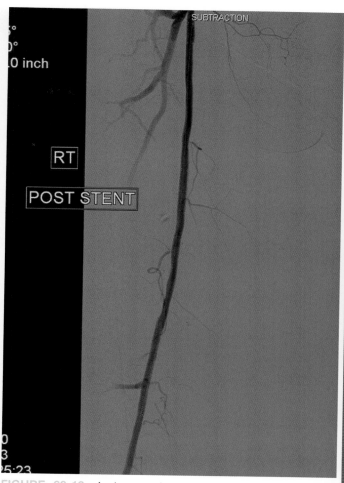

FIGURE 60-10. Angiogram of the mid-SFA obtained after stent deployment and postdilatation showing an excellent result.

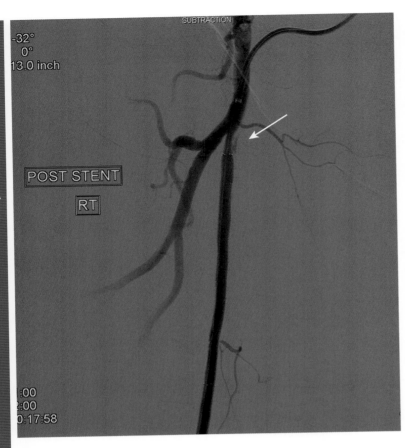

FIGURE 60-11. At the proximal edge of the stent, there is a dissection and residual stenosis in the right ostial SFA near the profunda femoris (*arrow*).

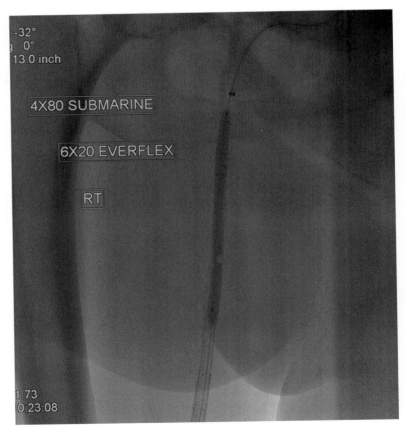

FIGURE 60-12. Placement of nitinol stent in the ostium of the right SFA.

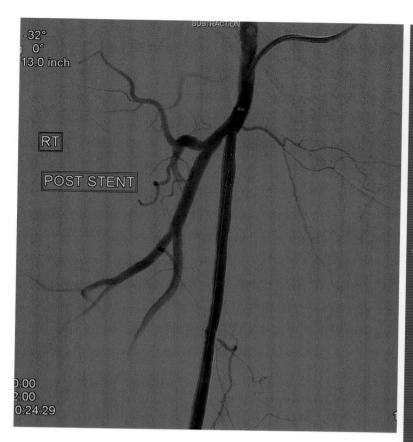

FIGURE 60-13. Final angiogram of the ostial SFA after stent placement.

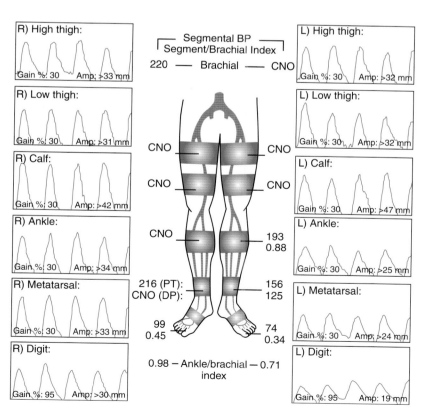

FIGURE 60-14. Postprocedure ABI/PVR showing normalization of the pressures and waveforms.

KEY CONCEPTS

1. SFA disease is very common among patients with peripheral arterial disease.

2. Peripheral vascular interventionalists should be familiar with a variety of access techniques including ultrasound guidance, anterograde access, and access of popliteal and pedal vessels.

3. Numerous devices and techniques are available to facilitate crossing chronically occluded femoral vessels.

4. Endovascular therapy is highly successful in the short term at improving symptoms but is limited by a high rate of restenosis, especially in the treatment of chronic total occlusions.

5. Patients with complex SFA disease treated with endovascular techniques need to be followed closely and treated with aggressive medical therapy. Repeat procedures are common.

Selected References

1. Creager MA, Loscalzo J: Vascular Diseases of the Extremities. In Fauci AS, Braunwald E, Kasper DL, Hauser SL, Longo DL, Jameson JL, Loscalzo J, editors: *Harrison's Principles of Internal Medicine*, ed 17, New York, NY, 2008, McGraw-Hill, pp 1568–1570.

2. Norgren L, Hiatt WR, Dormandy JA, Nehler MR, Harris KA, Fowkes FGR on behalf of the TASC II Working Group: Inter-Society consensus for the management of peripheral arterial disease (TASC II), *Eur J Vasc Endovasc Surg* 33:S1–S70, 2007.

3. Laird JR: Limitations of percutaneous transluminal angioplasty and stenting for the treatment of disease of the superficial femoral and popliteal arteries, *J Endovasc Ther* 13(Suppl II):II 30–II 40, 2006.

Index

Note: Page numbers followed by *b* indicate boxes, *f* indicate figures and *t* indicate tables.

Index

VERT catheter, 313, 316f
Vertebral artery, subclavian stenosis proximal to, 279f, 280–282
Vessel closure, acute, 93–94
   cardiac catheterization, 153–155, 153f, 154f, 155f, 156f, 157f
   case presentation, 153
   discussion, 156–158
   dissection and, 198–201, 201t
   key concepts, 158b
   non-IRA intervention in setting of STEMI and, 212–213
   postprocedural course, 155–156
   surgical backup and, 239–240, 242
   thrombus and, 88
   unsuccessful coronary intervention due to, 106

W
"Watermelon seed," 261
Wilkins score in mitral balloon valvuloplasty, 290, 293–294, 295t

X
X-sizer catheter, 88

Z
Zotarolimus-eluting stent for restenosis of sirolimus-eluting stent, 3, 6f